RESEARCH AND PERSPECTIVES IN ALZHEIMER'S DISEASE

Fondation Ipsen

P. M. Sinet Y. Lamour Y. Christen (Eds.)

Genetics and Alzheimer's Disease

Springer-Verlag
Berlin Heidelberg New York
London Paris Tokyo

Sinet, Pierre Marie, Dr.
Laboratoire de Biochimie Génétique

Lamour, Yvon, Dr.
INSERM U161, 75014 Paris, France

Christen, Yves, Dr.
Fondation IPSEN
pour la Recherche Thérapeutique
30, rue Cambronne
75737 Paris Cédex, France

ISBN-13: 978-3-642-73649-0 e-ISBN-13: 978-3-642-73647-6
DOI:10.1007/978-3-642-73647-6

Softcover reprint of the hardcover 1st edition 1988

Printed: Druckhaus Beltz, 6944 Hemsbach
Bookbinding: J. Schäffer, 6718 Grünstadt 1
2127/3140/543210 – Printed on acid-free paper

Preface

This volume contains the proceedings of the meeting *Genetics and Alzheimer's Disease* held in Paris, on March 25, 1988, by the Fondation Ipsen pour la Recherche Thérapeutique. This meeting was the second of the series of *Colloques Médecine et Recherche* devoted to Alzheimer's disease. The first one was held in Angers (France) on September 14, 1987; the proceedings of this meeting have already been published and are entitled *Immunology and Alzheimer's Disease* (1988, edited by A Pouplard-Barthelaix, J Emile, and Y Christen). The third *Colloque Médecine et Recherche,* organized in Montpellier on September 19, 1988, dealt with neuronal grafting; the proceedings of this last meeting will be published in early 1989 (*Neuronal Grafting and Alzheimer's Disease: Future Perspectives,* edited by F Gage, A Privat and Y Christen).

In each case, the Fondation Ipsen deliberately focuses attention on the most up-to-date themes, and sometimes the most controversial ones, from medical and scientific research. The genetic aspects of Alzheimer's Disease (AD) stands at the very forefront of research carried out in the last 2 years. It complements research using the formal approach, which has become possible thanks to the study of extended kindreds by J-F Foncin and other scientists.

The recent work on molecular and genetics biology has followed two main pathways:

1. The study of the gene(s) responsible for the familial form(s), which can be considered the AD gene(s). Several papers published in 1987 locate a gene of this type on chromosome 21. This location appears very interesting as (a) the question of the relationship between AD and Down's syndrome (trisomy 21) has been discussed for many years and (b) the gene encoding the precursor of the amyloid A4 protein or β protein (major component of senile plaques) is also located on chromosome 21, as several groups demonstrated in 1987.
   During this meeting of the Fondation Ipsen, researchers from Durham presented their findings, which indicated that the gene implicated in familial late-onset AD is not located on chromosome 21. More recently, scientists from Seattle have published other results also excluding chromosome 21 (Schellenberg GD, Bird TD, Wijsman EM, Moore DK, Boehnke M, Bryant EM, Lampe TH, Nochlin D et al.: Science, 1988, 242: 1507–1510). Therefore, it seems quite possible that AD may be an heterogenous disease and that, even for the familial forms, several loci located on different chromosomes are involved.
2. The amyloid A4 protein precursor (APP) gene. According to several authors, the amyloid formation (i.e., the A4 protein deposition) could be a crucial event for the clinical expression of dementia. Recent work on molecular genetics of APP gives a

better understanding of its function as a membrane protein probably involved in cell contact.

Morever, the finding in 1988 of longer forms of APP carrying an additional domain with protease inhibitor function raises a number of questions about this kind of protein. Some protease inhibitors are thought to control neurite extension. Therefore it is possible that longer forms of APP could control protease-dependant processes required for brain plasticity (and also tissue regeneration since the corresponding mRNAs are found not only in the brain but also in peripheral organs).

Thus, as we can see, all of this work not only provides a better understanding, of the mapping of the human genome, but also demonstrates a new approach – at the molecular level – about how to go from the gene to the lesion and to the disease. This is the main goal of the work described and gathered in this book.

The editors wish to thank Mrs. Mary Gage for her editorial assistance, Mrs. Jacqueline Mervaillie for the organization of the meeting in Paris, an Yves Agid, Claude Kordon, and Jacques Mallet for their collaboration as chairmen of the meeting.

Yves Christen
Vice-Président of the Fondation Ipsen pour la Recherche Thérapeutique

Contents

Contributors

Aalbo, J.
Massachussetts General Hospital and Harvard Medical School, Boston, MA 02114, USA

Alberts, M.J.
Department of Medicine, Division of Neurology, Duke University Medical Center, Durham, NC 27710, USA

Alpérovitch, A.
INSERM, U. 169, 16, avenue P.V. Couturier, 94807 Villejuif Cedex, France

Amaducci, L.
Instituto di Mallatie Nervose e Mentali, University of Florence, Florence, Italia

Anderton, B.H.
Department of Immunology, St. George's Hospital, Medical School, Cranmer Terrace, London SW17 0RE, UK

Backhovens, H.
University of Antwerp (U.I.A.), Departments of Biochemistry and Neurology, Ghent, Belgium

de Barsy, T.
Université Catholique de Louvain, Laboratoire de Neurochimie UCL 1352, Av. Hippocrate 10, B 1200, Bruxelles, Belgium

Bartlett, R.J.
Department of Medicine, Division of Neurology, Duke University Medical Center, Durham, NC 27710, USA

Beer, J.
Center for Molecular Biology, University of Heidelberg, Im Neuenheimer Feld 282, 6900 Heidelberg 1, W.-Germany

Berr, C.
INSERM, U 169, 16, avenue P.V. Couturier, 94807 Villejuif Cedex, France

Beyreuther, K.
Center for Molecular Biology, University of Heidelberg, Im Neuenheimer Feld 282, 6900 Heidelberg 1, W.-Germany

Blouin, J.-L.
Laboratoire de Biochimie Génétique, Hôpital Necker, 75015 Paris, France

Blume, A.J.
Lederle Laboratories, Pearl River, 10965 New York, USA

Boily, C.
Hôpital de Chicoutimi, Chicoutimi, Canada

Bouchard, G.
SOREP, Université du Québec à Chicoutimi, Chicoutimi, Canada

Bouchard, N.
Hôpital de la Baie, La Baie, Canada

Bouchard, P.
Hôpital de Jonquière, Jonquière, Canada

Bouchard, R.
Hôpital de l'Enfant-Jésus, Quebec, Canada

de Braekeleer, M.
SOREP, Université du Québec à Chicoutimi, Chicoutimi, Canada

v. Broeckhoven, C.
University of Antwerp (U.I.A.), Departments of Biochemistry and Neurology, Ghent, Belgium

Brucher, J.M.
Université Catholique de Louvain, Laboratoires de Neurochimie UCL 1352, Avenue Hippocrate 10, B. 1200, Bruxelles, Belgium

Bruni, A.C.
Servizio di Neurologia, USL 17, e Projetto SMID-SUD, Lamezia Terme, Italia

Bunke, D.
Center for Molecular Biology, University of Heidelberg, Im Neuenheimer Feld 282, 6900 Heidelberg 1, W. Germany

v. Camp, G.
University of Antwerp (U.I.A.), Departments of Biochemistry and Neurology, Ghent, Belgium

Ceballos, I.
Laboratoire de Biochemie Génétique, Hôpital Necker, 149 rue de Sèvres, 75015 Paris, France

Cholette, A.
Hôpital de Chicoutimi, Chicoutimi, Canada

Clark, C. M.
Department of Medicine, Division of Neurology, Duke University Medical Center, Durham, NC 27710, USA

Conneally, P. M.
Clinical Neuropharmacology Section, Medical Neurology, Branch National Institute of Neurological and Communicative Disorders and Stroke, Bethesda, MD 20892, USA

Creau-Goldberg, N.
INSERM U 173, CNRS, Hôpital Necker – Enfants Malades, 149, rue de Sévres, 75743 Paris, Cedex 15, France

Davous, P.
Hôpital d'Argenteuil, 95107 Argenteuil, France

Dawson, D. V.
Department of Community and Family Medicine, Division of Biometry and Medical Informatics, Duke University Medical Center, Durham, NC 27710, USA

Delabar, J.-M.
Laboratoire de Biochimie Génétique, Hôpital Necker, 149 rue de Sèvres, 75014 Paris, France

Doyon, L.-P.
Hôpital de Roberval, Roberval, Canada

Drachman, D.
Department of Neurology, University of Massachussetts Medical School and University of Massachussetts Medical Center, 55 Lake Avenue North Worcester, MA 01605, USA

Dumont, M.
Hôpital d'Alma, Alma, Canada

Dyrks, T.
Department of Pathology, University of Western Australia, Nedlands, 6009, Western Australia

Earl, N. L.
Department of Medicine, Division of Neurology, Duke University Medical Center, Durham, NC 27710, USA

Eisenmenger, J. P.
Center for Study of Aging and Human Development, Duke University Medical Center, Durham, NC 27710, USA

Epstein, C. J.
Department of Pediatrics, University of California, San Francisco, CA 94143, USA

Farrer, L.
Massachussetts General Hospital, Harvard Medical School, 10 Fruit Street, Boston, MA 02114, USA

Feldman, R. G.
Department of Neurology, Boston University Medical School, 80 East Concord Street, Boston, MA 02118, USA

Fischer, P.
Center for Molecular Biology, University of Heidelberg, Im Neuenheimer Feld 282, 6900 Heidelberg 1, W.-Germany

Folstein, M. F.
Department of Psychiatry and Behavioral Sciences, The Johns Hopkins University School of Medicine, Osler 320, Baltimore, MD 21205, USA

Foncin, J.-F.
Laboratoire de Neurohistologie, Ecole Pratique des Hautes Etudes et Unité 106, INSERM, La Salpètrière, 75651 Paris Cedex 13, France

Fournier, C.
Sanatorium Bégin, Lac Etchemin, Canada

Froda, S.
Université du Québec à Montréal, Montréal, Canada

Frommelt, P.
Kreiskrankenhaus Lemgo, Neurologische Abteilung, D 4920 Lemgo, West Germany

Fuller, S.
Department of Pathology, University of Western Australia and Department of Neuropathology, Royal Perth Hospital, Perth, Australia

Gajdusek, D. C.
CNS Studies Laboratory, NINCDS-NIH, Bethesda, MD 20892, USA

Gaskell, P. C.
Department of Medicine, Division of Neurology, Duke University Medical Center, Durham, NC 27710, USA

Gaudreault, M.
Hôpital de Chicoutimi, Chicoutimi, Canada

Gauthier, S.
McGill University, Montreal, Canada

Gautrin, D.
Institut National de la Recherche Scientifique (INRS-Santé), Pointe-Claire, QC H9R 1G6, Canada

Gauvreau, D.
Institut National de la Recherche Scientifique (INRS-Santé), Pointe-Claire, QC H9R 1G6, Canada

Gheuens, J.
University of Antwerp (U.I.A.), Departments of Biochemistry and Neurology, Ghent, Belgium

Gilbert, J. R.
Department of Medicine, Division of Neurology, Duke University Medical Center, Durham, NC 27710, USA

Goldgaber, D.
CNS Studies Laboratory, NINCDS-NIH, Bethesda, MD 20892, USA

de Grouchy, J.
INSERM U 173, CNRS, Hôpital Necker – Enfants Malades, 149, rue de Sèvres, 75743 Paris Cedex 15, France

Growdon, J.
Department of Neurology, Massachussetts General Hospital and Harvard Medical School, 32 Fruit Street, Boston, MA 02114, USA

Gusella, J.
Neurogenetics Laboratory, Massachussetts General Hospital, Harvard Medical School, 10 Fruit Street, Boston, MA 02114, USA

Haines, J. L.
Department of Medical Genetics, Indiana University, School of Medicine, Indianapolis, IN 46223, USA

Haynes, C. S.
Department of Medicine, Division of Neurology, Duke University Medical Center, Durham NC 27710, USA

Heyman, A. L.
Department of Medicine, Division of Neurology, Duke University Medical Center, Durham NC 27710, USA

Hilbich, C.
Center for Molecular Biology, University of Heidelberg, Im Neuenheimer Feld 282, 6900 Heidelberg 1, W.-Germany

v. Hul, W.
University of Antwerp (U.I.A.), Department of Biochemistry and Neurology, Ghent, Belgium

Hung, W.-Y.
Department of Medicine, Division of Neurology, Duke University Medical Center, Durham NC 27710

Huret, J.-L.
Laboratoire d'Hématologie, C.H.R.U. La Milétrie, 86021 Poitiers, France

Iqbal, K.
New York State Office of Mental Retardation and Developmental Disabilities, Institute for Basic Research in Developmental Disabilities, Staten Island, NY 10314, USA

Kishka, P.
Sanatorium Bégin, Lac Etchemin, Canada

König, G.
Center for Molecular Biology, University of Heidelberg, Im Neuenheimer Feld 282, 6900 Heidelberg 1, W. Germany

Kosik, K. S.
Center for Neurologic Diseases, Brigham and Women's Hospital, 75 Francis Street, Boston, MA 02115, USA

Lacoste-Royal, G.
Institut National de la Recherche Scientifique (INRS-Santé), Pointe-Claire, QC H9R 1G6, Canada

Lamour, Y.
INSERM U 161, 2 rue d'Alesia, 75014 Paris, France

Laterre, E. C.
Université Catholique de Louvain, Laboratoires de Neurochimie UCL 1352, Avenue Hippocrate 10, B. 1200, Bruxelles, Belgium

Lee, J. E.
Department of Psychiatry, Division of Child and Adolescent Psychiatry, Duke University Medical Center, Durham, NC 27710, USA

Macq, A. F.
Université Catholique de Louvain, Laboratoires de Neurochimie UCL 1352, Avenue Hippocrate 10, B. 1200, Bruxelles, Belgium

Maloteaux, J. M.
Université Catholique de Louvain, Laboratoires de Neurochimie UCL 1352, Avenue Hippocrate 10, B. 1200, Bruxelles, Belgium

Martins, R.
Department of Pathology, University of Western Australia, Nedlands 6009, Western Australia

Masters, C. L.
Department of Pathology, University of Western Australia, Nedlands 6009, Western Australia

Mathieu, J.
Hôpital de Chicoutimi, Chicoutimi, Canada

McHugh, P. R.
Department of Psychiatry and Behavioral Sciences, The John Hopkins University School of Medicine, Osler 320, Baltimore, MD 21205, USA

Mönning, U.
Center for Molecular Biology, University of Heidelberg, Im Neuenheimer Feld 282, 6900 Heidelberg 1, W. Germany

Mortimer, J.
University of Minneapolis, Minnesota, MN 55417, USA

Multhaup, G.
Center for Molecular Biology, University of Heidelberg, Im Neuenheimer Feld 282, 6900 Heidelberg 1, W.-Germany

Myers, R.
Department of Neurology, Boston University Medical School, 80 East Concord Street, Boston, MA 02118, USA

Nalbantoglu, J.
Institut National de la Recherche Scientifique (INRS-Santé), Pointe-Claire, QC H9R 1G6, Canada

Nee, L.
Clinical Neuropharmacology Section, Medical Neurology Branch National Institute of Neurological and Communicative Disorders and Stroke, Bethesda, MD 20892, USA

Nicole, A.
Laboratoire de Biochimie Génétique, Hôpital Necker, 149 rue de Sèvres, 75014 Paris, France

Octave, J. N.
Université Catholique de Louvain, Laboratorie de Neurochimie UCL 1352, Avenue Hippocrate 10, B. 1200, Bruxelles, Belgium

Okra Podrabinek, N.
Hôpital Charles Richet, 95400 Villiers le Bel, France

Ouellet, A.
Hôpital de Dolbeau, Dolbeau, Canada

Pericak-Vance, M. A.
Department of Medicine, Division of Neurology, Duke University Medical Center, Durham, NC 27710, USA

Piacentini, S.
Instituto di Mallatie Nervose e Mentali, University of Florence, Florence, Italia

Poissonnier, M.
Unité de Cytogénétique, Centre de Transfusion sanguine, 26, rue du Maréchal-Foch, 78000 Versailles, France

Polinsky, R.
Clinical Neuropharmacology Section, Medical Neurology, Branch National Institute of Neurological and Communicative Disorders and Stroke, Bethesda, MD 20892, USA

Pollen, D.
Department of Neurology, University of Massachussetts Medical School and University of Massachussetts Medical Center, 55 Lake Avenue North, Worcester, MA 01605, USA

Raeymaekers, G.
University of Antwerp (U.I.A.), Departments of Biochemistry and Neurology, Ghent, Belgiuim

Rahmani, Z.
Laboratoire de Biochimie Génétique, Hôpital Necker, 149 rue de Sèvres, 75014 Paris, France

Rapoport, S. I.
Laboratory of Neurosciences, National Institute on Aging, National Institutes of Health, Bethesda, MD 20892, USA

Rasool, C. G.
Lederle Laboratories, Pearl River, 10965 New York, USA

Robitaille, Y.
McGill University Montreal, Canada

Roses, A. D.
Department of Medicine, Division of Neurology, Duke University Medical Center, Durham, NC 27710, USA

Roudier, M.
Hôpital Charles Richet, 95400 Villiers-le-Bel, France

Roudier, P.
Hôpital Charles Richet, 95400 Villiers-le-Bel, France

Rumble, B.
Department of Pathology, University of Western Australia, Nedlands 6009, Western Australia

Salbaum, J. M.
Center for Molecular Biology, University of Heidelberg, Im Neuenheimer Feld 282, 6900 Heidelberg 1, W.-Germany

Salmon, D.
Institut National de Transfusion Sanguine, Paris, France

de Sauvage, F.
Université Catholique de Louvain, Laboratoire de Neurochimie UCL 1352, Avenue Hippocrate 10, B. 1200, Bruxelles, Belgium

Selkoe, D. J.
Harvard Medical School and Center for Neurological Diseases, Department of Medicine (Neurology), Brigham and Women's Hospital, Boston, MA 02115, USA

Siddique, T.
Department of Medicine, Division of Neurology, Duke University Medical Center, Durham, MC 27710, USA

Simms, G.
Department of Pathology, University of Western Australia, Nedlands 6009, Western Australia

Sinet, P.-M.
Laboratoire de Biochimie Génétique, Hôpital Necker, 149 rue de Sèvres, 75014 Paris, France

Sorbi, S.
Instituto di Mallatie Nervose e Mentali, University of Florence, Florence, Italia

Speer, M. C.
Department of Medicine, Division of Neurology, Duke University Medical Center, Durham, NC 27710, USA

St George-Hyslop, P. H.
Neurogenetics Laboratory, Massachussetts General Hospital, Harvard Medical School, 10 Fruit Street, Boston, MA 02114, USA

Stinissen, P.
University of Antwerp (U.I.A.), Departments of Biochemistry and Neurology, Ghent, Belgium

Tanzi, R.
Neurogenetics Laboratory, Massachussetts General Hospital, Harvard Medical School, 10 Fruit Street, Boston, MA 02114, USA

Teener, J. W.
CNS Studies Laboratory, NINCDS-NIH, Bethesda, MD 20892, USA

Trouet, A.
Université Catholique de Louvain, Laboratoire de Neurochimie UCL 1352, Avenue Hippocrate 10, B. 1200, Bruxelles, Belgium

Trofatter, J. A.
Department of Medical Genetics, Indiana University School of Medicine, Indianapolis, IN 46223, USA

Turleau, C.
INSERM U 173, CNRS, Hôpital Necker – Enfants Malades 149, rue de Sèvres, 75743 Paris Cedex 15, France

Vandenberghe, A.
University of Antwerp (U.I.A.), Department of Biochemistry and Neurology, Ghent, Belgium

Vitek, M. P.
Lederle Laboratories, Pearl River, 10965 New York, USA

Warren, A.
Department of Psychiatry and Behavioral Sciences, The John Hopkins University School of Medicine, Osler 320, Baltimore, MD 21205, USA

Watkins, P.
Integrated genetics Inc., 31 New York Avenue, Framingham, MA 02118, USA

Wehnert, A.
University of Antwerp (U.I.A.), Departments of Biochemistry and Neurology, Ghent, Belgium

Weidemann, A.
Department of Pathology, University of Western Australia, Nedlands 6009, Western Australia

de Winter, G.
University of Antwerp (U.I.A.), Departments of Biochemistry and Neurology, Ghent, Belgium

Wisniewski, H. M.
New York State Office of Mental Retardation and Developmental Disabilities, Institute for Basic Research in Development Disabilities, Staten Island, NY 10314, USA

Yamaoka, L. H.
Department of Medicine, Division of Neurology, Duke University Medical Center, Durham, NC 27710, USA

Genetics of Alzheimer's Disease: Current Status and Future Development of Research

B. H. Anderton

Alzheimer's disease appears at present to be heterogeneous in regard to genetic factors, as well as in other respects. It is generally agreed that Alzheimer's disease can show a familial tendency; however, it is not clear what proportion of cases are familial and how many are truly sporadic. This issue is not easy to resolve because of the uncertainty of establishing that deceased elderly family members had Alzheimer's disease or, more problematic still, whether they would have developed the disease had they lived longer. The earliest onset cases make familiality easier to establish, and it seems that the age of onset may be one of the factors that is genetically determined, as the age of onset is fairly consistent and typical for each affected family (Folstein, this volume).

This is one example of heterogeneity in Alzheimer's disease and more extensive epidemiological studies are required to establish the proportion of cases that exhibit a familial tendency. This has been emphasized by Alperovitch and Berr (this volume) who describe the methodological problems of studying a late onset disease, and conclude from an analysis of several epidemiological studies that there is still no clear epidemiological evidence of an increased familial risk of developing Alzheimer's disease in the general population; this is distinct from the rare familial early onset families, such as those investigated by Foncin and collaborators (this volume).

Heterogeneity of the disease is also an aspect of the variable clinical picture, and the clearly familial early onset Alzheimer's disease families usually have specific clinical features. Some of these early onset families for which large pedigrees are available have now been shown to exhibit a single autosomal dominant pattern of inheritance with the FAD (familial Alzheimer's disease) gene being located on chromosome 21 (St. George-Hyslop, this volume). Other much more common and later onset families with a history of Alzheimer's disease have not been found to be positively linked to a gene on chromosome 21 (Pericak-Vance and Roses, this volume). Further analysis is now required to establish whether alternative gene loci may lead to Alzheimer's disease in such families and to what extent other factors (e.g., environmental) may interact with a genetic predisposition towards Alzheimer's disease in producing the disease.

The FAD Gene

The excitement that was generated early in 1987 by the discovery that the FAD gene is located on chromosome 21 along with the gene for the amyloid beta-protein, and that trisomy of chromosome 21 in Down's syndrome gives rise to a brain pathology indistinguishable from Alzheimer's disease, has now been tempered by the demonstration that the FAD gene locus is not identical with the beta-protein locus (Kang et al. 1987; Goldgaber et al. 1987; St George-Hyslop et al. 1987; Robakis et al. 1987; Tanzi et al. 1987a, b; Van Broeckhoven et al. 1987). Nevertheless, interest in the beta-protein continues since understanding the mechanism of the deposition of amyloid could provide clues to the identity and function of the genetic defect. This also applies to the study of neurofibrillary tangle formation, including the production of their component paired helical filaments (PHFs).

The Beta-Protein Precursor

Recent reports that the mRNA for the beta-protein is expressed at elevated levels in neurones in Alzheimer's disease (Higgins et al. 1988; Cohen et al. 1988) may be related to the presence of a heat-shock consensus sequence in the promoter for the beta-protein precursor gene (Masters, this volume). However, unravelling the molecular mechanism for this apparent increased level of expression could be important for understanding the biochemical events that lead to neuronal death, just as working out the mechanism of precursor processing to produce amyloid deposits may also provide important insights into the molecular pathology of the disease. It remains to be seen, though, whether the colocalization of the FAD and beta-protein precursor genes on chromosome 21 has anything to do with these mechanisms of expression and processing of beta-protein or whether this is merely coincidental.

Another intriguing feature of the beta-protein precursor is the potential for alternative protein forms, some with an extra domain homologous with the Kunitz serine protease inhibitors (Goldgaber, this volume; Ponte et al. 1988; Tanzi et al. 1988; Kitaguchi et al. 1988). The significance of this finding is not yet apparent, but study of the expression and processing of alternative beta-protein precursor forms may be illuminating.

Paired Helical Filaments

The other area of considerable attention as far as molecular pathology is concerned is the composition of paired helical filaments (PHFs). There is general agreement that the microtubule-associated protein, tau, is consistently present and neurofilaments and ubiquitin are other components (Kosik, this volume). The presence of ubiquitin in PHF is indicative of abnormal posttranslational processing of cytoplasmic proteins that then give rise to PHFs.

One assumption frequently made is that amyloid deposition in senile plaques and the production of PHFs in tangles are tightly linked aspects of the pathology of Alzheimer's disease. This may not be the case, since tangles occur without plaques in several diseases (e.g., Guam ALS-parkinsonian-dementia complex, dementia pugilistica) and some cases of Alzheimer's disease exhibit areas of neocortex rich in senile plaques, but virtually free of tangles (Terry et al. 1987). These latter senile plaques seem not to contain PHFs in their neuritic elements, unlike senile plaques located in areas also containing tangles (Probst et al. 1988). Thus, it may be not only pragmatic but also scientifically sound to study separately the molecular mechanisms producing amyloid deposits and PHFs.

Conclusion

It is probably not yet feasible to construct a unifying and plausible hypothesis encompassing the possible aetiological factors for the known pathology of Alzheimer's disease. In the immediate future, we shall no doubt see considerable progress toward understanding these different aspects of this disease. However, for the present it would be unwise to predict how far apart are the genetic and pathological lines of investigation and how long it will be before we understand their relationships. In the meantime, working out the biochemical events that contribute to neuronal cell death may be very fruitful, since they could provide new targets for therapeutic intervention.

References

Cohen ML, Golde TE, Usiak MF, Younkin LH, Younkin SG (1988) In situ hybridisation of nucleus basalis neurons shows increased β-amyloid mRNA in Alzheimer disease. Proc Natl Acad Sci USA 85: 1227–1231

Goldgaber D, Lerman MI, McBride OW, Saffioti U, Gajdusek DC (1987) Characterisation and chromosomal localisation of a cDNA encoding brain amyloid of Alzheimer's disease. Science 23: 877–880

Higgins GA, Lewis DA, Bahmanyar S, Goldgaber D, Gajdusek DC, Young WG, Morrison JH, Wilson MC (1988) Differential regulation of amyloid-β-protein mRNA expression within hippocampal neuronal subpopulations in Alzheimer disease. Proc Natl Acad Sci USA 85: 1297–1301

Kang J, Lemaire H-G, Unterbeck A, Salbaum JM, Masters CL, Grzeschik K-H, Multhaup G, Beyreuther K, Müller-Hill B (1987) The precursor of Alzheimer's disease amyloid A4 protein resembles a cell-surface receptor. Nature 325: 733–736

Kitaguchi N, Takahashi Y, Tokushima Y, Shiojiri S, Ito H (1988) Novel precursor of Alzheimer's disease amyloid protein shows protease inhibitory activity. Nature 331: 530–532

Ponte P, Gonzalez-De Whitt P, Schilling J, Miller J, Hsu D, Greenberg B, Davis K, Wallace W, Lieberburg I, Fuller F, Cordell B (1988) A new A4 amyloid mRNA contains a domain homologous to serine proteinase inhibitors. Nature 331: 525–528

Probst A, Lautenschlager C, Brion J-P, Anderton BH, Ulrich J (1988) Differential pattern of senile plaque neurites immunoreactivity related to the presence or absence of neurofibrillary tangles in the neocortex. Interdisc Topics Geront, (in press)

Robakis NK, Ramakrishna N, Wolfe G, Wisniewski HM (1987) Molecular cloning and characterisation of a cDNA encoding the cerebrovascular and the neuritic plaque amyloid peptides. Proc Natl Acad Sci USA 84: 4190–4194

St George-Hyslop PH, Tanzi RE, Polinsky RJ, Haines JL, Nee L, Watkins PC, Myers RH, Feldman RG, Pollen D, Drachman D, Growdon J, Bruni A, Foncin J-F, Salmon D, Frommelt P, Amaducci L, Sorbi S, Piacentini S, Stewart GD, Hobbs WJ, Conneally M, Gusella JF (1987) The genetic defect causing familial Alzheimer's disease maps on chromosome 21. Science 235: 885–890

Tanzi RE, St George-Hyslop PH, Haines JL, Polinsky RJ, Nee L, Foncin J-F, Neve RL, McClatchey AI, Conneally PM, Gusella JF (1987a) The genetic defect in familial Alzheimer's disease is not tightly linked to the amyloid β-protein gene. Nature 329: 156–157

Tanzi RE, Gusella JF, Watkins PC, Bruns GAP, St George-Hyslop P, Van Keuren ML, Patterson D, Pagan S, Kurnit DM, Neve RL (1987b) Amyloid β protein gene: cDNA, mRNA distribution, and genetic linkage near the Alzheimer locus. Science 235: 880–884

Tanzi RE, McClatchey AI, Lamperti ED, Villa-Komaroff L, Gusella JF, Neve RL (1988) Protease inhibitor domain encoded by an amyloid protein precursor mRNA associated with Alzheimer's disease. Nature 331: 528–530

Terry RD, Hansen LA, De Teresa R, Davies P, Tobias H, Katzman R (1987) Senile dementia of the Alzheimer type without neocortical neurofibrillary tangles. J Neuropath Exp Neurol 46: 262–268

Van Broeckhoven C, Genthe AM, Vendenberghe A, Horsthemke B, Backhovens H, Raeymaekers P, Van Hul W, Wehnert A, Gheuens J, Cras P, Bruyland M, Martin JJ, Salbaum M, Multhaup G, Masters CL, Beyreuther K, Gurling HMD, Mullan MJ, Holland A, Barton A, Irving N, Williamson R, Richards SJ, Hardy JA (1987) Failure of familial Alzheimer's disease to segregate with the A4-amyloid gene in several European families. Nature 329: 153–156

Heterogeneity in Alzheimer's Disease: an Exercise in the Resolution of a Phenotype

M. F. Folstein, A. Warren, and *P. R. McHugh*

Summary

Clinical features related to age of onset, including amnesia, aphasia, apraxia, agnosia, depression, and fingerprint and platelet abnormalities, suggest heterogeneity in Alzheimer's disease. Since some of these features run in Alzheimer's disease families there could be genetic heterogeneity. Understanding the mechanisms which determine the age of onset and related features will be as important as the discovery of the genes, because delay of the age of onset could push it beyond the normal life span and thus eliminate expression of Alzheimer's disease in human populations even though the genes themselves and their possible beneficial effects would remain.

Knowledge of potential heterogeneity will aid in the design of linkage studies. Criteria must be constructed for the purpose of identifying probands and secondary cases in linkage studies in order to reduce the number of false positives. To put it another way, we must increase the predictive value of case detection methods, particularly regarding early cases, in linkage studies.

Introduction

Before we can understand how environmental and genetic factors determine the etiology and pathogenesis of Alzheimer's disease (AD), we must study phenotypic heterogeneity of AD to define accurate criteria for cases.

Importance of Variable Traits

AD is a complex clinico pathological entity that can be described in terms of clinical symptoms and laboratory tests during life and neuropathological examination after death. Accurate description of each of these features can divide the AD population into various subgroups. Clinically, the number and type of signs required for diagnosis will determine diagnostic subgroups; if more symptoms are required for diagnosis, such as amnesia and aphasia, then a different separation of cases from normals will result than if fewer symptoms are required, such as amnesia only. It is unclear which phenotypic features best define subgroups. The importance of the appropriate selection of phenotypic features to define cases is illustrated by the example of phenylketonuria: observation of hair color or intelligence does not clearly distinguish phenylketonurics from the general population, but the measurement of urine ketones does. Unfortunately, the pathognomonic protein abnormality in AD is unknown.

Three phenotypic features that may show heterogeneity in AD are (a) the cognitive syndrome itself, (b) the age of onset, and (c) the severity of dementia relative to neuropathology.

The Cognitive Syndrome

The cognitive syndrome of amnesia, aphasia, apraxia, and agnosia (AAAA) has been recognized to be a part of AD in descriptions even before Alzheimer's. J.C. Prichard and others recognized in the 19th century that the syndrome now called AD was something more than a prominent progressive loss of memory (Prichard 1837; Alzheimer 1907). Patients with amnesia due to AD can be divided into subgroups depending on the prominence of the additional cortical symptoms of aphasia, apraxia, and agnosia. For example, studies of aphasia in AD have suggested that this feature may characterize a subgroup of patients with early onset of dementia (Chui et al. 1985; Go et al. 1979; Appell et al. 1982; Seltzer and Sherwin 1983) and increased rate of progression of disease (Berg et al. 1984; Faber-Langendoen et al. 1988). We suggest that the presence of the clinical symptoms of amnesia, aphasia, apraxia, and agnosia delineate a group of subjects with AD who differ from normal elderly subjects and from subjects who have a dementia syndrome whose main feature is amnesia without prominent aphasia and apraxia, and that these differences are validated by differences in pathology and familial prevalence of AD.

AAAA May Be Associated with a Characteristic Pathology

Workers from Geneva and Sweden have demonstrated AAAA in a large proportion of cases of AD. They found that the presence of AAAA depends on duration of illness and on spread of the pathology to the neocortex (Larsson et al. 1963; Constantinidis et al. 1965). Positron emission tomography and single photon emission tomography have verified that in many cases of AD there is hypometabolism specifically in the temporal and parietal cortex, areas predicted to be affected in cases with aphasia and amnesia (Foster et al. 1987; Haxby et al. 1987; Jagust et al. 1987; Johnson et al. 1987).

AAAA Is Associated with a Defined Risk to Relatives of Dementia

Ten years ago we found that relatives of the probands with the AAAA syndrome had a higher risk for becoming demented than did the relatives of cases with the incomplete syndrome or a normal mental state (Folstein et al. 1981; Powell and Folstein 1984; Breitner and Folstein 1984). In this study all subjects had been ill for 6–7 years, a sufficient duration for AAAA to develop in susceptible individuals. The characteristics of individuals with the incomplete syndrome are similar to those cases that were described by Kraepelin as simple senile dementia. The prevalence of this condition is not clearly known since in most epidemiological surveys it is not separated from AD. Such a separation might be an important problem in genetic studies, but may exist primarily in studies of AD of late onset and long duration: subsequent studies of younger patients not in nursing homes show that the NINCDS ADRDA criteria for AD (which do not specify AAAA) are sufficient to identify a population whose first-degree relatives are at higher risk than nondemented controls (Mohs et al. 1987; Breitner et al. 1988; Huff et al. 1987; Martin et al. 1987).

Age of Onset

A second aspect of phenotypic heterogeneity in AD is age of onset. From its earliest description AD has been subclassified into the early onset or presenile form and the late onset or senile form. In recent years, however, clinicians and pathologists have proposed that these are one entity because of qualitative similarities of their neuropathologies. Although the unimodal distribution of age of onset supports this view, such evidence is inconclusive; for example, we know that familial factors can significantly modify the age of onset of Huntington's disease even in cases transmitted at the same locus.

Moreover, AD cases subdivided by age of onset differ in (a) psychological features, including severity of language disturbance and incidence of major depression; (b) somatic features, including platelet membrane fluidity and fingerprint pattern; (c) familial risk to relatives of early-onset AD; and (d) neuropathology.

Psychological Features

Several investigators have shown that early-onset cases have rapidly progressive language disturbance, and this difference in language function persists regardless of duration of illness in the cases (Chui et al. 1985). Cases of AD of early onset also seem to differ in certain noncognitive clinical symptoms, namely, the prevalence of a depressive syndrome that meets DSM III criteria. We have found that major depression defined by these criteria occurs in 15%–20% of cases of AD in contrast to less than 5% of the general population, and it tends to occur more often in the early-onset cases.

That this syndrome represents a variable phenotypic feature of disease rather than a reaction to the illness is supported by the finding of increased neuronal loss in the locus coeruleus in cases without depression (Rovner et al. 1988; Zweig et al. 1988). Furthermore, the depression appears to have a higher prevalence in the families of the cases, just as it does in Huntington's disease.

Somatic Features

In addition to these psychological signs of phenotypic heterogeneity related to age of onset, there are somatic signs which occur more often in the earlier onset cases. The fingerprints of early-onset cases have more ulnar loops and, therefore, more closely resemble the fingerprints of Down's syndrome (DS) patients than do the fingerprints of late-onset cases. The fingerprint abnormality has been found in a significant proportion of first-degree relatives of probands of early onset cases (Seltzer and Sherwin 1986; Weinreb 1985; Nee 1987). The platelet membrane fluidity of early-onset cases is more frequently abnormal than in late-onset cases. This abnormality is also found in a significant proportion of relatives, even if they are as yet unaffected with illness (Zubenko et al. 1987).

Familial Risk to Relatives of Early-Onset AD

Like these somatic features which have a higher prevalence in families of cases, the early age-of-onset form of AD also carries with it the risk for an early age of onset of disease in the relatives, as demonstrated by cases from Drs. Brown, Masters, and Gadjusek, and our own autopsy and clinical cases. Over a wide range the age of onset is more similar within families than between families (Fig. 1). The age of onset is not affected by sex of the parent, as children of affected fathers or affected mothers have similar ages of onset.

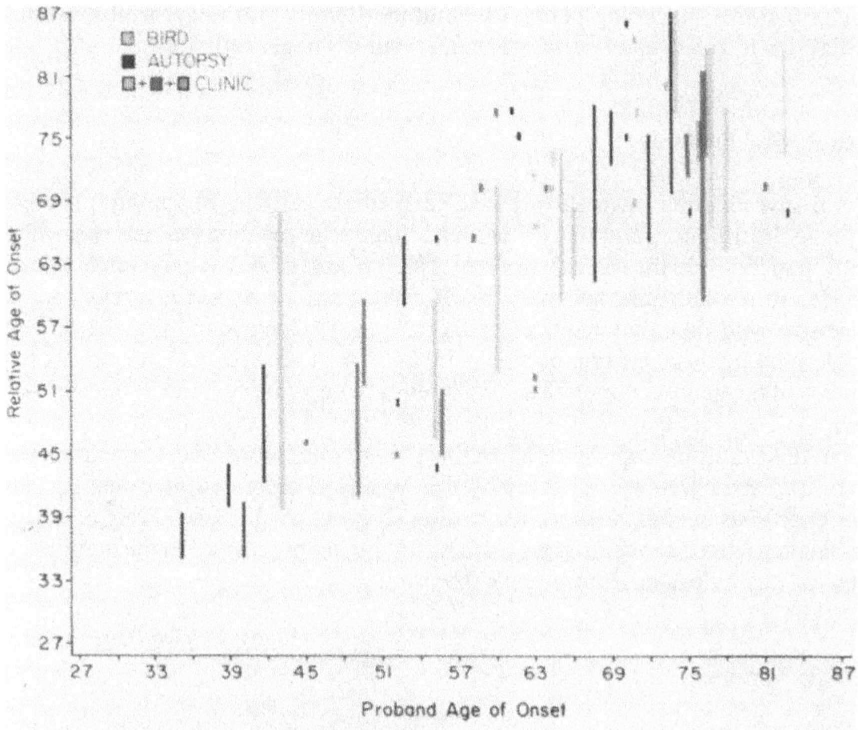

Fig. 1. Age of onset of Alzheimer's disease in 59 families

Neuropathology

Cases with early onset of AD have increased numbers of neuritic plaques and tangles, compared with cases with late onset, and decreased numbers of neurons in the locus coeruleus (Constantinidis 1978; Bondareef et al. 1981). These differences might be due to a longer duration of illness in the younger group.

In summary, clinical features related to age of onset including AAAA, depression, fingerprints, and platelet abnormalities suggest heterogeneity in AD. Since some of these features are found with an increased prevalence in AD families, they could represent genetic heterogeneity. Since a dementia syndrome of long duration but without AAAA does not increase risk to relatives, it may be a phenocopy.

Severity of Dementia Relative to Neuropathology

Although the degree of dementia observed clinically usually correlates with the severity of neuropathology of AD observed after death, individuals have been described who had no evidence of dementia but displayed the neuropathology of AD (Fitch et al. 1988; Katzman et al. 1988). These results have been discussed in terms of a requirement for the severity of neuropathology to exceed a threshold value before symptoms of dementia emerge (Fitch et al. 1988); such a threshold may differ between individuals, and might explain the apparent lack of correlation between dementia and neuropathology in individuals with DS (Wisniewski et al. 1985; Eisner 1983).

Several investigations have demonstrated a high if not universal prevalence of the pathology of AD in DS cases over the age of 40 (Jervis 1948; Malamud 1973; Wisniewski et al. 1985). However, only a small proportion of cases appeared to deteriorate cognitively before death, even though they showed the neuropathological changes of AD (Wisniewski et al. 1985; Eisner 1983; Dalton and Crapper 1984). Since these initial studies were conducted retrospectively it seems quite likely that the patients had deteriorated, but that deterioration was not detected. However, several subsequent studies have been conducted prospectively; the cases were very carefully examined and a significant proportion of cases with DS did not appear to deteriorate (Dalton and Crapper 1984). These results must still be viewed cautiously because a large study has not yet been conducted in which cases are examined prospectively until death and then autopsied. However, the autopsy studies suggest that the majority of cases do have the pathology of AD at death. If we assume that only 20%–30% of cases develop the clinical syndrome by age 50, this would still be a rate many times higher than that in the general population, but certainly not 100%. An interesting speculation is that one result of trisomy 21 is protection from the clinical signs of AD even in the presence of part of the neuropathology. Given this possible protective factor, either a particularly high number of plaques and tangles must be present to cause deterioration or a critical feature of the pathology of AD is not present in DS. The study of cognitive deterioration of individuals with partial translocation DS might clarify the chromosomal location of such a protective factor. Partial translocations are rare and study of them is difficult, but we have begun to look for them. A collaborative effort to collect and study partial translocations would be rewarding.

Understanding the mechanisms which determine the age of onset and its related features will be as important as the discovery of the genes responsible for AD, because delay of the age of onset could push it beyond the normal life span and thus eliminate the expression of AD in human populations.

Accurate Definition of the AD Phenotype is Important for Genetic Linkage studies

The important problem remains of establishing the location of the genes responsible for AD. Knowledge of phenotypic heterogeneity will aid in the design of linkage studies. Criteria must be constructed for the purpose of identifying probands and secondary cases in linkage studies in order to reduce the number of falsely diagnosed cases. To put it another way, we must increase the predictive value of case detection methods in linkage studies.

Predictive value depends on sensitivity, specificity, and prevalence. Current AD diagnostic criteria have sensitivity approaching 90% and specificity somewhat lower for cases followed for many years and then autopsied. Accuracy of diagnosis of cases earlier in the course of illness is not as high, but might be improved by the application of neuroimaging, platelet membrane tests, and fingerprint analysis in a manner subsequently modified by autopsy verification, although this would also increase the cost of studies. The predictive value is also increased if the prevalence of the condition in the study population is high. Thus, families chosen for linkage studies should have high rates of AD diagnosed by rigorous criteria, and low rates of phenocopies. These would include families with a high proportion of cases with amnesia, aphasia, apraxia, and agnosia and exclude families with possible presbyophrenia or vascular disease. Families with younger age of onset should thus be studied first since those families have higher rates of amnesia and aphasia and lower rates of simple senile dementia and stroke. Another way of improving accuracy and reducing heterogeneity of families and cases in linkage studies rests on the common-sense suggestion that we should understand one thing thoroughly before trying to divide it into two things. Perhaps we should devote our efforts to finding the gene in the families already linked and then use this gene as a diagnostic test in other families. This process would be facilitated if the cell lines from the families already linked and the probes near the locus were available for general use.

Acknowledgements. The work and many of the ideas in this presentation are the results of a collaboration with many others, mostly psychiatrists, including Doctors Breitner, Powell, Ross, Rovner, Chase, Murphy, Zweig, and Price. Grant support includes: American Philosophical Society, Alzheimer's Disease and Related Disorders, American Federation for Aging Research, Alzheimer's Disease Research Center (NIA AG-05146), John Douglas French Foundation, Meridian Healthcare Systems, Huntington's Disease Center Without Walls (NINCDS-16735), Impact of Mental Morbidity on Nursing Home Experience (NIA RO1 MH41570-02), Consolidated Gift Fund for Dementia Research, and Research Training in the Dementias of Aging (T32 AG00149).

References

Alzheimer A (1907) Über eine eigenartige Erkrankung der Hirnrinde. Allgemeine Zeitschrift für Psychiatris und Psychisch-Gerichtliche Medicin 64: 146–148

Appell J, Kertesz A, Fisman M (1982) A study of language functioning in Alzheimer patients. Brain Lang 17: 73–91

Berg L, Danziger WL, Storandt M, et al. (1984) Predictive features in mild senile dementia of the Alzheimer type. Neurology 34: 563–569

Bondareef W, Mountjoy OQ, Roth M (1981) Selective loss of neurons of origin of adrenergic projection to cerebral cortex (nucleus locus ceruleus) in senile dementia. Lancet I: 783–784

Breitner JCS, Folstein MF (1984) Familial Alzheimer's disease: a prevalent disorder with specific clinical features. Psychol Med 14: 63–80

Breitner JC, Silverman JM, Mohs RC, Davis KL (1988) Familial aggregation in Alzheimer's disease: comparison of risk among relatives in successive generations. Neurology 38: 207–212

Chui HC, Teng EL, Henderson VW, Moy AC (1985) Clinical subtypes of dementia of the Alzheimer type. Neurology 35: 1544–1550

Constantinidis J (1978) Is Alzheimer's disease a major form of senile dementia? Clinical, anatomical, and genetic data. In: Katzman R, Terry RD, Bick KL (eds) Alzheimer's disease: senile dementia and related disorders (Aging, vol 7). Raven Press, New York, pp 15–25

Constantinidis J, Garrone G, Tissot R, DeAjuriaguerra J (1965) L'incidence familiale des alterations neurofibrillaires corticales d'Alzheimer. Psychiat Neurol (Basel) 51: 330–344

Dalton AJ, Crapper DR (1984) Influence of memory deterioration in aging persons with Down's Syndrome. In: Berg JM (ed) Perspectives and progress in mental retardation. Biomedical aspects, vol 2. University Park Press, Baltimore, pp 55–62

Eisner D (1983) Downs syndrome and aging: Is senile dementia inevitable? Psychol Rep 52: 119–124

Faber-Langendoen K, Morris JC, Knesevich JW, LaBarge E, Miller JP, Berg L (1988) Aphasia in senile dementia of the Alzheimer type. Ann Neurol 23: 365–370

Fitch N, Becker R, Heller A (1988) The inheritance of Alzheimer's disease: or new interpretation. Ann Neurol 23: 14–19

Folstein MF, Breitner J (1981) Language disorder predicts familial Alzheimer's disease. Johns Hopkins Med J 21: 686–689

Foster NL, VanDerSpek AF, Aldrich MS, Berent S, Hichwa RH, Sackellares JC, Gilman S, Agranoff BW (1987) The effect of diazepam sedation on cerebral glucose metabolism in Alzheimer's disease as measured using positron emission tomography. J Cereb Blood Flow Metab 7: 415–420

Go RCP, Todorov AB, Elston RC, Constantinidis J (1979) The malignancy of dementias. Ann Neurol 3: 559–561

Haxby JV, Grady CL, Duara R, Schlalageter N, Berg G, Rapoport SI (1987) Neocortical metabolic abnormalities precede nonmemory cognitive defects in early Alzheimer-type. Arch Neurol 43: 882–885

Huff FJ, Auerbach J, Charavarti A, Boller F (1988) Risk of dementia in relatives of patients with Alzheimer's disease. Neurology 38: 786–790

Jagust WJ, Budinger TF, Reed BR (1987) The diagnosis of dementia with single photon emission computed tomography. Arch Neurol 44: 258–263

Jervis GA (1948) Early senile dementia in mongoloid idiocy. Am J Psychiatry 105: 102–106

Johnson KA, Mueller ST, Walshe TM, English RJ, Holman BL (1987) Cerebral perfusion imaging in Alzheimer's disease. Use of single photon emission computed tomography and iofetamine hydrochloride I 123. Arch Neurol 44: 165–168

Katzman R, Terry R, DeTeresa R, Brown T, Davies P, Fuld P, Renbing X, Peck A (1988) Clinical, pathological and neurochemical changes in dementia: a subgroup with preserved mental status and numerous cortical plaques. Ann Neurol 23: 138–144

Larsson T, Sjogren T, Jacobson G (1963) Senile dementia. Acta Psych Scand (Copenh) [Suppl 167] 39: 1–259

Malamud N (1972) Neuropathology of organic brain syndromes associated with ageism. In: Gaitz CM (ed) Aging and the brain. New York, Plenum, pp 63–87

Martin RL, Gerteis G, Gabrielli WF (1987) A family-genetic study of dementia of Alzheimer type.

Mohs RC, Breitner JC, Silverman JM, Davis KL (1987) Alzheimer's disease. Morbid risk among first-degree relatives approximates 50% by 90 years of age. Arch Gen Psychiatry 44: 405–408

Nee LE (1987) Fingerprint patterns in subjects at risk for inherited Alzheimer's disease. International Symposium of Familial Alzheimer's Disease, Tulsa, Oklahoma 1987
Powell D, Folstein MF (1984) Pedigree study of familial Alzheimer's disease. J Neurogenetics 1: 189–197
Prichard JC (1837) A treatise on insanity and other disorders affecting the mind. Haswell, Barnington and Haswell, Philadelphia, pp 69–80
Rovner BW, Broadhead J, Spencer M, Carson K, Folstein MF (1988) Depression and Alzheimer's disease. Am J Psychiatry (in press)
Seltzer B, Sherwin I (1983) A comparison of clinical features in early- and late-onset primary degenerative dementia: one entity or two? Arch Neurol 40: 143–146
Seltzer B, Sherwin I (1986) Fingerprint pattern differences in early- and late-onset primary degenerative dementia. Arch Neurol 43: 665–668
Weinreb HJ (1985) Fingerprint patterns in Alzheimer's disease. Arch Neurol 42: 50–54
Wisniewski KE, Wisniewski HM, Wen GY (1985) Occurrence of neuropathological changes in dementia of Alzheimer's disease in Down's syndrome. Ann Neurol 17: 278–282
Zweig RM, Ross CA, Hedreen JC, Steele C, Cardillo JE, Whitehouse PJ, Folstein MF (1988) The neuropathology of aminergic nuclei. Ann Neurol 24: 233–242
Zubenko GS, Wusylko M, Cohen BM, Boller F, Teply I (1987) Platelet membraned fluidity in Alzheimer's disease. Science 238: 539–542

Extended Kindreds as a Model for Research on Alzheimer's Disease

J.-F. Foncin, D. Salmon, and *A. C. Bruni*

Summary

This chapter reviews the methods used to gather, organize and analyse the data, and explains how we used the information provided by large kindreds in which Alzheimer's disease occurs with very high incidence, drawing primarily from our experience with a southern Italian extended family (family "N"). About 4000 subjects, 60 of whom were affected with Alzheimer's disease, are identified in this pedigree, with the common ancestor of all affected subjects being identified as a woman born in 1715. Exploration of municipal and parish records on a blanket basis was fundamental to establish the pedigree, mental (state) hospital records were used to establish diagnosis, and Bayesian probabilities permitted an estimate of status for subjects for whom age at death was known and genotype probability was known or estimated. Segregation ratio and thence mode of transmission may be established within narrow confidence limits from large bias-free pedigrees; these are the only ones for which Mendelian dominant autosomal transmission, to the exclusion of environmental effects, has been established. Large pedigrees have been decisive in recent progress in the molecular genetics of Alzheimer's disease. The nosological relationship between the disease expressed in those kindreds and that appearing sporadically or in small clusters is a matter under discussion. What seems certain is that large kindreds are one of the most powerful models at our disposal for research on Alzheimer's disease.

Introduction

The quasi explosive developments in research on Alzheimer's disease in recent years have largely been due to progress in molecular genetics. Extended families, or kindreds, in which Alzheimer's disease occurs with very high incidence have been fundamental to that endeavor, in spite of the comparatively small number which have been adequately described. In the present paper we first review the methods used to gather and organize the data needed for a useful description of large kindreds. Most papers describing large Alzheimer's disease pedigrees do not, for obvious reasons of space limitation, go into detail about the methods used by the authors; this is regrettable, however, inasmuch as hidden bias in data collection and retention may impair the validity of statistics and, consequently, of conclusions. We will therefore, draw largely on our own experience with the study of the southern Italian family "N" (Foncin et al. 1973, 1985, 1986; Bruni et al. 1987).

The second part of the paper deals with the mathematical and statistical treatments which allow a demonstration of the genetic character and mode of transmission of Alzheimer's disease in affected families, that is, the formal genetics stage.

Once the formal genetics are established, the stage is set for molecular genetics studies: how material gathered from Alzheimer's disease families with large pedigrees has been and may be used for that purpose is the third theme of this chapter. Problems such as the relevance of large pedigree studies to Alzheimer's disease in general and speculations about future directions of research are dealt with in a concluding section.

Gathering the Data

Obviously, the first step in any study of extended kindreds with Alzheimer's disease is awareness of cluster occurrence of the disease in the family of patients examined for the first time. This information is most often obtained through a conventional familial history obtained from relatives. So important is the detection of familial Alzheimer's disease for progress in Alzheimer's disease research in general, and so much depends on the collaborative attitude of the next of kin, that every effort must be made to establish a positive rapport during the first interview with relatives of any patient with possible cognitive impairment. The demonstration of interest on the part of the physician, afforded by thorough family history taking, is an important step in that direction. On psychological as well as scientific grounds, however, it is important for the interviewer to project a neutral but kind attitude. Direct interrogation about "other cases of the same illness in the family," as the question is often worded by junior staff wishing to go straight to the heart of the matter, may be counterproductive in two ways. As an effect of (often unconscious) reactive denial, the interviewer is perceived negatively and instances of Alzheimer's disease in the family are "forgotten," and the occasion is lost for the detection of familial Alzheimer's disease. On the other hand, a halo effect may lead to spurious "overdiagnosis" by the relatives. From the start, systematic inquiry about matters of public record concerning every relative in memory (even if presumably unaffected) should be pursued, avoiding direct questions concerning mental illness. The data that are registered are full names, date and place of birth; maiden name, date and place of marriage; employment; intervening illnesses with names and addresses of attending physicians and hospitals; apparent cause, date and place of death, and whether an autopsy was done. Of course, spontaneous indications regarding cases of dementing illness in the family are recorded, but without unduly stressing their importance.

Such an inquiry may be sufficient to give an indication about possible clustering of Alzheimer's disease in the patient's family, giving additional elements for a diagnosis of the same disease in the patient himself. Recording yet another familial cluster of Alzheimer's disease is, however, not an aim in itself. When a number of them are grouped into one study, such clusters may be, and have been, used in well-planned studies, starting with the detection of a large number of index cases. Examples are the studies of Sjögren et al. (1952), Heston and Mastri (1977), Heston and White (1978), the Geneva school (Constantinidis 1965) and the Folstein group (Chase et al. 1983). To go further within one family, with the aim of providing a pedigree as extensive and as free of bias as possible, and thus suitable as a basis for further applications, more extended inquiries have to be made, which are by nature quite different from usual clinical history taking. As we know from personal experience, a decision to follow a kindred to its remotest branches and to establish a reliable pedigree may mean starting a multi-year endeavor. Criteria have to be determined for the selection of families to be studied with the best hope for useful results.

The first criterion is, of course, the cooperation of family members, which depends on a number of factors: the first contact with the medical team may be decisive, as stressed above. A prolific family is an important plus, representing more significant statistics and less chance for interruption of transmission in any given branch. Under the same heading of reproductive mores, we stress the importance of strict monogamy in the population to be studied. In fact, HLA typing and molecular biology studies failed to show any instance of paternity exclusion in family "N." In the same kindred we found only one instance of Alzheimer's disease clinically identical with the familial form and which had to be explained either by sporadic occurrence or by adultery. By contrast, when studying a family with Gerstmann Sträussler Scheinker disease originating from the mining country in northern France (Foncin et al. 1982), we found a large proportion of illegitimate births, and were stopped, while tracing upwards the transmission of the disease, when we found both legal parents of the affected grandmother to be out of risk by reason of their longevity. In fact, Lefebvre and Tauzin (unpublished data) recently found a recorded suspicion that the postman had been the biological father of the obligate transmitter. The postman's phenotype remains unknown.

A second set of favorable conditions falls under the heading "accessibility." Records grouped in one place are easier to gather and to compare; field trips to many places are costly and time-consuming. Stable families within traditional, rural societies tend to be more favorable in all those respects. Families with roots in countries where public records were not kept during the nineteenth century, or where records are inaccessible, such as Soviet Russia (Goudsmit et al. 1981), or were destroyed during wars, such as much of central Europe, often lead to frustrating deadends. Local legal conditions for access to records may also vary.

These factors are not specific for familial Alzheimer's disease research; they were prominent in two recent "success stories" of molecular genetics, namely Huntington's disease in Venezuela (Gusella et al. 1983) and manic-depressive illness among the Amish in the U. S. A. (Egeland et al. 1987). What is specific to Alzheimer's disease is its wide clinical spectrum. Clear-cut forms of the disease are, of course, easier to trace in old records; they may be marked by early onset, and thence early death, detectable in civil records, and/or by distinct symptoms, detectable in medical records. "Simple" senile dementia, dismissed as a normal phenomenon due to aging, usually went, and often still goes, unrecorded. The unsolved question of the relevance of results obtained on (early onset) familial Alzheimer's disease models to (mainly late-onset) Alzheimer's disease in general (see last section of this paper) ought, nevertheless, to induce researchers to try tracing late onset Alzheimer's disease pedigrees, in spite of the inherent difficulties.

Even if a cooperating aged relative with a good memory and interest in family affairs is available, data obtained from interviews with members of the nuclear family of the proband are only a small beginning, both from the point of view of reliability and of extension. Visits to the homes of more distant relatives are useful, but still limited in scope. Other methods have to be used, which are outlined below. Many of these methods are not specific to familial Alzheimer's disease research, and derive from those which have been developed for the tracing of private genealogies, a hobby which has been recently made popular by books such as *Roots*. Clubs and societies of persons interested in genealogy exist, and useful tips and introductions may often be obtained from them. Members of such groups are usually happy to see their hobby considered as serious scientific business. Membership in a genealogical society is often an asset for workers engaged in medical pedigree tracing.

The first sources to be consulted are the municipal registers of births, marriages and deaths (in France, *Etat-Civil;* in Italy, *Stato Civile*) which were organized in most of Europe under Napoleonic influence. In southern Italy, these registers date back to 1809, during the reign of Murat. Records dating back more than 100 years may be consulted by all comers and freely copied from the registers. Copies of more recent records may be legally obtained by members of the family (if the existence and date of the document are known); permission for use of recent registers for our study has been granted by authorities without difficulty in view of the fact that a public research organization was involved. When dealing with records of a population in which the relative density of members of the kindred is low, such as in localities distant from the cradle of the family, it may be cost-efficient to take copies only of those records which are in evident relationship with the family under study, that is, to use a "tracing" method. According to this method, records in which one participant is already known are copied. It favors the patrilinear link because surnames are more discriminating that given names, and in this way introduces bias; moreover, when new surnames in matrilinear ascent/descent are identified, further runs of the registers are needed. In using the registers in the cradle town of the family, we have instead preferred a "blanket" approach, aiming to take substantial copies of every record in which a surname appears that is known in the intermarrying population to which the family under study belongs. The creation of a computer database incorporating all of the registers would be the ultimate in blanket coverage. This has been done for parts of Quebec (in that case mostly from parish books, Etat Civil being a recent institution in the province) and is put to use by the IMAGE project (Gauvreau et al., this volume). The Church of Jesus-Christ of Latter Day Saints maintains such a database for religious reasons, covering various parts of Europe and America. We have no personal experience, however, in using this database, which under French law might require special authorization.

Other registers may be used which cover the nineteenth and twentieth centuries. Registers of emigration, kept in Italian municipal offices, are a link between research in the family's hometown and research on emigrated branches. Recent church records may be useful for two reasons: although people nowadays tend to be born and die away from home, baptism and burial take place at their own parish, providing a better concentration of documents. Moreover, in countries with no established church, parish books are not covered by restrictions of public access to recent government records. We have found most useful the Status Animarum, which used to be written up by parish priests at fixed intervals. This record of all the households in the parish contained a wealth of data on all parish members, including the names of the parishioners' parents and whether they were alive of dead. For records before the nineteenth century, parish books usually constitute the only available source. Extent and quality of records vary considerably according to country and even province. In Switzerland, for instance, civic records kept in ancient cities often go back to the fifteenth century. In France, although King François I enjoined parish priests to keep records of baptisms (1539) and King Henri III did the same for marriages and burials (1579), complete records are often available only for the eighteenth century. In southern Italy, records regularly cover the eighteenth century, occasionally the seventeenth century and, rarely, the late sixteenth century. The difficulty of reading ancient handwriting, the irregular form of the entries, and haphazard variations in spelling make their use awkward for the nonspecialist. Dr. Gei, a scholar in modern Italian history, has recently tackled the eighteenth century parish records of the town of N..., the cradle of family "N," and of neighboring villages from which the carrier of the Alzheimer's disease gene may have come in the early eighteenth century. In collaboration with Dr. Gei (unpublished results) we could identify the nearest common affected ancestor, twelve generations removed, of two Alzheimer's disease patients examined in N... by A.C. Bruni. This common ancestor proved to be a woman named G... Vittoria, who was born in 1715 and died at 43 years of age. This finding confirms the clinical diagnoses and, more importantly, the value of the methods we had used for retrospective diagnosis of affected (carrier) subjects (see below). It testifies to the value of systematic exploration of very old records as a tool for human genetics.

A specific source in medical pedigree tracing is, of course, medical records. Copies of records of patients within living memory may be obtained from attending physicians or from hospitals. More specifically, in the case of dementing illness, the records of the State Mental Hospital system have proven valuable, partly because they were, by law, kept for 100 years. They may be approached in various ways. From the time of the institution of death certificate transcription – that is, a mention of date and place of death in the margin of the birth certificate – the mention of a locality with a State Mental Hospital (often a small community with little other population movement) as the place of death is a presumption of fatal mental illness, and subsequent tracing of the record is an easy task. Using this procedure we located the record of a long-lost member of the above-cited family with Gerstmann Sträussler Scheinker disease (Foncin et al. 1982). Records of the State Mental Hospital serving the town of N... were studied first for patients with surnames known in family "N"; later an attempt was made to study the records of all patients who died within the age range at death of affected members of family "N". Unfortunately, an Italian law aiming to abolish mental illness by abolishing the State Mental Hospital system is now putting in jeopardy the continued accessibility and even existence of these precious records.

The mode of definition of subject status is a recurring question in familial Alzheimer's disease work. The usual definitions of possible, probable, and proven Alzheimer's disease diagnosis are not applicable to familial Alzheimer's disease. If genetic transmission is demonstrated and one case in the genetic chain is proven, a priori probability for Alzheimer's disease may be orders of magnitude higher for at-risk subjects, as compared with the general population, especially in the case of early-onset forms. Bayes' theorem (Bayes 1763) applied to conditionally "possible" cases then results in an a posteriori probability equivalent to quasicertitude. Mistakes are still possible, arising from erroneous evaluation of conditional probabilities, as we experienced in our own study. Two brothers of the family "N" proband were hospitalized at the same time in a university neurological clinic for evaluation. Both were diagnosed as having Alzheimer's disease. The elder one subsequently died with dementia, the younger one recovered, is now in good health past the maximum age of manifestation of familial Alzheimer's disease in family "N", and is retrospectively believed to have presented pseudodementia as a manifestation of depression reactive to his brother's illness.

Bayesian probabilities are fundamental in estimating the status of subjects who lived at times for which no medical records are available and, moreover, in which dementia, not to speak of Alzheimer's disease, was not a valid category. This point requires elaboration, because problems about status definition are often raised in discussions about the validity of extended kindreds reaching more than two centuries into the past as a model to be used in Alzheimer's disease research. Patients with early-onset familial Alzheimer's disease die within a well-defined age span, and mortality of familial Alzheimer's disease patients may be compared for each age group with mortality of not-at-risk subjects in the same population (spouses and their families). An a posteriori probability for familial Alzheimer's disease may be computed for subjects with known age at death and known or estimated a priori genetic risk. In family "N", a posteriori probability of Alzheimer's disease in subjects at first-degree risk who died between ages 45 and 55 is quite high, approaching 0.9. Compound probabilities applied to sibships may lead to still higher figures. Conversely, no subject with (empirically ascertained) affected or carrier status died older than age 66. As is often the case with Bayesian probabilities, the main difficulty lies in estimating a priori probability when the genetic relationship of the subject under study with known affected subjects, that is genetic risk, is not precisely known. An estimate may in these instances be obtained by taking advantage of the heredity of surnames (Crow and Mange 1965). At a time in our research (1984) when subject no. 18, M... Pietro Salvatore, who was born in 1803 and died at age 45, was the earliest known common ancestor of all affected subjects, the surname M... was borne by 33 sibships in the file as it stood. Of these, three were affected, that is with at least one affected member, and 20 were "controls," that is without any known gene identity by descent with affected subjects. The remainder were of undefined status. The a priori risk for an M... sibship could therefore be estimated at $3/23 = 0.13$. Applying the method we just outlined to the sibship born in the second quarter of the nineteenth century out of subject no. 1259, M... Giuseppe (a sibship without any known gene identity by descent with affected subjects known to us at that time), we found a 0.70 probability for that sibship to have been affected. As it happened, this result was soon afterwards confirmed by the rediscovery of subject no. 1259 as an ancestor of a patient affected by Alzheimer's disease, with age at onset and clinical presentation identical to those of previously known members of family "N". It has been definitely proven by the recent discovery (see above) of the affected common ancestor. Consequently, combining Bayesian probabilities for inclusion, and exclusion of subjects who died older than the empirical cut-off age of 66 years, we could trace the transmission of Alzheimer's disease in family "N" for 12 generations, back to the early eighteenth century. This limit could probably be pushed back further by research in seventeenth-century archives.

Organizing the Data

Avoiding bias in pedigree construction means that any subject identified through the procedures indicated in the preceding section, and linked to the proband through the transitive set of relationships (consanguinity, marriage), is to be included in the pedigree, being an element of a connected net (generalized genealogical tree) which includes the proband. This method obviously leads to storage of information regarding people without any apparent genetic relationship with the proband. When applied, however, to approximately closed communities such as the ones most favorable for pedigree tracing, it leads to the description of a population, in the population genetics meaning of the term. We have often found that later discovery of new subjects leads to a change in the status of previously recorded relatives by marriage to that of blood relatives, of primary interest for Mendelian genetics purposes. These subjects would have been lost if not recorded in the first place as an application of the "blanket" method. Another and more fundamental advantage of the "blanket" method is that it does not inject, via the gathering and recording of data, any hypotheses about the mode of transmission, the testing of which is one of the aims of the study. Obviously, a pedigree restricted to carriers and their descendants has a built-in bias in favour of dominant transmission and cannot be used to test, for instance, polygenic hypotheses. Another reason for the systematic recording of "spouses" and their ancestry is to provide an internal demographic standard, as demonstrated above.

Handling such a rapidly growing mass of data (the "N" family pedigree now numbers more than 4000 subjects) obviously necessitates the use of computer facilities. In fact, we almost stopped working on the "N" pedigree in the mid-1970s, during the period between the first data gathering by J. F. Foncin and the introduction of computer treatment by D. Salmon. Most of the researchers working on large pedigrees certainly also use some form of computer aid, but the methods they use are seldom clear from the Methods sections of their published papers. Therefore, we will outline here our own experience. Our way of handling the data reflects the changes in technology during the long period we have been working with computers, and certainly would not be the same if designed today. The core of a subject's entry had been modeled on the 80-column IBM punched card standard which was the usual link between user and (mainframe, of course) computer in the early 1970s. A free commentary was later added, taking advantage of the remaining space on a standard printer line, when it became obvious that paper notes would become useless because of their mass. Essential in this set-up is an arbitrary but unique subject serial number, usually given by order of entry. One should avoid the designation of subject by combined generation (vertical) and horizontal number, such as VI-34, which is inevitably ambiguous in large kindreds where any numbering of generations is bound to be arbitrary, as a result of consanguinous marriages between people belonging to different generations in respect to one or many founders. The serial number is the main identification tool for any given subject, because of the extensive homonymy of surnames in closed communities and of the lack of imagination of nineteenth century parents for given names. Serial number of parents (0 for "founders" or original parents, i. e., subjects whose parents are, at the time, not yet recorded) and code numbers for gender and status are the other essential data. The best way to record a marriage without known children is to enter a fictitious child of the couple, with an appropriate code number in lieu of gender.

In contrast with the early dependence of mainframe computers, database programs implemented on personal computers are a more modern approach to family studies. We "repatriated" the family "N" file via modem in the form of an Apple Works database file (configuration, Apple IIe with 512K memory extension and hard disk). This minimal setup enables one to permanently check with the file to incorporate new subjects or to update previous entries. Printouts sorted according to various criteria are used primarily for field work and for communication with other workers on the same project, for instance, molecular biologists. Ancillary programs, which handle a simplified ASCII version of the database, detect inconsistencies in entries, such as a masculine mother or a father who died as an infant. Other programs list all the ancestors or all the descendants of a given subject, and detect consanguinity with respect to a given ancestor. The latter program is useful for the detection of possible homozygotes for the familial Alzheimer's disease genetic anomaly (see below). Marriage between cousins used to be rare and consciously avoided in the "N" family. We detected a few instances of consanguinity with respect to G... Vittoria, the common affected ancestor; none, however, could be an instance of homozygocy, at least one of the parents being separated from the common affected ancestor by an "escapee". Another series of programs was run on the mainframe computer (Landre et al. 1972) with, as a final output, the automatic drawing of genealogical trees on paper. These trees have been very useful to enable one to form a mental image of the family, but their future role, except for teaching and publication, is in doubt. Our last complete tree was drawn in 1982, at a time when the number of known members of family "N" was about one-third of the present one; the drawing was already about 10 m long. Since then, only partial trees have been drawn, destined for field work or for communication with colleagues working on other aspects of the genetics of family "N". The future probably lies in more powerful and specially adapted database systems, which are already in use by other teams, for instance in the above-cited IMAGE project, and which give the user instant fingertip access to all the relationships of any subject.

Analyzing the Data

Analyzing the data provided by a large Alzheimer's disease pedigree, be it with the aid of elaborate mathematical tools or by simple inspection of a tree, confronts us with problems quite different from those usually met in human mathematical genetics, which usually deal with multiple small pedigrees. The first task, of course, is segregation analysis, the results of which are fundamental in order to decide whether transmission is Mendelian or not, and if in the affirmative, to determine the type of transmission. Thirty years ago, segregation analysis in the human was limited to the constant segregation ratio of Mendelian traits and neglected vertical nongenetic transmission, cultural inheritance, and polygeny. The polygenic model, on the other hand, which underlies the concept of susceptibility to disease, neglected the major loci. The development of computer treatment allowed generalization of these models into the mixed model which hypothesizes a major locus and both polygenic and environmental effects. Implementation of large kindreds on these programs, however, is difficult and expensive in terms of computer time, in spite of the ingenious methods developed by Elston and Stewart (1971) to condense pedigree information. On the other hand, very large kindreds may lend themselves to conclusive analysis of problems without the need for computer treatment. For instance, a branch of family "N" which emigrated to the U. S. A. at the end of the nineteenth century, and had been independently described by Feldman et al. (1963), has been followed up by the same author (Foncin et al. 1985) and by L. Nee (unpublished data). Clinical manifestation, age at onset, and apparent segregation ratio are identical in the European and American branches, in spite of the marked differences in environment, dietary habits, and style of living between middle-class northeastern Americans and rural southern Italians. This fact alone is enough to rule out any environmental effect in the determination of Alzheimer's disease in family "N".

Precise calculation of the segregation ratio, with determination of confidence intervals, is a well-known source of pitfalls in human genetics studies, which nearly all lead to overestimation of the segregation ratio. The so-called segregation of a Mendelian trait follows a binomial distribution. The expected number of affected individuals in an at-risk sibship is thereby easily formulated. Another parameter is relevant, however: namely, the ascertainment probability, which is defined as the conditional probability that an affected member of the population can be detected as a proband, independently from his relatives. The first proband to be ascertained is called the propositus or index case. Serious bias results if other probands are treated as true secondary cases. Elaborate (and computer time-consuming) quantitative methods have been developed (Lalouel and Morton 1981) to deal with this problem. Qualitatively, they may be roughly explained as a generalization of the rule eliminating the index case when calculating a segregation ratio by hand. In family "N", we deal with three probands: the index cases of the American and of the European branches, and the patient who confirmed the calculated carrier status of subject no. 1259 (see above). Apart from these clear-cut cases, however, when ascertainment probability is low, the probability that a sibship can be ascertained is nearly proportional to the number of its affected members. This entails considerable bias towards sibships with an excess of affected subjects, and is more likely to occur when dealing with Alzheimer's disease, the ascertainment probability of which, especially in late onset forms, is certainly lower than that of, for instance, Huntington's disease.

The methods of data gathering for the description of such very large pedigrees and their sheer size, however, make the application of theoretically correct methods more difficult, more costly, and less necessary, With a few exceptions, the notion of secondary proband becomes ill-defined. Ascertainment of pedigree members through the exploitation of municipal records does not introduce bias in favour of affected subjects, as opposed to conventional history taking. Bias is introduced, however, when a subject is ascertained (as distinct from his status being determined) through his presence on hospital records. Status estimation through Bayesian methods using the age at death (or determination of the escapee status of subjects dying past the cut-off age) is not subject to the same errors. We once felt (Foncin et al. 1985) that the uncorrected calculation of a 0.65 (significantly different from 0.5) segregation ratio from near exhaustively known sibships, subjects with unknown status being rated as unaffected, would be bias-free, and even speculated that increased fitness of Alzheimer's disease carriers during infancy could account for the difference. In fact, calculations from the present state of the pedigree (Bruni et al. 1987), incorporating about three times as many subjects and a more thorough study of all the at-risk sibships, show a segregation ratio not significantly different from 0.5, in conformity with the null hypothesis of autosomal dominant Mendelian transmission with complete penetrance. A lesson to be drawn from this experience is that the use of uncorrected results for segregation ratio calculation is only warranted when starting from very large pedigrees and objective (that is, independent from informant intervention) ascertainment.

Using the Data

Our main endeavor has been to provide the basis for molecular biology studies intended to cast light on fundamental problems of Alzheimer's disease. Implicitly, an aim of the same general nature motivated researchers who studied Alzheimer's disease with the methods of family tracing, even before it could be apparent that the way from family tracing to formal genetics to molecular genetics would be decisive for progress in the study of a disease which had eluded the usual types of modeling. Of course, it was even more apparent from the time it became obvious that the model set up by Gusella et al. (1983) would be of general value (Wexler et al. 1985).

Large pedigrees are useful in other ways, however. Bayesian probabilities, either explicitly or implicitly used, make possible a quasicertain diagnosis of Alzheimer's disease in subjects with early symptoms which would at most entail a "possible" diagnosis according to established criteria. The prerequisite is a quantitatively defined a priori probability, which is to be calculated from a known segregation ratio and a simple relationship to a "confirmed" case of Alzheimer's disease in the family, both of which are attainable in well-studied large kindreds. This provides an opportunity, and a unique one as long as positive biological diagnosis of oligosymptomatic Alzheimer's disease is not possible, to test various diagnostic procedures applicable to early Alzheimer's disease (Polinsky et al. 1987), and, hopefully, to evaluate therapeutic measures which obviously would require, for efficacy, a stage of the disease at which neurone loss is not irreversible. Another application of large Alzheimer's disease kindreds should be the identification and study of homozygotes for the familial Alzheimer's disease genetic anomaly, as has been done for Huntington's disease (Wexler et al. 1987). Their phenotype would significantly constrain the mechanism of action of that anomaly; for instance, a phenotype identical with that of heterozygotes would rule out a gene dosage effect and further differentiate Alzheimer's disease from Down's syndrome.

It is not our purpose to enter into details concerning the results in the molecular biology domain obtained through the use of data and material originating from large Alzheimer's disease kindreds. The role of the field researchers, as people working with the families may be characterized, is firstly to provide reliable data relative to the formal genetics of Alzheimer's disease in the families under study, and to the status of individuals in the families, as described above. Secondly, they must obtain biological material, that is DNA sources, from key individuals. A major problem is that few affected subjects are alive at a given time even in the largest Alzheimer's disease kindreds known at present. This situation may not always be palliated by genome reconstitution using surviving parents, spouses, and children. This is an incentive for further enlarging the pedigrees, and tracing downwards new branches which, once followed down to the present time, may yield new, informative nuclear families. A positive relationship of investigators with family members is an indispensable asset for the collection of material. We feel that the patient-physician relationship is the best adapted to the circumstances; utmost care should be given to preserving it and to preventing the intrusion of people resented by the families as outsiders.

Four such kindreds were the basis of the mapping of the FAD gene, defined as cosegregating with Alzheimer's disease phenotype in these families, to the proximal part of the long arm of chromosome 21 (St George-Hyslop et al. 1987 a). The kindreds referred to in that paper have been reported: FAD1 by Nee et al. (1983); FAD2 by Frommelt et al. (1987); FAD3 by Goudsmit et al. (1981; FAD4 is family "N" (see above). In spite of the large kindreds used for the study, the number of informative meioses was too small in each family to reach the conventional +3 lod score within a single family. The highest single point-single family LOD score – +2.46 for linkage with the D21S16 locus at 0.00 recombination fraction – was observed in the "N" family. Multipoint analysis and combination of the four families were necessary to attain a +4.25 peak lod score. Van Broeckhoven et al. (this volume) found in one of two large Belgian families a lod score suggestive of linkage between FAD and the D21S13 locus, which itself is tightly linked to D21S16, thus confirming the proximal situation of the FAD locus on the long arm of chromosome 21.

The four families referred to above have been used again by St George-Hyslop et al. (1987 b) and Tanzi et al. (1987). The first of these two papers used sporadic and small-cluster Alzheimer's disease instances as well as the large pedigrees to demonstrate that gene duplication is at most exceptionally found on chromosome 21 in cases with Alzheimer's disease. This conclusion has been independently reached by other investigators studying "sporadic," "probable" (Furuya et al. 1988), or "confirmed" cases (Murdoch et al. 1988). It shows that the relationship between Alzheimer's disease and Down's syndrome, while having successfully pointed to chromosome 21 as the right candidate for carrying the FAD gene, is not an easy one to define. The second paper used the four large pedigrees to show that, contrary to early speculation, a defect in the AP gene encoding the precursor protein of beta amyloid could not be causal for familial Alzheimer's disease, the AP gene not being linked with Alzheimer's disease transmission itself. The same conclusion was simultaneously reached by van Broeckhoven et al. (1987) using as material the two large Belgian families referred to above, together with several smaller, clinically diagnosed clusters. We may be allowed to add parenthetically that this result was not unexpected (and indeed could be predicted) by the neuropathologist who sees, at the ultrastructural level, axone terminal degeneration occurring as an apparently primary phenomenon in plaque formation, in the absence of visible amyloid (Foncin and Le Beau 1965; Gonatas and Gambetti 1970). Isolated accumulation of amyloid, by contrast, has traditionally been deemed characteristic of the late, "burnt out" plaque (Terry and Wisniewski 1970). Amyloid deposits are then easily explained as an unspecific residue of the degradation of the transmembrane protein (Kang et al. 1987; Masters et al., this volume) released by the destruction of degenerated axone terminals.

A Model for Alzheimer's Disease

Extensively studied large kindreds have, as we have just shown, provided important results on both the positive side (mapping the FAD gene) and the negative side (disproving an enticing hypothesis). A critical question is then whether conclusions drawn from very rare instances, that is, from the small number of very large Alzheimer's disease pedigrees to have been described and used, are relevant to Alzheimer's disease in general.

The first question to be addressed is whether familial occurrence of Alzheimer's disease is common or not. The question may be approached in a variety of ways. The first approach is the clinical one, that is routine family history taking, as described above. This approach tends to underestimate the proportion of familial occurrence of Alzheimer's disease. Family "N" is a case in point: the index patient had been, successively, under the care of a general practitioner, psychiatrist, neurologist, and neurosurgeon, before the familial nature of her condition was recognized when a neuropathologist interviewed her husband. The reasons for underreporting familial occurrence of fatal diseases are multiple, beyond simple laziness. One is probably the bad reputation that medical genetics still has in some quarters, due to crimes which had nothing to do with science. (One of us a few years ago was an invited guest to a meeting of psychiatrists. Asked what psychiatrists could do to participate in research on mental diseases, he answered, "Take careful family histories." He was then called a fascist.)

Another approach is the epidemiological one, exemplified by the contribution of Alperovitch and Berr to this volume. We cannot go into any detail about results from this type of work beyond the general conclusions that dementia cases are found significantly more frequently among the relatives of patients with Alzheimer's disease, and that no clue for an environmental factor has been unequivocally identified, in contrast, for instance, with multiple sclerosis.

The second question is the relative numerical importance of genetic causation of Alzheimer's disease. This question is distinct from the preceding one, inasmuch as familial clustering may be due to vertical or lateral transmission of a causative agent, and/or to other environmental factors, as we are reminded by the Kuru story (Harper 1977). Association, as distinct from linkage, cannot demonstrate a genetic causation of disease. It is not necessary to cite the numerous papers devoted to association between Alzheimer's disease and various phenotypically detectable polymorphisms, particularly in the major histocompatibility system. Shortly before FAD was mapped to chromosome 21, it was shown that histocompatibility and complement loci are not linked to Alzheimer's disease in family "N" (Muller et al. 1986; Clemenceau et al. 1986). This was a trivial result in retrospect, the major histocompatibility loci being, of course, mapped to chromosome 6. For the same reason, the statistical association of an Apo C2 allele (mapped to chromosome 19) with familial Alzheimer's disease in small pedigrees (Schellenberg et al. 1987) is impossible to interpret.

The key to an answer, short of significant cosegregation, is the determination of the segregation ratio, which, if internally consistent and moreover consistent with an established model of Mendelian transmission, is a strong indication for the latter. We indicated earlier in this paper the problems with segregation ratio determination in large pedigrees. These problems nevertheless may be overcome and the null hypothesis of a 0.5 segregation ratio may be shown to be acceptable concerning those pedigrees. Small pedigrees, on the other hand, do not allow a calculation within a confidence interval small enough for the result to be of practical significance. The standard answer to that problem is the simultaneous treatment of a number of independent pedigrees. This approach, however, may be incorrect when dealing with Alzheimer's disease, because we have no a priori certitude that genetic transmission is causal in all instances of familial clustering, nor that the same transmission mode is involved in all instances of genetic transmission. It has nevertheless been attempted by Breitner et al. (1984, 1986, 1988). The central feature of this type of work is the use of correction by actuarial methods to take into account the fact that, especially in late-onset forms, death from other causes may occur before Alzheimer's disease could be phenotypically apparent in subjects with the Alzheimer's disease genotype (Chase et al. 1983). Overall results show a (corrected) 50% risk for Alzheimer's disease among first-degree relatives of probands, pointing to a 0.5 segregation ratio for late-onset as well as early-onset forms, which, of course, would be indicative of Mendelian autosomal transmission with complete penetrance. Methodological criticism has been directed at this type of work. Most of the error sources, such as errors in the diagnosis of Alzheimer's disease in probands, would add noise, and thus lower the apparent segregation ratio. Other sources of error, such as preferential ascertainment and overdiagnosis of secondary cases, would tend to increase that ratio. It is just possible that the two types of error would compensate for each other in order to reach a spurious apparent 0.5 segregation ratio. Nevertheless, these findings are an interesting indication in favour of genetic transmission in an important proportion of Alzheimer's disease instances.

There are other sides to the picture, however. We discount the "consensus" opinion about the prevalence of sporadic cases: its roots lie mainly in clinical opinion, whereas we have seen the practical limits of clinical family histories. Artifacts arising from the death of genotypically affected subjects before age of clinical onset could account for the commonly held notion that early-onset Alzheimer's disease is genetic, whereas late-onset "senile dementia of the Alzheimer type" is not. Twin studies, on the other hand, apparently pose severe limitations to the prevalence of genetic forms of Alzheimer's disease (Nee et al. 1987). In this study, the concordance rate was 41% in monozygotic twins and 40% in dizygotic twins: such figures are exactly of the order expected for an environmental factor active during infancy or early childhood. At any rate, to account for those results while retaining a genetic hypothesis, one would have to admit a widely scattered age-at-onset in subjects with identical genotype, and consequently an incomplete dependence of phenotype to genotype. Note that we did not find in family "N" any instance of at-risk twins of either kind (in the population and the period under study, moreover, most twins died in early infancy).

All the above question marks lead to a currently much debated problem, that is the one of homogeneity vs heterogeneity of Alzheimer's disease. Although heavy with problems in semantics and theoretical nosology, the problem may be approached from several operative sides. It has been claimed, in particular, that genetic heterogeneity in Alzheimer's disease might be detected by neuropsychological evaluation, "aphasic" forms of the disease being the ones showing Mendelian-like segregation among first-degree relatives (Folstein and Breitner 1982; Breitner and Folstein

1984). Methodological problems, however, weigh heavily on these questions (Knesevich et al. 1985; Breitner 1985; Knesevich 1985).

Are large Alzheimer's disease kindreds instances of one, or perhaps many, separate entities which ought to be radically distinguished from "ordinary" cases occurring sporadically or in small clusters? Inasmuch as the definition of confirmed Alzheimer's disease – associating progressive dementia with the three landmarks of "neuritic plaques," "neurofibrillary tangles," and "granulovacuolar degeneration" – is fulfilled in each kindred for at least one (and generally many) subjects, no formal diagnostic problem should arise. On the face of it, however, features of individual cases of Alzheimer's disease occurring in large kindreds are different from those of most "ordinary" cases. First, they are early-onset forms. Second, they often present, at least at a late stage of evolution, distinct neurological symptoms such as rigidity, myoclonus, and epileptiform seizures. One of the Van Bogaert et al. (1940) families featured paraplegia. However, apparent distinction of "Mendelian Alzheimer's disease," as defined by large pedigrees, from "ordinary Alzheimer's disease," as defined by apparently sporadic cases, with cases occurring in small clusters somewhere in between, may be mainly due to bias in selecting families to be extensively studied (as noted earlier in this paper) and to uneven success in data gathering. The odds for success in Alzheimer's disease pedigree tracing are heavily loaded in favor of early-onset forms. The same bias runs particularly in favor of forms of Alzheimer's disease with clear neurological symptoms. Whether this bias alone is responsible for the widely held notion that early-onset Alzheimer's disease is much more commonly genetic that late-onset forms is not clear.

On the neuropathological side, cases from large Alzheimer's disease families sometimes show atypical features, such as amyloid plaques in the molecular layer of the cerebellum (Pro et al. 1979). The neuropathological picture may vary from one case to another in the same family (Frommelt et al. 1987), which may show that neuropathology is not strictly determined by genotype, and may recall the situation in Gerstmann Sträussler Scheinker disease (Boellaard and Schlote 1980). We do not know at present which clinical or neuropathological characteristics may be important from a genetic point of view, or indeed whether any of them is important. What seems certain is that simple statements in the Material and Methods sections of research papers, on the model of "the patients fulfilled such and such (internationally accepted, of course) criteria for diagnosis of Alzheimer's disease," do not allow a critical interpretation of results, since the implicitly postulate homogeneity of Alzheimer's disease. A full clinical and neuropathological description ought to be given in each instance. Since this would be impractical in most journals, a wise practice would be to use only previously recorded pedigrees; a reference would then be sufficient.

A much debated point is now whether heterogeneity of Alzheimer's disease means that genetic forms are themselves heterogeneous and, specifically, whether loci are multiple (Pericak-Vance et al., this volume). This hypothesis is by no means improbable. A typical precedent would be the thalassemia group, which a generation ago was considered as one disease with a small number of clinical variants, and is now ascribed to two loci on two different chromosomes, with multiple alleles on the beta locus, corresponding to almost all the possible defects from deletion to nonsense codon to defective promoter and many others. Alzheimer's disease, however, is far from the degree of analysis which made possible such a detailed description, which, incidentally, arose mainly through the classical path from protein to gene, and in the simple setting of recessive disease with its straightforward relationship of defective gene to abnormal, insufficient, or absent protein. We have to keep in mind that, contrary to the above-mentioned example, genetic transmission is by no means established in the majority of Alzheimer's disease cases, even though they may be found in clusters, and that, moreover, the high incidence of the disease in the older age groups makes heterogeneity within one cluster a distinct possibility and the necessary assumptions about gene frequency questionable. A demonstration of the mode of transmission within a family is necessary before molecular genetics can be used to disprove linkage with a given marker. Adding LOD scores calculated using separate clusters while genetic transmission and its mode are not established in each instance only adds uncertainties. In our opinion, multiplicity of loci is to be demonstrated by the same methods which led to the mapping of a first locus, that is, starting from large pedigrees.

In fact, we do not consider these problems as very important at the present time, which is the beginning of a new period in Alzheimer's disease research. From the time of its definition, successful research on Alzheimer's disease had been of the descriptive kind only. Since a consensus has been reached on a "disease" (as distinct from "aging") paradigm for Alzheimer's *disease,* and since the demise of the cholinergic hypothesis as a general explanation of that disease, no model, and particularly no experimental model, could be used to construct hypotheses which could in turn be tested on the real thing. In at least a few kindreds, however, a condition which has at least some points in common with "ordinary" Alzheimer's disease is transmitted in a dominant autosomic Mendelian fashion with full penetrance. This constitutes a simple model, amenable to the methods of molecular biology, which are the most promising for research on the causes and mechanisms of disease when no direct clue is available. Once molecular mechanisms are elucidated through "reverse genetics" methods using information obtained from large kindreds, their validity is going to be tested in other instances of Alzheimer's disease. We do not know the time that will be necessary to reach that goal; the Huntington's disease story is there to remind us it may be long. We have hold, however, of one end of the chain; we ought to take a firm grip. It is sure to lead us into uncharted regions – the results are certainly going to transcend our present schematic notion of what Alzheimer's disease really is.

Acknowledgements. We thank Prof. J. Le Beau, who made possible a diagnosis in the index case of family "N"; Dr. J.E. Gruner, whose encouragements were decisive in the first phase of the work on that family; Mr. C. Molinaro, who guided us in the archives he oversees; Dr. Fragola, formerly director of the provincial mental hospital; Dr. Caruso, in charge of the Servizio di Neurologia, USL17; Mr. K.H. El Hachimi, who originated the reference file. We acknowledge with thanks aid from Echanges et Recherche Medicale and from Fondation pour la Recherche Medicale. This work has been supported for various periods by INSERM, CNRS, Ministère de l'Industrie et de la Recherche and Faculté de Médecine Pitié-Salpêtière. J.F.F. is currently a recipient of Réseau INSERM 48 60 11 under contract with Mutuelle Générale de l'Education Nationale; A.C.B. is a Fellow of the John Douglas French Foundation.

References

Bayes T (1763) Essay toward solving a problem in the doctrine of chances. Phil Trans (London); reprinted in Bioimetrika (1958) 45: 293–315

Boellaard JN, Schlote W (1980) Subakute spongiforme Encephalopathie mit multiforme Plaquenbildung: „Eigenartige familiär-hereditäre Krankheit des Zentralnervensystems (spinocerebellare Atrophie mit Demenz, Plaques und plaqueähnlichen Ablagerungen im Klein- und Großhirn" (Gerstmann, Sträussler, Scheinker). Acta Neuropathol (Berl) 49: 205–212

Breitner JCS (1985) Dementia of the Alzheimer type: methodological comments. Psychiatry Res 16: 263–264

Breitner JCS, Folstein MF (1984) Familial Alzheimer dementia: a prevalent disorder with specific clinical features. Psycholog Med 14: 63–71

Breitner JCS, Folstein MF (1984) Familial nature of Alzheimer's disease. N Engl J Med 14: 63–80

Breitner JCS, Folstein MF, Murphy EA (1986) Familial aggregation in Alzheimer dementia. I: A model for the age-dependent expression of an autosomal dominant gene. J Psychiatr Res 20: 31–43

Breitner JCS, Murphy EA, Folstein MF (1986) Familial aggregation in Alzheimer dementia. II: Clinical genetic implications of age-dependent onset. J Psychiatr Res 20: 44–45

Breitner JCS, Silverman JM, Mohs RC, Davis KL (1988) Familial aggregation in Alzheimer's disease: Comparison of risk among relatives of early- and late-onset cases, and among male and female relatives in successive generations. Neurology 38: 207–212

Bruni AC, Salmon D, Montesi MP, Foncin JF (1987) Malattia di Alzheimer familiare: progressi di uno studio. Atti XXV Congresso Nazionale della Società Italiana di Neurologia

Chase GA, Folstein MF, Breitner JCS, Beaty TH, Self SG (1983) The use of life tables and survival analysis in testing genetic hypotheses, with an application to Alzheimer's disease. Am J Epidemiol 117: 590–597

Clemenceau S, Foncin J-F, Muller JY, Halle L, Hauptmann G, Seger J, Salmon Ch (1986) Absence de liaison entre la maladie d'Alzheimer et les marqueurs du complément. CR Acad Sc Paris Série III, 303: 149–154

Constantinidis J (1965) L'incidence familiale des lésions cérébrales vasculaires et dégénératives de l'age anvancé. L'Encéphale 54: 204–239

Crow JF, Mange AP (1965) Measurement of inbreeding from the frequency of marriages between persons of the same surname. Eugenics Q 12: 199–203

Egeland JA, Gerhard DS, Pauls DL, Sussex JN, Kidd KK, Allen CR, Hostetter AM, Housman DE (1987) Bipolar affective disorders linked to DNA markers on chromosome 11. Nature 325: 783–786

Elston RC, Stewart J (1971) A general model for the genetic analysis of pedigree data. Hum Hered 21: 523–542

Feldman RG, Chandler KA, Levy LL, Glaser GH (1963) Familial Alzheimer's disease. Neurology 13: 1402–1421

Folstein MF, Breitner JCS (1982) Language disorder predicts familial Alzheimer's disease. Aging 19: 197–205

Foncin J-F, Cardot JL, Martinet Y, Arnott G (1982) Maladie de Gerstmann-Stràussler-Scheinker: étude anatomo-clinique et généalogique. Rev Neurol (Paris) 138: 123–135

Foncin J-F, Le Beau J (1965) Ultrastructure des plaques séniles. Rev Neurol (Paris) 112: 61–62

Foncin J-F, Supino-Viterbo V (1973) Maladie d'Alzheimer familiale: histopathologie ultrastructurale, étude généalogique. International Congress of Neurology, Barcelona. Excerpta Medica International Congress Series 296: 63–64

Foncin J-F, Salmon D, Bruni AC (1986) Genetics of Alzheimer's disease: a large kindred with apparent Mendelian transmission; possible implications for a linkage study. In: Briley M, Kato A, Weber M (eds) New Concepts in Alzheimer's Disease. Macmillan, London, pp 242–256

Foncin J-F, Salmon D, Supino Viterbo V, Feldman RG, Macchi G, Mariotti P, Scoppetta C, Caruso G, Bruni AC (1985) Démence présénile d'Alzheimer transmise dans une famille étendue. Rev Neurol (Paris) 141: 194–202

Frommelt P, Schnabel R, Manz F, Nee L, Polinsky RJ (1987) Neuropathological heterogeneity within a family with dominantly inherited Alzheimer's disease. International Symposium on Alzheimer's disease, Amsterdam, 7–9 May

Furuya H, Sasaki H, Goto I, Wong CW, Glenner GG, Sakaki Y (1988) Amyloid B protein gene duplication is not common in Alzheimer's disease: analysis by polymorphic restriction fragments. Biochem Biophys Res Commun 150: 75–81

Gonatas NK, Gambetti P (1970) The pathology of the synapse in Alzheimer's disease. In: Wolstenholme GEW, O'Connor M (eds) Alzheimer's disease and related conditions. Churchill, London, pp 169–180

Goudsmit J, White BJ, Weitkamp LR, Keats BJB, Morrow CH, Gajdusek DC (1981) Familial Alzheimer's disease in two kindreds of the same geographic and ethnic origin. A clinical and genetic study. J Neurol Sc 49: 79–89

Gusella JF, Wexler NS, Conneally PM, Naylor SL, Anderson MA, Tanzi RE, Watkins PC, Ottina K, Wallace MR, Sakagushi AY, Yong AB, Shoulson I, Bonilla E, Martin JB (1983) A polymorphic DNA marker genetically linked to Huntington's disease. Nature 306: 234–238

Harper PS (1977) Mendelian inheritance or transmissible agent? The lesson of Kuru and the Australia antigen. J Med Genet 14: 379–398

Heston LL, Mastri AR (1977) The genetics of Alzheimer's disease. Associations with hematologic malignancy and Down's syndrome. Arch Gen Psychiatry 34: 976–981

Heston LL, White J (1978) Pedigrees of 30 families with Alzheimer's disease: association with defective organisation of microfilaments and microtubules. Behav Genet 8: 315–331

Kang J, Lemaire HG, Unterbeck A, Salbaum JM, Masters CL, Grzeschik K-H, Multhaup G, Beyreuther K, Muller-Hill B (1987) The precursor of Alzheimer's disease amyloid A4 protein resembles a cell-surface receptor. Nature 325: 733–736

Knesevich JW, Toro FR, Morris JC, LaBarge E (1985) Aphasia, family history, and the longitudinal course of senile dementia of the Alzheimer type. Psychiatry Res 14: 255–264

Knesevich JW (1985) The author replies. Psychiatry Res 16: 263–264

Lalouel JM, Morton NE (1981) Complex segregation analysis with pointers. Hum Hered 31: 312–321

Landre MF, Vallat MT, Jutier P (1972) Reconnaissance automatique des liens de parenté. Tracé automatique d'arbre généalogique. MIS 10 Villeurbanne, SIMEP

Muller JY, Clemenceau S, Foncin J-F, Salmon D, Halle L, Castellano F, Salmon Ch (1986) Absence de liaison entre la maladie d'Alzheimer et le système HLA. CR Acad Sc Paris. Serie III, 303: 105–108

Murdoch GH, Manuelidis L, Kim JH, Manuelidis EE (1988) Beta-amyloid gene dosage in Alzheimer's disease. Nucleic Acid Res 16: 357

Nee LE, Eldridge R, Sunderland T, Thomas CB, Katz D, Thompson KE, Weingartner H, Weiss H, Julian C, Cohen R (1987) Dementia of the Alzheimer type: clinical and family study of 22 twin pairs. Neurology 37: 359–363

Nee LE, Polinsky RJ, Eldridge R, Weingartner J, Smallberg S, Ebert M (1983) A family with histologically confirmed Alzheimer's disease. Arch Neurol 40: 203–208

Polinsky RJ, Noble H, Di Chiro G, Nee LE, Feldman RG, Brown RT (1987) Dominantly inherited Alzheimer's disease: cerebral glucose metabolism. J Neurol Neurosurg Psychiatry 50: 752–757

Pro JD, Sumi M, Smith CH (1979) Amyloid plaques in the cerebellum in presenile familial Alzheimer's disease. Neurology 29: 538–539

Sjögren T, Sjogren H, Lindgren H (1952) A genetic study of Morbus Alzheimer and Morbus Pick. Acta Psychiatr Scand 82: [Suppl 9]

Schellenberg GD, Deeb SS, Boehnke M, Bryant EM, Martin GM, Lampe TH, Bird TD (1987) Association of an apolipoprotein CII allele with familial dementia of Alzheimer type. J Neurogenetic 4: 97–108

St George-Hyslop PH, Tanzi RE, Polinsky RJ, Haines JL, Nee L, Watkins PC, Myers R, Feldman RG, Pollen D, Drachman D, Growdon J, Bruni A, Foncin J-F, Salmon D, Frommelt P, Amaducci L, Sorbi S, Piacentini S, Stewart GD, Hobbs WJ, Conneally PM, Gusella JF (1987a) The genetic defect causing familial Alzheimer's disease maps on chromosome 21. Science 235: 885–890

St George-Hyslop PH, Tanzi RE, Polinsky RJ, Neve RL, Pollen D, Drachman D, Growdon J, Cupples LA, Nee L, Myers R, O'Sullivan D, Watkins PC, Amos JA, Deutsch CK, Bodfish JW, Kinsbourne M, Feldman RG, Bruni A, Amaducci L, Foncin J-F, Gusella JF (1987b) Absence of duplication of chromosome 21 genes in familial and sporadic Alzheimer's disease. Science 238: 664–666

Tanzi RE, St George-Hyslop PH, Haines JL, Polinsky RJ, Nee L, Foncin J-F, Neve RL, McClathey AI, Conneally PM, Gusella JF (1987) The genetic defect in familial Alzheimer's disease is not tightly linked to the amyloid beta-protein gene. Nature 329: 156–157

Terry RD, Wisniewski H (1970) The ultrastructure of the neurofibrillary tangle and the senile plaque. In: Wolstenholme GEW, O'Connor M (eds) Alzheimer's disease and related conditions. Churchill, London, pp 145–165

Van Bogaert L, Maere M, De Smedt E (1940) Sur les formes familiales précoces de la maladie d'Alzheimer. Monatschr Psych Neurol 102: 247–301

Van Broeckhoven C, Genthe AM, Vandenberghe A, Horsthemke B, Backhovens H, Raeymaekers P, Van Hul W, Wehnert A, Gheuens J, Cras P, Bryuland M, Martin JJ, Salbaum M, Multhaup G, Masters CL, Beyreuther K, Gurling HMD, Mullan MJ, Holland A, Barton A, Irving N, Williamson R, Richards SJ, Hardy JA (1987) Failure of familial Alzheimer's disease to segregate with the A4-Amyloid gene in several European families. Nature 329: 153–155

Wexler NS, Conneally PM, Houseman D, Gusella JF (1985) A DNA polymorphism for Huntington's disease marks the future. Arch Neurol 42: 20–24

Wexler NS, Young AB, Tanzi RE, Travers H, Starosta-Rubinstein S, Penney J, Snodgrass SR, Shoulson I, Gomez F, Ramos Arroyo MA, Penchaszadeh GK, Moreno H, Gibbons K, Faryniarz A, Hobbs W, Anderson MA, Bonilla E, Conneally PM, Gusella JF (1987) Homozygotes for Huntington's disease. Nature 326: 194–197

Familial Aggregation of Dementia of Alzheimer Type: Analysis from an Epidemiological Point of View

A. Alpérovitch, and *C. Berr*

Summary

Familial risk in dementia of Alzheimer type (DAT) can be investigated by either or both genetic and epidemiological studies. The main objective of these latter studies is to examine whether an increased familial risk does exist. Case-control studies have yet to provide clear evidence for familial aggregation of DAT. The inconclusiveness of these results is due to the very small number of studies with positive results and to methodological problems which are present in studies of both positive and negative outcome. Both positive and negative findings must be carefully discussed and bias, such as the difference in age distributions of relatives or recall bias in information obtained from respondents, must be considered for either type of result. Negative findings must be interpreted in the context of data quality and sample size. The compatibility of positive findings with epidemiological characteristics of DAT in the general population must be verified.

Introduction

Because about 3% of individuals over 65 years of age show signs of dementia of the Alzheimer type (DAT), DAT has been one of the main public health concerns in developed countries since the late 1970s. While neurologists have been interested in this dementing illness for several decades, their long-standing debate over the existence of two distinct diseases, presenile and senile (Newton 1948), has now shifted to other controversies.

Most authors agree that there are two types of Alzheimer's disease, sporadic and familial (Kay 1982). However, the sporadic variant of DAT is regarded as a specific disease, a simple acceleration of the aging process, or a stage of normal brain aging in late-onset DAT cases. The familial type of the disease is sometimes referred to as genetic DAT. But genetic and familial are not synonymous and, until now, genetic factors that might be involved in familial DAT have not been described with certainty (Tanzi et al. 1987; St. Georges-Hyslop et al. 1987a, b; Delabar et al. 1986; Van Broeckoven et al. 1987)

When combined with extensive research using molecular genetic techniques, clinical and epidemiological studies can help clarify heterogeneity in Alzheimer's disease. Familial risk can be investigated using either classical epidemiological methods or techniques of genetic epidemiology (Khoury et al. 1986). The main purpose of genetic epidemiology studies is to suggest a possible model of disease inheritance. Such models can be defined either or both by analyzing the pattern of transmission in large pedigrees or testing various genetic hypotheses in a sample of families with multiple cases of the disease.

Even if it had been demonstrated with certainty that, in some families, DAT is genetically determined, it is nevertheless uncertain whether increased familial risk exists in the general population. Indeed, if the genetic variant of the disease were rare, familial risk in DAT would not be substantially increased at the epidemiological level. The main objective of epidemiological studies is to examine whether this familial risk does exist. Additional objectives are to investigate possible familial associations between DAT and other pathological conditions and to suggest environmental factors that might be responsible for familial risk in DAT.

Within the past two decades, several reports on familial factors in Alzheimer's disease have been published. The purpose of the present paper is to analyze the most recent of these reports, with respect to possible epidemiological models for DAT and to discuss problems which remain to be resolved in further epidemiological studies.

Epidemiological Studies on Familial Risk in Dementia of the Alzheimer Type: Discussion of Material and Methods

Study Design

Familial risk in DAT is investigated through case-control studies. In rare instances, rates of DAT in relatives of probands have been compared with the prevalence of DAT in the general population and, for obvious reasons, findings of such studies are not very reliable.

Many of the problems encountered in case-control studies on familial risk in DAT are almost unsolvable. Some of these problems are not specific to studies on familial risk; they are common to all epidemiological studies in DAT and have already been extensively discussed.

Identification of Probands

Dementia of the Alzheimer type is defined in terms of both clinical and pathological features and it is very difficult to meet both criteria in epidemiological studies. Error rates in clinically diagnosed DAT ranging from 10% to 30% have been reported (Sulkava et al. 1983). False-positive and false-negative error rates obtained by using the criteria for "probable DAT" proposed by the NINCDS-ADRDA Work Group (McKhann et al. 1984) have not yet been precisely estimated.

As pointed out by Breitner and Folstein (1984) the neuropathological diagnosis of DAT may itself be nonspecific, but, so far, very little information is available on interobserver and intraobserver variations in diagnosing DAT from pathological features.

Selection of Controls

In most studies, nondemented controls are selected from the general population or from a hospital population. Despite the interesting potential of using a control group consisting of "non-DAT" demented individuals, controls are rarely recruited among groups of patients with multi-infarct dementia or other types of dementing illness.

Controls are matched to a case by sex and age. Moreover, as in the study by Chandra et al. (1987), the surrogate respondent for each control should be matched to the surrogate respondent for each case by relationship. This is because spouses, offspring, and siblings are likely to differ in their recall of familial history and past events in the subject's life.

Data Collection

Information on potential familial risk factors is obtained from a structured interview. It is advisable to assess the reliability of the procedure for data collection prior to the study. This validation can be done by giving the questionnaire to nondemented subjects and to their next of kin (Pickle et al. 1983). By comparing the answers of these two groups, investigators are able to identify and eliminate questions based on factors for which the next of kin respondent cannot provide reliable information.

The main concern is to identify cases of dementia in relatives and to define the etiology of dementia. Interviewers must follow very strict guidelines and be blind with respect to the categorization of the respondent. Respondents are usually unaware of the purpose of the study. This is more easily accomplished if a large number of factors are examined in the questionnaire. A drawback of this extended interview strategy is that the greater the number of questions, the lower the reliability of answers.

To ascertain whether or not the respondents are truly unaware of the aim of the study, they can be asked, at the end of the interview, their supposition of its aim. If the true purpose is more often guessed by relatives of cases than by relatives of controls, there is a major bias which must be carefully discussed.

However, even if surrogate respondents for cases are unaware of the purpose of the study, they are often unable to ignore the fact that one of their very close relatives is demented. Consequently, they may feel particularly anxious by questions about dementing illness and their responses reflect this. Paradoxically, one wonders if it might not be preferable to inform both case and control surrogate respondents of the aim of the study. Thus, surrogate respondents for the controls might be induced to make a special effort to provide reliable data on dementia cases in the family.

As in the study by Chandra et al. (1987), information of greater reliability can be obtained if the definition of family is restricted to first-degree relatives. In addition, this restriction permits verification of the comparability of families in cases and controls in terms of the number of members at risk, their age and sex. These data are not easily obtained from respondents, even if the definition of family is restricted to first-degree relatives. The importance of comparable families must be stressed because it is often overlooked or underestimated in many studies.

Statistical Design and Analysis

An estimate of the number of first-degree relatives required for each group must be calculated prior to the study. The required sample size depends on the assumed value for the rate of DAT in controls. This value must be defined with regard to the age of "at risk" relatives who are included in the study: the younger this age, the lower the expected rate of DAT. The required number of relatives also depends on the expected rate of DAT in relatives of cases. Lastly, the *P*-value which is considered statistically significant and the study power must both be defined in order to calculate adequate sample size.

Many authors, such as Prusiner (1984), have suggested that about 15% of DAT cases are familial. Thus, when making assumptions on the rate of DAT in relatives of cases, it must be considered that most probands – about 85% – have probable sporadic DAT. The following example illustrates some consequences of this remark.

Let us assume that the frequencies of occurrence of DAT in "at risk" relatives of cases (both familial and sporadic DAT) and controls are 15% and 5%, respectively. Based on a one-sided test with a *P*-value of 0.05 as statistically significant and a power value of 0.95, statistical design requires about 180 relatives in each group. Among the 180 relatives of cases, we assume, as suggested by Prusiner (1984), that about 27 (15%) are related to probands with familial DAT. Thus, 153 relatives (180−27) are related to probands with sporadic DAT. Consequently, they have about the same risk of DAT as relatives of controls (5%). Thus the expected numbers of DAT cases are, respectively, 8 in the 153 relatives of sporadic cases, and 9 in the 180 relatives of controls.

We can now calculate how many DAT cases should occur in the 27 relatives of probands with familial DAT to verify the initial assumption of an overall rate of 15% of DAT in the 180 relatives of cases. The result of this calculation is 19 ($n = (180 \times 0.15) - (153 \times 0.05) = 27 - 8 = 19$). Such a high frequency of occurrence (70%) seems very unlikely and the initial model should be revised with different basic estimates.

If: P is the proportion of familial DAT, p_s is the frequency of occurrence of DAT in relatives of sporadic cases, and p_f is the frequency of occurrence of DAT in relatives of familial cases, then the expected frequency of occurrence of DAT in relatives of proband cases, both familial and sporadic is:

$$(P \times p_f) + ((1 - P) \times p_s)$$

Thus, by changing estimates for P, p_s, and p_f within a reasonable range of possible values, epidemiological models can be defined and the sample size can be calculated according to selected models. The range of possible values must be compatible with the prevalence rate of DAT that is observed in the general population and with other general features of this disease (Chase et al. 1983). Also, even if familial DAT was actually related to an autosomic dominant genetic factor, the crude frequency of occurrence of DAT observed in families would probably be considerably less than the 50% theoretical rate. This point must be taken into consideration to define an estimate for p_f.

Matching

A close matching of controls to cases by sex, age, and relationship to surrogate respondent does not ensure that characteristics of first-degree relatives of cases are similar to those of controls. Therefore, rates of DAT in relatives of cases and controls must be adjusted for the number of members in each group, their age, and sex. As the incidence of DAT increases very quickly with age, small differences in age distributions have an important effect upon the frequency of occurrence of this disease in families.

Statistical Analysis

Data analysis raises methodological difficulties. With regard to the preceding remarks, the matched-pair method of analysis is not totally appropriate. The classical calculation of odds ratio to estimate the relative risk in families of cases over families of controls does not take into account that the group consisting of N relatives of n cases (or controls) is not identical to the group of N independent subjects.

The power of statistical tests is affected by misclassifications of both proband cases and DAT cases in relatives. The magnitude of this effect is difficult to estimate.

In interpreting the significance of an increased familial risk of DAT in relatives of cases, the distribution of these secondary cases in families must be considered. Indeed, this interpretation will be different according to whether or not aggregation of cases is restricted to a few pedigrees with multiple cases.

Studies on Familial Risk in Dementia of the Alzheimer Type: Results

Familial risk in DAT has been investigated in a very small number of epidemiological studies (Breitner and Folstein 1984; Chandra et al. 1987; Chase et al. 1983; Heston et al. 1981; Heyman et al. 1984; Amaducci et al. 1986; Whalley et al. 1982; Shalar et al. 1987). In most of these studies, cases were compared with controls for various potential risk factors, including family history of dementia. The present paper focuses on the results of four recent reports which are presented in Table 1 (Breitner and Folstein 1984; Chandra et al. 1987; Amaducci et al. 1986; Shalar et al. 1987). In one of these reports, the frequency of occurrence of DAT in first-degree relatives was not separately available (Schalar et al. 1987). Two studies (Breitner and Folstein 1986; Schalar et al. 1987) reported an increased rate of dementia in families of patients with DAT compared with families of controls. The two other studies found no increase (Chandra et al. 1987; Amaducci et al. 1986).

In two studies, the frequencies of occurrence of DAT in relatives have been calculated. In one of these studies (Breitner and Folstein 1984) the frequency in cases (8.5%) was significantly greater than the frequency in controls (2.6%); in the other (Chandra et al. 1987) the frequencies did not differ (6.6% and 6.8%). In two studies, these frequencies could not be calculated because the number of relatives was not known (Amaducci et al. 1986; Shalar et al. 1987).

Table 1. Results of recent case-control studies on familial risk in DAT

Reference	Probands/controls (*n*)	Increased risk in first-degree relatives	Comments
Breitner and Folstein (1984)	54/ 33	Yes	Rates of secondary DAT cases: 8.5/2.6
Amaducci et al. (1986)	116/116	No	Number of relatives not known
Chandra et al.[a] (1987)	64/ 64	No	Rate of secondary DAT cases 6.8/6.6
Shalat et al.[b] (1987)	98/162	Yes	Number of relatives not known

[a] Late onset DAT
[b] Men only, and all relatives

One (Chandra et al. 1987) of the two negative studies was restricted to case probands with late-onset dementia (after age 70), while it has been suggested that genetic factors may be more important in young-onset cases. It is of interest to note that, in this study, the authors reviewed 175 cases of dementia to obtain their study sample. Of these cases, only 74 met the diagnostic criteria of the NINCDS-ADRDA Work Group (McKhann et al. 1987) for "probable Alzheimer's disease" and in most of them (70), the onset of illness was after age 70.

Negative findings do not mean that familial risk does not exist. Factors that must be taken into account in interpreting negative results are extensively discussed in the paper by Chandra et al. (1987). These authors also examine the significance of a positive family history of dementia. To illustrate additional epidemiological speculations which can be made from positive findings, we will discuss the paper by Breitner and Folstein (1984).

Breitner and Folstein found an increased risk of dementia among first-degree relatives (aged 60 years and above) in DAT probands (8.46%) compared with controls (2.55%). The rate in controls is comparable with the prevalence of DAT observed in the general population over age 60. Further interpretation of the significance of their findings depends on the proportion of DAT probands with the familial type of this disease. Despite the 15% rate for familial DAT suggested by some authors, there is no reliable estimate for this proportion and we will examine three different values: 10%, 20%, and 30%.

The problem that we want to resolve is the following: assuming a given rate (10% to 30%) of the familial variant of DAT in case probands, is it possible to obtain from observed data an estimate for the frequency of occurrence of DAT in relatives of probands with the familial variant of DAT? An estimate can be calculated if we assume that the average frequency of occurrence of DAT in relatives of both controls and sporadic DAT probands is the same. This assumption seems reasonable. Calculations are presented in Table 2. Crude frequencies of 61.5% and 32.1%, which correspond with assumed proportions of the familial variant of DAT equal to 10% and 20%, respectively, are very high when compared with the 50%, 90-year lifetime incidence which is expected with an autosomal dominant pattern of inheritance

Table 2. Epidemiological analysis of data presented by Breitner and Folstein (1984)

Data: Cases, 22 DAT patients among 260 first-degree relatives (rate, 8.46%); controls, 4 DAT patients among 157 first-degree relatives (rate, 2.55%)

Assumed proportion of case probands with familial DAT (%)	10	20	30
Expected number of relatives proband cases with			
familial DAT *(a)*	26	52	78
sporadic DAT *(b)*	234	208	182
Expected number ($c = b \times 0.0255$) of DAT in relatives of case probands with sporadic DAT	6.0	5.3	4.6
Expected number ($d = 22 - c$) of DAT in relatives of case probands with familial DAT	16.0	16.7	17.4
Frequency of occurrence (d/a) of DAT in relatives of case probands with familial DAT (%)	61.5	32.1	22.3

(Breitner and Folstein 1984). The third estimate (22.3%) and the corresponding underlying model are, at first view, more likely. But, further computations are needed to verify whether this epidemiological model is compatible with the prevalence rate of DAT observed in the general population.

A similar analysis can be made from the findings of Shalat et al. (1987). However, as the number of relatives is not known, some additional assumptions are required to interpret the significance of this positive study. Analysis leads to questions similar to those resulting from the discussion of the results of Breitner and Folstein.

Conclusion

Both negative and positive results on familial risk in DAT must be carefully discussed. Positive findings must be examined with respect to possible underlying epidemiological models. So far there is no strong epidemiological evidence that an increased familial risk in DAT exists. This uncertainty is due to the very small number of studies with positive results, some methodological problems which were present in both positive and negative studies, and the lack of discussion about the epidemiological significance of findings.

Therefore, there is a need for further epidemiological studies with improved methodology to answer questions which remain to be resolved on familial risk in DAT. Does an increased familial risk exist in the general population and what is the relative risk in families of cases over families of controls? What is the prevalence of the familial variant of DAT in the general population? Is familial aggregation – if demonstrated – due to either or both genetic and environmental factors (Khoury et al. 1988)?

Different epidemiological studies, particularly longitudinal studies in non-demented individuals, and twin studies can be used to approach these problems. Longitudinal studies permit analysis of whether a positive familial history of DAT is a risk factor for developing this dementing illness. From studies comparing monozygotic and dizygotic twins (Hrubec and Robinette 1984), it is possible to discuss whether concordant pairs are likely to be due to shared genes, shared environment, or both. Nevertheless, epidemiological studies are not capable of providing a precise estimate of the prevalence of familial DAT without reference to any biological (or clinical) marker for the diagnosis of this form of dementia.

References

Amaducci LA, Fratiglioni L, Rocca WA, Fieschi C, Livrea P, Pedone D, Bracco L, Lippi A, Gandolfo C, Bino G (1986) Risk factors for clinically diagnosed Alzheimer's disease: a case-control study of an Italian population. Neurology 36: 922–931

Breitner JCS, Folstein MF (1984) Familial Alzheimer dementia: a prevalent disorder with specific clinical features. Psychol Med 14: 63–80

Chandra V, Phillipose V, Bell PA, Lazaroff A, Schoenberg BS (1987) Case-control study of late onset "probable Alzheimer's disease." Neurology 37: 1295–1300

Chase GA, Folstein MF, Breitner JCS, Beaty TH, Self SG (1983) The use of life tables and survival analysis in testing genetic hypotheses with an application to Alzheimer's disease. Am J Epidemiol 117: 590–597

Delabar JM, Goldgaber D, Lamour Y, Nicole A, Huret JL, de Grouchy J, Brown P, Gajdusek DC, Sinet PM (1987) β-amyloid gene duplication in Alzheimer's disease and karyotypically normal Down syndrome. Science 235: 1390–1392

Heston LL, Mastri AR, Anderson E, White J (1981) Dementia of the Alzheimer type: clinical genetics, natural history, and associated conditions. Arch Gen Psychiatry 38: 1085–1090

Heyman A, Wilkinson WE, Stafford JA, Helms MJ, Sigmon AH, Weinberg T (1984) Alzheimer's disease: a study of epidemiological aspects. Ann Neurol 15: 335–341

Hrubec Z, Robinette CD (1984) The study of human twins in medical research. N Engl J Med 310: 435–441

Kay DWK (1987) Heterogeneity in Alzheimer's disease: epidemiological and family studies. Trends Neurosc 10: 194–195

Khoury MJ, Beaty TH, Cohen BH (1986) The interface of genetics and epidemiology. J Chron Dis 39: 963–978

Khoury MJ, Beaty TH, Liang KY (1988) Can familial aggregation of disease be explained by familial aggregation of environmental risk factors? Am J Epidemiol 137: 674–683

McKhann G, Drachman D, Folstein M, Katzman R, Price D, Stadlan EM (1984) Clinical diagnosis of Alzheimer's disease: report of the NINCDS-ADRDA Work Group under the auspices of Department of Health and Human Services Task Force on Alzheimer's disease. Neurology 34: 939–944

Newton RD (1948) The identity of Alzheimer's disease in a large mental hospital. J Ment Sci 94: 225–249

Pickle LW, Brown LM, Blot WJ (1983) Information available from surrogate respondents in case-control interview studies. Am J Epidemiol 118: 99–108

Prusiner SB (1984) Some speculations about prions, amyloid and Alzheimer's disease. N Engl J Med 310: 661–663

Shalat SL, Seltzer B, Pidcock C, Baker EL (1987) Risk factors for Alzheimer's disease: a case-control study. Neurology 37: 1630–1633

St. George-Hyslop PH, Tanzi RE, Polinsky RJ, Haines JL, Nee L, Watkins PC, Myers RH, Feldman RG, Pollen D, Drachman D, Growdon J, Bruni A, Foncin J-F, Salmon D, Frommelt P, Amaducci L, Sorbi S, Piacentini S, Stewart GD, Hobbs WJ, Conneally PM, Gusella JF (1987a) The genetic defect causing familial Alzheimer's disease maps on chromosome 21. Science 235: 885–890

St. George-Hyslop PH, Tanzi RE, Polinsky RJ, Neve RL, Pollen D, Drachman D, Growdon J, Cupples LA, Nee L, Myers RH, O'Sullivan D, Watkins PC, Amos JA, Deutsch CK, Bodfish JW, Kinsbourne M, Feldman RG, Bruni A, Amaducci L, Foncin J-F, Gusella JF (1987b) Absence of duplication of chromosome 21 genes in familial and sporadic Alzheimer's disease. Science 238: 664–666

Sulkava R, Haltia M, Paetau A, Wikström J, Palo J (1983) Accuracy of clinical diagnosis in primary degenerative dementia: correlation with neuropathological findings. J Neurol Neurosurg Psychiatr 46: 9–13

Tanzi RE, Gusella JF, Watkins PL, Bruns GAP, St. George-Hyslop P, van Keuren ML, Patterson D, Pagan S, Kurnit DM, Neve RL (1987) Amyloid β-protein gene: cDNA, mRNA distribution, and genetic linkage near the Alzheimer locus. Science 235: 880–884

Van Broeckhoven C, Genthe AM, Vandenberghe A, Horsthemke B, Backhovens H, Raeymaekers P, Van Hul W, Wehnert A, Gheuens J, Cras P, Bruyland M, Martin JJ, Salbaum M, Multhaup G, Masters CL, Beyreuther K, Gruling HMD, Mullan MJ, Holland A, Barton A, Irvin N, Williamson R, Richards SJ, Hardy JA (1987) Failure of familial Alzheimer's disease to segregate with the A4-amyloid gene in several European families. Nature 329: 153–155

Whalley LF, Carothers AD, Collyer S, DeMey R, Frackiewicz A (1982) A study of familial factors in Alzheimer's disease. Br J Psychiatry 140: 249–256

The IMAGE Project: A Geographical Laboratory for the Integration of Multidisciplinary Data

D. Gauvreau, R. Bouchard, S. Gauthier, J. Mathieu, C. Boily, A. Cholette, Y. Robitaille, P. Bouchard, N. Bouchard, L.-P. Doyon, M. Gaudreault, A. Ouellet, M. Dumont, P. Kishka, C. Fournier, J. Nalbantoglu, G. Lacoste-Royal, D. Gautrin, S. Froda, M. de Braekeleer, G. Bouchard, and *J. Mortimer*

Summary

The absence of an adequate experimental model constitutes a significant barrier to the study of Alzheimer's disease (AD). The establishment of a population-based registry of Alzheimer cases was initiated in the Province of Quebec with a view to combining the analytical techniques from various disciplines, including descriptive epidemiology, biostatistics, genetic epidemiology, and molecular genetics. The search for a model to permit the integration of multidisciplinary data has led to the creation of a large geographical laboratory in the Saguenay-Lac-Saint-Jean area. As a field of study, this area possesses unique features; among others, its parish registries are completely computerized, allowing for retrospective genealogical analyses over 145 years. The different research components planned for the IMAGE project include measurement of the clinical and neuropathological features of AD, the genealogical study of AD families, various putative risk factors involved in the development of the disease, the sociogeographic distribution of cases over the field of study, the caretaking of patients, the environmental toxicology of the target territory and the molecular genetics of the disease in large extended families.

Key Questions, Caveats and Conceptual Problems in the Study of Alzheimer's Disease

Regardless of personal feelings over the exact nature of Alzheimer's disease (AD), there is no question that AD research scientists face significant hurdles in trying to discover the origins of the disease. First and foremost, there is no clear-cut "operational" definition of AD: in the absence of any biological marker, the clinical-neuropsychological criteria currently used by neurologists and geriatricians around the world to describe the disease and the neuropathological criteria used to definitively corroborate a clinical diagnosis of AD are poor second-bests (McKhann et al. 1984). For the time being, the definition of AD suffers from the inherent circularity between these two sets of criteria (Tierney et al. 1986). Moreover, the variety of patterns in the clinical evolution of AD, as well as in the distribution of plaques and tangles across specific areas of the brain, suggest, the existence of a certain number of subtypes (Mayeux et al. 1985). These could in fact represent different diseases from an etiological point of view, and AD may in reality be a syndrome.

The enormous variability in the expression delay of the disease constitutes another significant caveat in the study of AD, and in trying to set the conditions for defining the experimental model (Breitner et al. 1988). Are AD lesions "normal" features of the aging brain? Is AD merely an amplification of the age-related modulation of those phenomena that usually underlie the otherwise limited appearance of such lesions? Or does it represent a complete loss of control in these age-related modulations (Berg 1985)? If age modulation is to be accounted for, it would seem that penetrance plays a part in the interaction between the factors that lead to the development of the disease.

Furthermore, it remains to be seen whether the fact that AD seems to run in some families (an observation which points to a strong genetic etiological factor) contradicts the fact that discordance for the disease has been observed in many sets of identical twins (which suggests that environmental factors play a significant role in the development of AD; Nee et al. 1987).

In considering the study of AD, we have to accept that there may be numerous "missing links" between what we want to define as the primary etiological factors and what constitutes the most obvious and observable expression of the disease in the brain per se (i. e., plaques, tangles, changes in the concentrations of neurotransmitters, and as yet undetermined features of cerebral metabolism). And, indeed, no linkage has been measured between the disease trait and the genes already known to be implicated in the production of AD lesions (Tanzi et al. 1987; Van Broeckhoven et al. 1987); a certain number of chromosome 21 probes have also been tested but the studies have not produced conclusive evidence (St George-Hyslop et al., this volume). Obviously, we may not have yet characterized all of the constituents of typical AD lesions and it can be argued that the study of the molecular genetics of this disease has only recently begun. We continue to hope, however, that one of these "etiological gaps" does not extend beyond the target organ, the brain itself. If for the sake of analogy we describe the brain as the "battlefield" of the disease, we must not exclude the possibility that the "commander's headquarters" are elsewhere in the body.

To sum up, the caveats that constitute, in our opinion, important considerations in the study of AD are:

1. Lack of disease definition, with a large gray area in correlations to be established between current clinical and neuropathological measurements
2. Wide time-window for the manifestation of the disease, with consideration given to whether or not one assumes AD types I and II, and normal aging to be all one and the same from the point of view of lesions and etiology – notwithstanding the validity of this assumption, AD is a condition from which one seems to be generally protected during development and in the first phases of adulthood
3. Likelihood of a multifactorial etiology (perhaps even in its causal "digits"), with a complex blend or a variable combination of some genetic predisposition, age-related genes or phenomena, and different environmental triggering factors
4. Unspecificity of AD neuropathological lesions

In an overall schematic approach to AD, some of the key questions concern:

1. *Disease Heterogeneity and Subtypes.* Is there a familial or genetic heterogeneity of risk? In diagnostic terms, can we define who is a familial case and who is a sporadic case? What is the mean age of onset in familial cases? More concretely, what is the

degree to which clustering of the disease occurs in families? For linkage studies, how many and which types of informative families can we identify?

2. *Genetic Assessment and Other Pathological Associations*. What is the interaction between the genetics of AD (or of other associated diseases) and the aging phenomena? Are different genes involved in this disease? Do familial factors become more or less important with age? Is there early mortality and does it cluster in relatives of familial cases?
3. *Attributable Risk or the Proportion of Variance Associated with Familial Factors*. What are the relative contributions of genetic and environmental factors in the development of AD? Are the genetic factors arising from multigenerational vertical transmission or are alterations in the genotype occurring in only one generation?

The degree of apparent etiological complexity of this disease is complicated by the absence of an animal model, representing a major obstacle in establishing an experimental design to investigate the pathological phenomenon in a step-by-step mechanistic fashion. Although the data on the etiology of AD remain somewhat sketchy, we would argue that the directions for working towards the definition of a research model are more obvious. The principal considerations are:

1. Since heterogeneity seems to characterize AD, if not in its basic causes, at least in the combination and relative contribution of etiological factors as well as in the consecutive degree or intensity of neurodegeneration, a prospective design is patently called for. It should include an intrinsic ability to perform detailed clinicopathological studies and allow for retrospective analyses and reclassification of cases (if need be), and ultimately even redefinition of the Alzheimer syndrome and its subtypes.
2. If aging genes or age-related modulating factors play a significant role in the development of AD, covering the entire "at-risk period" or "vulnerability timespan" for AD constitutes a vital feature of the research model that we are seeking to develop.
3. As environmental influences or exposures (e.g., occupational or geographical characteristics) can obviously not be disregarded outright in the search for the various causal digits leading to the development of AD, the milieu also needs to be carefully monitored.
4. Whatever the cellular or physiological steps are that lead to what we currently use as diagnostic criteria from a neuropathological viewpoint, attempts should certainly be made to try to correct for the lack of a systemic history of the disease. As this cannot easily be carried out on a case-by-case basis, large families offer an obvious alternative for assessing other pathological conditions possibly associated with AD.

As mentioned above, it may be that this disease is actually multifactorial with a complex polygenic basis, in which case a simple telescopic approach can only provide fragmentary information on its cause(s) and clinical subtypes. And indeed, with the data obtained so far in a "disciplinary" fashion – a situation that is currently translating into a collection of elements for which one has little idea of where each piece fits into the overall puzzle – we possess in reality very few clues as to which key physiological or cellular systems might interact to bring about, in the first instance, the outbreak of the disease. We believe that a longitudinal approach, founded on a human population-based registry over a large field, provides the best way (albeit incomplete and imperfect) to correct for the conceptual problems illustrated by the few caveats briefly discussed above. Since in all likelihood AD is more than just a "one-factor disease," perhaps considerably more complex than a single-gene disease, a research model that is as comprehensive and as exhaustive as possible in scope is probably called for. This model should represent a resource to test for numerous combinations of etiological factors.

The IMAGE Concept: A Multimatrix Model for the Study of Alzheimer's Disease

The realization that a comprehensive and longitudinal approach to the study of this disease in a well-defined human population provides the best chances for discovering the differenct factors involved in its etiology has constituted the seed for launching the IMAGE project. The objective for establishing a case registry over a whole area of the Province of Quebec is to create an extended research laboratory, one in which it will be possible to simultaneously combine analytical techniques in epidemiology, biostatistics, and population genetics as well as cellular and molecular biology from a series of measurements, all based on a single population. Conceptually, the project can be defined as a set of disciplinary research matrices to be examined in a continuum. Through integration of its collective data, IMAGE provides an opportunity for truly interdisciplinary studies of the etiology, natural history, and management of the disease. We believe that what is original about the IMAGE concept is the likelihood of creative "feedforward" or feedback inferences between the different matrices, and in the inherent synergic effect that constructive relationships should in turn have on scientific queries within each research matrix. Moreover, the IMAGE project possesses a registry that is eminently suited for investigating the relationships between, and the relative importance of, genetic and environmental factors that are suspected to interact in the etiology of AD.

Short Introduction to the IMAGE Project

A registry of AD cases is currently being established for the Saguenay-Lac-Saint-Jean (SLSJ) region of the Province of Quebec. The targeted field is situated between the longitudes of 70° and 75°, and between latitudes 48° and 49° north (see Fig. 1). The SLSJ area, the centre of which is located some 200 km north of the city of Quebec, covers approximately 225 km from east to west and about 100 km from north to south. It is interesting to note an historical feature characteristic of SLSJ, namely its relative isolation from the rest of the Province of Quebec. Until the end of the nineteenth century, access was rendered virtually impossible because of extremely poor roads; the only other means of communication and transportation was the Saguenay River, which is navigable as far as Chicoutimi. However, the river is frozen for 4 or 5 months of the year, which meant, to all intents and purposes (and

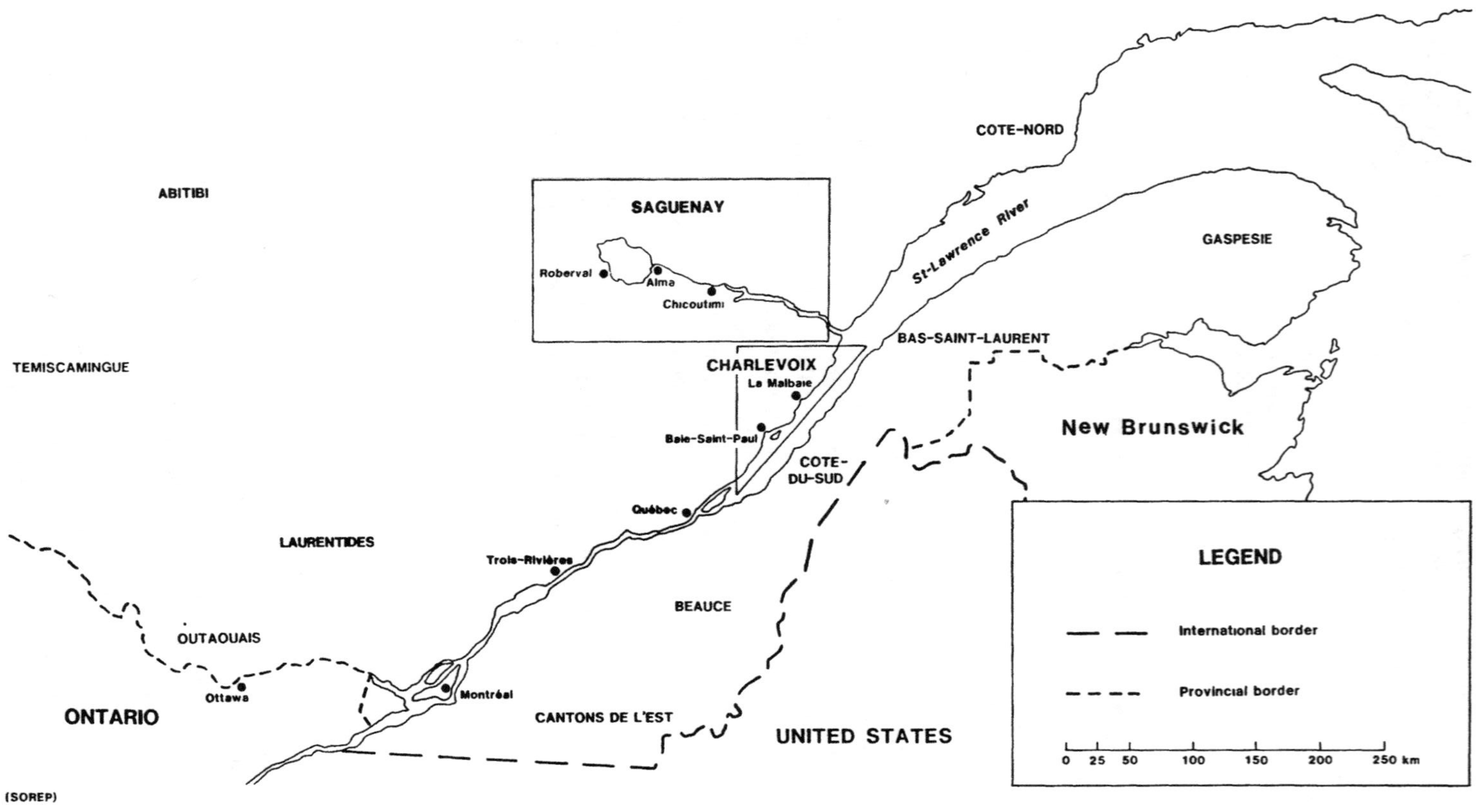

Fig. 1. The Saguenay-Lac-Saint-Jean (SLSJ) territory, selected as field of study for the IMAGE project. SLSJ is located north of the city of Quebec; it covers an area of approximately 22 500 km^2, with a population of approximately 290 000 persons

apart from limited access by railway), that the area was isolated from the rest of Quebec from early December until the end of April. This relative isolation obviously had a direct bearing on the composition of genetic stocks that are found in SLSJ today. The total population of SLSJ is approximately 290000, with an estimated 25000 at risk for developing AD.

The IMAGE project has been in progress since late 1985 and has secured the cooperation and participation of a large number of specialists and key-informants in the field of study. The project has grown into a population-based study of AD designed to investigate by means of a multidisciplinary approach the etiology, epidemiology, and natural history of this disease. The research structure of IMAGE is composed of eight (8) matrices, pertaining to:

1. Clinicopathological correlational studies
2. Population genetics, including derivation of genealogical indices of the population
3. Analytic case-control epidemiological studies of AD, employing all of the cases in a defined geographical region
4. Sociogeographical distribution of cases
5. Study of caretaking and case management in the field
6. Environmental and toxicological data relevant to the AD etiology
7. Molecular genetics underlying the etiology of AD
8. Physiocellular analyses of gene products affecting the expression of the disease condition

Characteristic Features of the IMAGE Field of Study

A variety of important features have led to the choice of SLSJ as the field of study for IMAGE. We believe that the study of this region provides scientists with an opportunity to investigate simultaneously genetic, environmental, and sociogeographic factors related to AD in a manner that is unique. The basic strength of the IMAGE registry of AD cases is that investigators can access a computerized database of all the parish registries, currently dating back to 1842, in collaboration with the SOREP Consortium at the University of Quebec at Chicoutimi (SOREP stands for Centre interuniversitaire de recherches sur les populations, and is constituted as a tri-university consortium in human genetics, involving Laval University (Quebec), McGill University (Montreal), and the University of Quebec at Chicoutimi). In its capacity for rapid and automatic reconstruction of family pedigrees, this special database offers a unique tool for studying in detail the demographic and genetic evolution of the SLSJ community. The SOREP database currently includes all civil records in the field of study for the past 145 years; soon it will be extended into the Charlevoix area just south of SLSJ. It is estimated that 70%–80% of the gene pool of SLSJ comes from Charlevoix, meaning that IMAGE will be in a position to trace the ancestors of cases back to the seventeenth century. This database possesses information on place and date of birth, place and date of death, as well as residential and professional histories of the constituents. Anyone having spent his or her life in SLSJ appears on average 10 times in the database.

In addition to this genealogical database, there is also a computerized database of the geographical and socioeconomic characteristics of SLSJ (based on the information obtained from Statistics Canada through periodic census), providing a tool for street-by-street analysis of the spatial distribution of cases.

The area per se also lends itself well to the investigation of the relative influence of environmental factors in the etiology of the disease. SLSJ is divided into two distinct regions, a clearly demarcated agricultural section and a concentrated industrial area. The two sections roughly correspond to rural and urban concentrations, with small villages in the first, and medium-size cities in the second. The territorial limits are very reasonable from a management point of view with respect to travelling within the field of study (i. e., size of the region), as well as with respect to air transport from the cities of Montreal and Quebec. Because of the ethnic homogeneity of the population and the strong degree of cooperation from the residents, SLSJ provides a basis for establishing an adequate network of collaborators and key-informants, as well as for frequent contacts with the different hospitals, nursing homes, and medical specialists. There is also in the area a major hospital center with modern diagnostic equipment and biochemical laboratories. IMAGE headquarters in the field, as well as links with computer facilities in the laboratories in Montreal and Chicoutimi, are provided through the University of Quebec network by the University of Quebec at Chicoutimi.

Furthermore, there is in the area a major aluminum-producing plant that was established in the early part of this century (1926). In view of the low mobility and rather homogeneous nature of the population, this feature constitutes a special means for testing the etiological hypothesis of aluminum in AD.

Most important, IMAGE provides through this field an opportunity for geneticists to identify at least three generations of living AD cases. The average family size between 1880 and 1940 was approximately 12 members, among the largest on record in the world. In dealing with very large families in successive generations, the odds are therefore very high that IMAGE will simultaneously locate a proband with affected children or nieces and nephews as well as uncles or aunts (i. e., cases of AD in different generations, who are all *alive*). Such a combination is only possible in very large families with births spread over a long period (25 or so years) and overlapping successive generations. This special feature of the IMAGE field is especially important with regard to the genetic study of the etiology of AD. Indeed, as AD would appear to develop on the basis of a multifactorial matrix of more than one combination of different factors (with some gene regulation operating on the expression of those factors), large numbers of cases in nuclear families will probably not be sufficient to provide the linkage necessary for identifying the "one causal" gene. In fact, in the case of AD, it seems more likely that measuring tight linkage to establish the identity of the different genetic factors will require very large isolates or extended families. Furthermore, because AD likely results from a combination of genetic and environmental factors, understanding the genetic-environmental interaction depends on a study of large numbers of blood relatives separated geographically to allow for the discrimination between environmental influences and genetic factors. Such a study requires very large families coupled with the ability to trace distant relatives efficiently.

Preliminary Results on Yearly Birth Distribution

Figure 2 shows the yearly birth distribution of the first 125 Alzheimer's patients in the IMAGE registry. Most of the current cases were found to be born between 1900 and 1920. The project was not initiated until 1985, so most of the putative patients born before 1900 had already died, and therefore could not be screened; most of the individuals born after 1920 who may develop AD have obviously not yet been diagnosed. The distribution was found to be highly uneven with 2- or 3-year cycles (peaks in 1904, 1906–1908, 1911–1913, 1916, and 1919). We are now studying on a yearly basis the distribution of mortality of all individuals born between 1891 and 1930 as well as the yearly distribution of stillbirth and infant mortality.

Although it clearly is too early to draw definite conclusions from the yearly birth distribution, showing an alternation of peaks and depressions and a periodicity of 2 to 3 years, different working hypotheses can be generated from these results. The general suggestion is that it would appear that genetic factors or specific exposures acting during the gestation period or at birth could play a crucial role in the etiology of AD. Different possibilities could explain such a phenomenon. For example, a deleterious modification of the genome by viral DNA might occur during intrauterine life; gene function would only be disrupted in a later period of life if prompted by some other environmental or genetic factor(s). This model perhaps applies more readily to the sporadic form of the disease. On the other hand, one could also hypothesize that viral infection or some exposure to an environmental toxin during intrauterine life causes a significant phenomenon of selective cell depletion in cerebral areas; the loss of cells would not interfere specifically with the development or functions of the brain

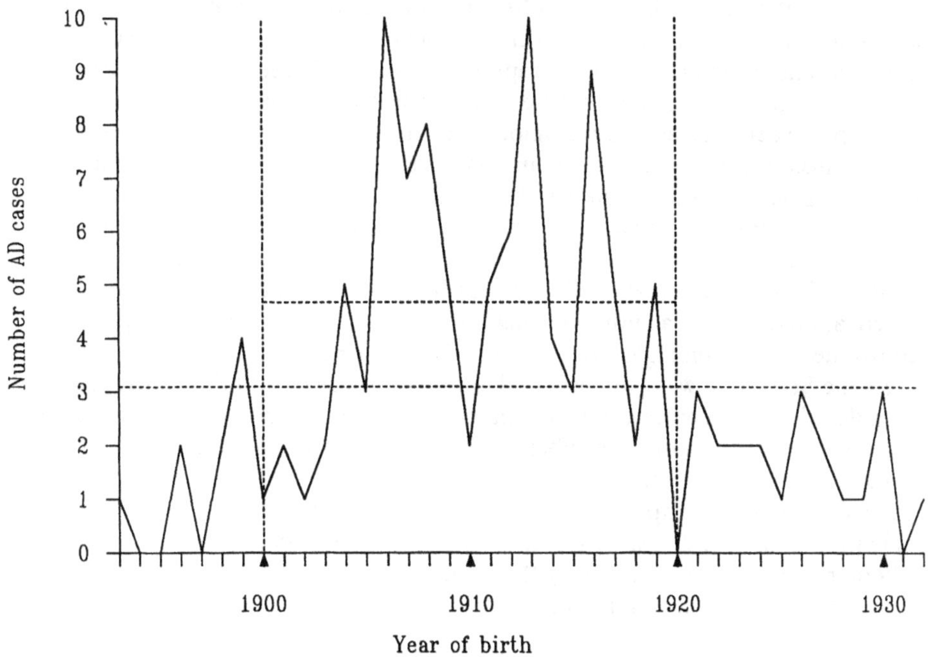

Fig. 2. Yearly birth distribution in cases of Alzheimer's disease from the IMAGE project registry

but, as a result of progressive aging, the number of active cells in the particular locus of the original scar could fall below that of the threshold number of cells required to preserve vital cerebral functions. Hence, severe reduction of cells in some subcortical nuclei may lead rapidly to a situation where coping with normal physiological requirements becomes impossible, leading to a cascade of pathological events.

Sartwell's incubation period model has been used by Horner as a tool to study the question of the relative importance of genetic and environmental factors in AD (Horner 1987). Sartwell has demonstrated that the incubation period for infectious diseases usually fits a log-normal distribution; therefore, if genetic factors are predominant in the development of a disease, age at disease onset is considered the incubation period. In an analysis of four series of AD cases, Horner has established that age at onset consistently follows a log-normal distribution. Despite a number of inherent limitations in the method, this finding would support the hypothesis of a genetic etiology; however, it may also suggest that the search for environmental risk factors should focus on the prenatal period of the cases. On the other hand, the fact that AD is widespread throughout any given population would appear to suggest that its causal factor(s) is (are) ubiquitous. On the basis of the initial results obtained from the IMAGE registry, and in particular the observation that the yearly distribution of births of the AD patients follows periodic cycles, it could be postulated that a common virus may act in a deleterious fashion on the central nervous system (or the brain per se) during intrauterine life or the neonatal period. In fact, many viruses (e.g., measles, varicella) are known to recur in epidemics at specific and regular intervals in the population. Assuming that this hypothesis were correct, one can only speculate at this stage on the exact mechanism of action of any candidate viruses in the developing or neonatal brain. Whether it is as mentioned above, by direct insertion of novel genomic material, or through a phenomenon of molecular mimicry initiated by antiviral antibodies, or reactivation after preservation in a latent or persistent state of a few virions, it would obviously represent a very "discreet cellular or anatomical alteration"; this modification would clearly not disturb the normal metabolic pathways up to a certain stage past development. It would in fact represent a change that the organism can easily cope with during the greater part of its life, not leading to any obvious clinical manifestation well before aging exposes or reactivates the original viral scar. Herpes viruses have already been suggested as likely primary causal factors in Alzheimer's disease, since they have an affinity for the cells of ectodermal origin (Ball 1982; Roberts et al. 1986). According to the hypothesis discussed above, reactivation of a virus acquired during intrauterine life or the neonatal period could constitute the real biological onset of the disease condition.

As the SLSJ area was quite isolated during the early part of this century, it can be considered as an appropriate geographical test-tube to validate such an hypothesis. However, we have not been able so far to reconstruct a reliable history of the epidemics in SLSJ for the most common viruses affecting children (i.e., measles, varicella, rubella, mumps, influenza, etc.) from 1900 to 1920. As our results are still only preliminary findings, larger numbers of cases are required to clearly establish whether or not it is worth pursuing this viral trail by identification of genomic material through hybridization techniques.

Development of the IMAGE Project

The network of collaborators and key-informants in the IMAGE project currently extends throughout the field of study through its nursing homes and hospitals, involving pathologists, neurologists, and general practitioners in the area. Its structure has already been described in detail elsewhere (Gauvreau et al. 1988). It is providing numerous services to both families and medical professionals (e.g., headquarters in the field, a newsletter on IMAGE, videos, family information booklets, bibliographical services, Alzheimer CT scan clinics, etc.). The infrastructure for a prospective and longitudinal study is effectively in place, and we expect to be able to identify at least 90% of the 600 anticipated cases in the area.

The scientific opportunities offered by this project are numerous, and the intrinsic qualities of the IMAGE field of study open a variety of investigative avenues. At the same time as developing an operational model for establishing a population-based registry of AD cases, the project should permit validation of clinical diagnostic criteria against quantitative neuropathological observations in order to improve criteria for the selection of AD cases. Furthermore, relationships between clinical, neuropsychological, and neuropathological data may allow for the concrete characterization of Alzheimer subtypes. IMAGE provides a tool to investigate genetic-environmental relationships contributing to the development of AD in a manner heretofore impossible. The availability of a computerized population database opens the way for measurements on a variety of genealogical indices in the AD population within SLSJ, and for randomly selecting reliable control groups based on any appropriate combination of matching variables. From ascending and descending reconstructions of familial pedigrees, it may in fact be possible to infer the existence of a founding effect, in order, among other things, to identify subjects most likely to possess a genetic predisposition to the development of the disease. Based on the results of family medical history surveys, we hope to select extended families in order to study linkage with any number of molecular probes to determine the specific genetic factors involved in the etiology of AD and to further characterize the genetic predisposition to the disease and the age-related modulating factors involved in its development. Finally, the IMAGE field of study offers a very special opportunity to assess the existence of social gradients in the distribution of cases and to establish the Alzheimer cartography in an area clearly separated into agricultural and industrial districts, laying the groundwork for future studies of putative environmental risk factors.

References

Ball MJ (1982) Limbic predilection in Alzheimer dementia: Is reactivated herpes virus involved? Can J Neurol Sci 9: 303–306

Berg L (1985) Does Alzheimer's disease represent an exaggeration of normal aging? Arch Neurol 42: 737–739

Breitner JCS, Murphy EA, Silverman JM, Mohs RC, Davis KL (1988) Age-dependent expression of familial risk in Alzheimer's disease. Am J Epidemiol 128: 536–548

Gauvreau D, Bouchard R, Gauthier S, Mathieu J, Boily C, Cholettte A, Robitaille Y, Bouchard P, Bouchard N, Doyon LP, Gaudreault M, Ouellet A, Dumont M, Kishka P, Fournier C, Nalbantoglu J, Lacoste-Royal G, Gautrin D, Froda S, deBraekeleer M, Bouchard G (1988) The IMAGE project: A multmatrix model for the study of Alzheimer's disease. In: Blass JP, Miner G, Miner

LA, Richter RN, Valentine JL (eds) Familial Alzheimer's disease: molecular genetics, clinical aspects and societal prospects. Dekker, New York, (in press)

Horner RD (1987) Age at onset of Alzheimer's disease: Clue to the relative importance of etiologic factors? Am J Epidemiol 126: 409–414

Mayeux R, Stern Y, Spanton S (1985) Heterogeneity in dementia of the Alzheimer type: evidence of subgroups. Neurology 35: 453–461

McKhann G, Drachman D, Folstein M, Katzman R, Price D, Stadlan EM (1984) Clinical diagnosis of Alzheimer's disease: report of the NINCDS-ADRDA work group under the auspices of the Department of Health and Human Services Task Force on Alzheimer's disease. Neurology 34: 939–944

Nee LE, Eldridge R, Sunderland T, Thomas D, Katz KE, Thompson H, Weingartner HW, Julian C, Cohen R (1987) Dementia of the Alzheimer type: clinical and family study of 22 twin pairs. Neurology 37: 359–363

Roberts GW, Taylor GR, Carter GI, Johnson JA, Bloxham C, Brown R, Crow TJ (1986) Herpes simplex virus: a role in the etiology of Alzheimer's disease? J Neurol Neurosurg Psychiatry 49: 216–219

Tierney MC, Reid DW, Zorzitto ML, Snow WG, Fisher RH, Campbell-Taylor I, Lewis A (1986) The differential diagnosis of Alzheimer's disease: conceptual and methodological issues. Can J Neurol Sci 13: 424–426

Tanzi RE, St George-Hyslop PH, Haines JL, Polinsky RJ, Nee L, Foncin J-F, Neve RL, McClatchey AI, Conneally PM, Gusella JF (1987) The genetic defect in familial Alzheimer's disease is not tightly linked to the amyloid β-protein gene. Nature 329: 156–157

Van Broeckhoven C, Genthe AM, Vandenberghe A, Horsthemke B, Backhovens H, Raeymaekers P, Hul WV, Wehnert A, Ghevens J, Cras P, Bruyland M, Martin JJ, Salbaum M, Masters CL, Beyreuther K, Gurling HMD, Mullan MJ, Holland A, Barton A, Irving N, Williamson R, Richards SJ, Hardy JA (1987) Failure of Alzheimer's disease to segregate with the A4-amyloid gene in several European families. Nature 329: 153–155

Dermatoglyphic Patterns in Senile Dementia of Alzheimer's Type

N. Okra Podrabinek, M. Roudier, Y. Lamour, and *J. de Grouchy*

Summary

Several reports suggest a genetic relationship between senile dementia of the Alzheimer type (SDAT) and Down's syndrome. We analyzed fingerprints and palmar patterns in an elderly female population comprising a group of 34 patients with probable SDAT, a group of 20 patients with other dementias, and a group of 20 nondemented controls. A bilateral Sydney line was found to be significantly more frequent in the SDAT group than in the two other groups ($P < 0.01$, sensitivity 30%, specificity 95%, positive predictive value 91%, negative predictive value 61%). A bilateral Sydney line is as common in SDAT as in Down's syndrome. A limit value of the index of transversality equal or superior to 31, which is considered as a feature of Down's syndrome, was significantly more frequent in the SDAT group than in the two other groups (right-hand $P < 0.05$, left-hand $P < 0.02$). A bilateral discriminant value of this index was also significantly more frequent in the SDAT group than in the two other groups ($P < 0.02$), as was an index of transversality higher than 31 on at least one hand ($P < 0.01$).

In contrast with other reports, we have not found significantly different frequencies of digital ulnar loops and true hypothenar patterns between the SDAT group and the two others.

Introduction

Alzheimer's disease is the most frequent dementia in the population over the age of 65. Its cause is unknown. Patients with Down's syndrome who survive more than 35 years (Oliver and Holland 1986) present the same neuropathological features found in Alzheimer's disease (senile plaques, neurofibrillary tangles, granulovacuolar degeneration). The discovery of patients with a Down's syndrome phenotype and a normal karyotype but with duplications of a short segment of chromosome 21, and the duplication of the 21 q 22 1 region found in sporadic Alzheimer's disease by certain authors (Delabar et al. 1986; Blanquet et al. 1987) but not by others (Tanzi et al. 1987; Podlisny et al. 1987; St George Hyslop et al. 1987) suggest the existence of genetic relationships. In Down's syndrome, the dermatoglyphic patterns are characteristic and of practical use in establishing diagnosis (Turpin and Lejeune 1953; Walker 1957; Plato et al. 1973; Smith and Berg 1976). The dermatoglyphic features in Down's syndrome are independent of sex, laterality, race, and ethnic origin: ulnar loops on fingertips, hypothenar ulnar loops, Simian crease, distal axial triradius, and high value of the index of transversality are more frequent in Down's syndrome than in the normal population. It is known that dermatoglyphic patterns are under genetic control, but the mechanisms of inheritance involved are not fully known (Schaumann and Alter 1976). Identification of patients who have a genetic predisposition to Alzheimer's disease might have important implications for an eventual prophylaxis.

For Alzheimer's disease, several authors (Weinreb 1985; Seltzer and Sherwin 1986; Ghidoni et al. 1987) studied only fingerprint patterns. The study of fingerprint and palmar patterns was reported by Luxenberg et al. (1987), who found no difference between SDAT patients and controls, and by Weinreb (1987) who found a significantly higher frequency of true hypothenar patterns, Simian crease, and digital ulnar loops.

Thus, in keeping with the hypothesis of a common genetic background for Down's syndrome and Alzheimer's disease, we studied the fingerprints and palmar patterns in a population of elderly patients suffering from probable senile dementia of the Alzheimer type (McKhann et al. 1984) as well as in patients with other dementias and in a control group without dementia.

Patients and Methods

Patients

The patients were from a geriatric unit in the Paris area. All were women, there being too few men to form a group. The men were not included in the female population, because some dermatoglyphic variations are sex-related.

A Mini Mental State Examination (MMSE; Folstein et al. 1975) permitting a rapid assessment of cognitive functions, was performed for each patient. Three groups were then formed (Table 1).

Group 1

A group of 34 patients with senile dementia of the Alzheimer type (SDAT), ranging from 70 to 92 years old (mean age 82.8 ± 7.6 years), was given a complete, detailed

Table 1. Ages and MMSE scores in the three groups under study

	SDAT (n = 34)	Controls (n = 20)	OD (n = 20)
Age (years)			
Mean ± SD	82.7 ± 7.6	80.9 ± 6	83.8 ± 6.9
Range	70 – 92	68 – 88	74 – 98
MMSE score			
Mean ± SD	8 ± 5	24.2 ± 3	11.85 ± 5.6
Range	0 – 18	20 – 30	2 – 19

SDAT, senile dementia of the Alzheimer type; OD, other dementias

neurological examination, in particular, a complete neuropsychological examination (Boller and Hecaen 1979; Roudier et al. 1986), when the patient's understanding was not too impaired. This was completed using the usual biological tests, thyroid function tests, serologic tests for syphilis, EEG, and cerebral CT scan.

Two neurologists diagnosed probable SDAT based on criteria defined by the Diagnostic and Statistical Manual (DSM III, 1980) and the National Institute of Neurological Communicative Disorders and Strokes (McKhann et al. 1984). In this group the MMSE scores ranged from 0 to 18 (8 ± 5). All these patients were included in a long-term study with repeated assessments and pathological investigation of lesions of the brain after death. Certain diagnoses were then corrected, there being a risk error of 20% between SDAT and other dementias (Boller et al. 1988).

Group 2

There were 20 control patients, ranging in age from 68 to 88 years (mean age: 80.9 ± 6 years), hospitalized for orthopedic, rheumatologic, or cardiovascular diseases, or for social reasons. All these patients were free of all signs of dementia. Their MMSE scores ranged from 20 to 30 (24.2 ± 3).

Group 3

A group of 20 patients suffering from dementia of other etiology (other dementias: OD) was formed. They ranged in age from 74 to 98 years (mean age: 83.8 ± 6.9). Of these 20 patients, 10 suffered from vascular dementia, which was diagnosed by using the score of modified ischemia, superior to 4 (Loeb and Gandolfo 1983); five patients suffered from psychiatric dementia; and five patients suffered from dementia associated with hypothyroidism. The MMSE scores ranged from 2 to 19 (11.85 ± 5.6).

Patients with Parkinson's disease, with or without dementia, were not included; neither were patients with hand deformities that would make the investigation of complete dermatoglyphic patterns impossible.

Methods

The dermatoglyphic patterns of palms and all fingertips were recorded for both hands by pressing the inked hand on a thin sheet of paper supported by foam rubber (Alter 1966). The impressions were taken one or several times for each patient, depending on the quality of the prints. The following parameters were studied with reference to the classical nomenclature (Lafourcade and Rethoré 1967; Holt 1968): the existence of a Simian crease and of a Sydney line (Schaumann and Alter 1976); the position of the axial triradii in t (proximal position), t′ (intermediate position), or t″ (distal position) (Cummins and Midlo 1943); the value of the index of transversality, conventionally defined by the sum of the exit numbers of the mainlines issued from the four digital triradii (Cummins and Midlo 1943); true hypothenar patterns (radial and ulnar loops); and the digital patterns classified as arches, whorls, radial loops, ulnar loops, and combined patterns. The index described by Turpin and Lejeune (1953) was also studied.

Defined empirically, this index is obtained by summing up the coefficients attributed to the transversality index when it is equal or superior to 31 (+1), to the presence of a hypothenar ulnar loop (+1), of a Simian crease (+4), of a hypothenar radial loop (−2), and to the position of the axial triradius in t″ (+2). The index obtained by adding the indexes of each hand allows the exact classification of 95% of patients with Down's syndrome when it is superior to 4. Moreover, our results were compared with dermatoglyphic norms for females according to Turpin and Schutzenberger (1949), as well as with dermatoglyphic characteristics of Down's syndrome, according to Turpin and Lejeune (1953) and Smith (1976).

For statistical analysis we used the chi^2 test with Yate's correction for small groups, nonpaired Student's coefficient t and the table of standard deviations (Schwartz 1963).

Results

The Simian Crease

No Simian crease or equivalent pattern was observed in the three study groups. In Down's syndrome the Simian crease is unilateral right in 8.6%, unilateral left in 6.4%, and bilateral in 26.3% (Turpin and Lejeune 1953).

The Sydney Line

The Sydney line is an extension of the proximal transverse crease across the entire palm, rather than stopping short of the ulnar border (Table 2). A Sydney line was observed in the SDAT group but not significantly ($P < 0.10$), compared with the control group and the OD group, respectively: SDAT group, 13/34 in the right hand and 11/34 in the left hand; control group, 2/20 in the right hand and 4/20 in the left hand; OD group, 4/20 in the right hand and 4/20 in the left hand.

A bilateral Sydney line is more frequent, near significance, in the SDAT group than in the control group ($0.10 < P < 0.05$). It is significantly more frequent in the SDAT group (10/34) than in the OD group (0/20; $P < 0.02$). It is significantly more frequent in the SDAT group than in the two other groups combined: SDAT group, 10/34; control and OD groups, 1/40 ($P < 0.01$) with a 30% sensitivity, a 95% specificity. The positive predictive value is 91% and the negative predictive value is 61%.

A Sydney line is significantly more frequent in the SDAT group (right hand, 38%; left hand, 32%) than in Down's syndrome (right hand, 8.6%; left hand, 6.4%; $P < 0.01$), but a bilateral Sydney line is found with the same frequency in the SDAT group (30%) and in Down's syndrome (26.3%).

Table 2. Percentage frequencies of Sydney line and of position of axial triradius in SDAT patients, controls, other dementias (OD), Down's syndrome, and normal population

		SDAT (n = 34)	Controls (n = 20)	OD (n = 20)	Down's syndrome[a]	Normal population
		n %	n %	n %	%	% Right and left combined[b]
Sydney line	Right hand	13/38[c]	2/10	4/20	8.8[f]	11
	Left hand	11/32[d]	4/20	4/20	6.4[f]	
	Bilateral	10/30[e]	1/5	0/0	26.3[g]	
Position of axial triradius	Right hand					Right and left combined[a]
	t	25/73	14/70	16/80	27[h] (t + t′)	93.9 (t + t′)
	t′	7/20	6/30	4/20		
	t″	2/6	0/0	0/0	72.8[i]	6.1
	Left hand					
	t	24/74	27/65	18/90	27[h] (t + t′)	
	t′	9/23	7/35	2/10		
	t″	1/3	0/0	0/0	72.8[i]	

[a] From Turpin and Lejeune (1953)
[b] From Fraser and Nora (1986)
[c] $P < 0.05$ in SDAT vs controls + OD
[d] NS < 0.30 in SDAT vs controls + OD
[e] $P < 0.01$ in SDAT vs controls + OD
[f] $P < 0.01$ in Down's syndrome vs SDAT
[g] NS in Down's syndrome vs SDAT
[h] $P < 0.01$ in Down's syndrome vs SDAT, controls, OD, normal population
[i] $P < 0.01$ in Down's syndrome vs SDAT, controls, OD, normal population

The Axial Triradius

The incidences of axial triradii in t, t′, t″ are not different in the three study groups, in particular in triradius t″ (Table 2). In Down's syndrome, an axial triradius in t″ is frequent (72%) while an axial triradius in t′ is very rare (1%; Turpin and Lejeune 1953).

The Index of Transversality

The mean value of the index of transversality is not significantly different in the SDAT group (right hand, 29.6 ± 2.4; left hand, 28.6 ± 2.8), in the control group (right hand, 27.9 ± 3; left hand, 27.05 ± 2.8) and in the OD group (right hand, 27.5 ± 2.2; left hand, 26.8 ± 3.4); (Table 3). When the value of this index is equal or superior to 31, it is considered a feature of Down's syndrome with a sensitivity of 75% and a specificity of 81% (Turpin and Lejeune 1953).

An index superior or equal to 31 was significantly more frequent in the SDAT group than in the control group or in the OD group, with a sensitivity of 62% and a specificity of 80%. An index of transversality superior or equal to 31 was significantly more

Table 3. Value of the index of transversality and frequency of index ≥ 31 in SDAT, controls, OD (other dementias), and Down's syndrome

Index of transversality		SDAT (n = 34)	Controls (n = 20)	OD (n 20)	Down's syndrome[a]
Mean value ± SD	Right hand Left hand	29.6 ± 2.4 28.6 ± 2.8	27.9 ± 3 27.05 ± 2.8	27.5 ± 2.2 26.8 ± 3.4	30.95 ± 0.24 30.12 ± 0.25
Frequency of index of transversality ≥ 31	Right hand Left hand Bilateral	18[b] 15[c] 13[c]	4 2 2	2 3 1	
Frequency of at least one index of transversality ≥ 31 on at least one hand		21[d]	4	4	

[a] From Turpin and Lejeune (1953)
[b] $P < 0.05$ SDAT vs controls and OD
[c] $P < 0.02$ SDAT vs controls and OD
[d] $P < 0.01$ SDAT vs controls and OD

frequent in the SDAT group (13/34) than in the control group (2/20) and in the OD group (1/20) ($P < 0.02$). An index of transversality superior or equal to 31 on at least one hand is more frequent in the SDAT group (21/34) than in the control group (4/20) as well as in the OD group (4/20), and highly significantly so ($X^2 = 7.98$, df = 1, $P < 0.01$).

Patients having a bilateral Sydney line and at least one index of transversality superior or equal to 31 are significantly more common in the SDAT group (7/34) than in the two other groups (0/40; $P < 0.01$).

The True Hypothenar Patterns

No difference was found in the frequency and in the distribution of true hypothenar patterns between the three groups, and in particular no difference was found for bilateral hypothenar patterns (Table 4). Moreover, radial loops were observed in the SDAT group, while they are almost never observed in Down's syndrome.

The Fingertip Patterns

No significant difference was found in the frequencies of fingertip patterns in the three groups (Fig. 1), in particular of ulnar loops (62.7% in the SDAT group, 54% in the control group, and 60% in the OD group). The frequency of ulnar loops in Down's syndrome, estimated at 79% (Smith 1967), is significantly higher than in the SDAT group ($P < 0.02$). The frequency of patients having at least 8 ulnar loops on 10 fingers

Table 4. True hypothenar patterns: percentage frequencies[a] in SDAT, controls, OD, Down's syndrome and normal population.

	SDAT ($n = 34$) %	Controls + OD ($n = 40$) %	Down's syndrome[b] %	Normal population[b] %
Right hand				
Radial loops	26.4	20	0	23
Ulnar loops	6	2.5	54	10
Left hand				
Radial loops	12	15	0	20
Ulnar loops	8	10	46	13
Bilateral				
Radial loops + Ulnar loops	8.8	12.5	57	30

[a] The frequencies are significantly different from SDAT patients and Down's syndrome for radial loops in right hand ($P < 0.001$), in left hand ($P < 0.05$), for ulnar loops in right and left hands ($P < 0.01$), from controls plus OD and Down's syndrome for radial loops in left and right hands ($P < 0.05$), and for ulnar loops in left and right hands ($P < 0.01$)

[b] From Turpin and Lejeune (1953)

is higher, but not significantly so ($P < 0.10$), in the SDAT group (13/34) than in the control group (3/20) and the OD group (5/20).

The Index of Turpin and Lejeune

The mean value of the Turpin and Lejeune index in the SDAT group (0.62 ± 2.04, m ± SD) is not significantly different from the mean value of the indexes of the two other groups (control group, −0.23 ± 1.4; OD group, −0.26 ± 1.48).

Discussion

Our results show apparent discrepancies with those of other authors. Their meaning will be discussed later. While Luxenberg et al. (1987) found no difference in the dermatoglyphic patterns between SDAT patients and controls, other authors found, with a significantly higher frequency, digital ulnar loops (Weinreb 1985; Seltzer and Sherwin 1986; Ghidoni et al. 1987), true hypothenar patterns, and a Simian crease (Weinreb 1986; Table 5).

The only dermatoglyphic traits with a significantly different incidence between the SDAT group and the two other groups were the existence of a bilateral Sydney line and an index of transversality equal or superior to 31. There was no difference between the control group and the OD group, so that SDAT is distinguishable among the dementias. The control group was similar to a normal female French population

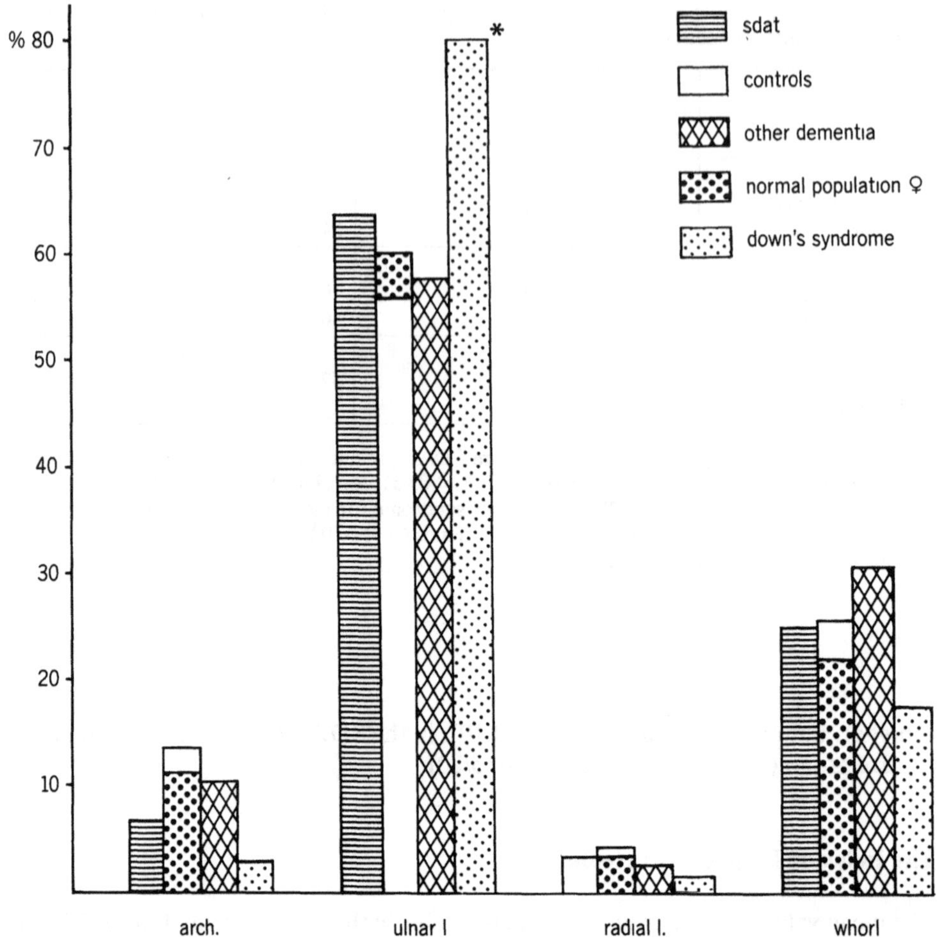

Fig. 1. Percentage distribution of fingerprint patterns in SDAT, controls, other dementias, normal population (Turpin and Schutzenberger 1949), and Down's syndrome (Smith 1967). * $P < 0.01$ Down's syndrome vs all other groups

(Turpin and Schutzenberger 1949). The frequency of the Sydney line (Table 2) in the normal population was estimated to be approximately 11% (Fraser and Nora 1986).

A Sydney line was significantly more frequent in the SDAT group than in the other two groups as well as in Down's syndrome (Turpin and Lejeune 1953).

The frequency of the Sydney line in Down's syndrome seemed lower than in the normal population. This could be explained by a higher frequency in Down's syndrome patients of a Simian crease, which can include a Sydney line. Weinreb (1986) also found, with a higher, but not significant, frequency, the existence of a Sydney line in the Alzheimer's disease group as compared with the control group; moreover, he found, with a significantly higher frequency, the existence of a Simian crease, which we did not find in our patients. The existence on both hands of a Sydney line was

Table 5. Percentage frequencies of dermatoglyphic traits in Alzheimer's disease patients and control patients, in different studies

	Weinreb (1986)	Seltzer and Sherwin (1986)		Ghidoni et al. (1987)		Luxenberg et al. (1987)	Our results
Features of patients	$n = 50$ 33 ♂ 17 ♀	$n = 82$ EAAO 47 ♂	 LAAO 35 ♂	$n = 65$ 38 ♂	 27 ♀	$n = 56$ 29 ♂ 27 ♀	$n = 34$ ♀
Ulnar loops on fingertips	72 S	68.5 S	51.4 NS	54.5 S	59.7 NS	NS	62.7 NS
True hypothenar patterns	50 S						26 NS
Sydney line	10 $P < 0.10$						Right hand S Left hand NS Bilateral S
Simian crease	11 S						0

EAAO, early age at onset; LAAO, late age at onset; S, significantly different from controls ($P < 0.05$); NS, not significantly different from controls

significantly more frequent in the SDAT group as compared with the other two groups, with a good specificity (95%), a good positive predictive value (91%), and a rather good negative predictive value (61%). A bilateral Sydney line in the SDAT group was as frequent as in Down's syndrome.

Whereas the mean value of the index of transversality was not different in the three groups, the value of 31 on the index allowed a discrimination between the SDAT group and the other two groups, with a good specificity (80%) and a good sensitivity (62%).

A bilateral discriminant value in the SDAT group had a good positive predictive value (81%) and a quite good negative predictive value (64%). Therefore, the index discriminant value was of great help in establishing the diagnosis of SDAT, especially as its existence on at least one hand was significantly more frequent in the SDAT group than in the other two groups.

An axial triradius in t″, which is a major feature of Down's syndrome (Turpin and Lejeune 1953), was not found in the three studied groups. The variations in the position of the axial triradius were identical in the three groups and similar to those of a normal population, in particular the intermediate position (t′), which is extremely rare in Down's syndrome.

The distribution of the digital ulnar loops was not significantly different in the three groups, in particular there was not a significantly higher frequency of digital ulnar loops, such as has been described in Down's syndrome (Smith 1967) and found by certain authors in Alzheimer's disease. Seltzer and Sherwin (1986) found this higher frequency of digital ulnar loops in a male population only with early-onset primary degenerative dementia but not with late-onset primary degenerative dementia. Ghidoni et al. (1987) found this result only in the male but not female SDAT group; while Weinreb (1986) found this result in a mixed, predominantly male, population whose mean age was slightly lower than both our SDAT and control groups. Therefore, the differences of sex and age at the onset on dementia in all the groups studied could explain the discrepancies with our results. Seltzer and Sherwin (1986) suggested that the early-onset and late-onset dementias were distinct pathological entities. Neither the existence of at least 6 digital ulnar loops on both hands (Seltzer and Sherwin 1986), nor the existence of at least 8 digital ulnar loops (Weinreb 1985) found with a significantly higher incidence in SDAT patients compared with controls, was of help in our study.

The distribution and the bilateral existence of true hypothenar patterns was not different in the three groups. Weinreb (1986) found a higher frequency of bilateral true hypothenar patterns in the Alzheimer's disease group than in the control group and a similar frequency in the Alzheimer's disease and Down's syndrome groups; however, he found a great number of hypothenar radial loops, which were extremely rare in Down's syndrome.

In Down's syndrome, the index of Turpin and Lejeune (1953), when superior to 4, was of great help in establishing diagnosis, while in our study this index was of no help in distinguishing between the SDAT group and the other two groups. In fact, if the frequent existence of an index of transversality equal or superior to 31 raised the index of Turpin and Lejeune, the similarly frequent existence of radial hypothenar loops lowered it.

Thus, the dermatoglyphic characteristics of SDAT patients were similar to those with Down's syndrome, as seen in the frequent existence on both hands of the Sydney line and the frequent existence of a high index of transversality, in particular on both hands; however, they differed, among other traits, in the existence of radial hypothenar loops.

The etiological diagnosis of different dementias is actually impossible before death. Therefore, the discovery of a biological or clinical marker would represent a major breakthrough. The neuropathological examination of the brains of our patients, after death, should permit more accurate results, by confirming or correcting certain diagnoses. This preliminary study will be pursued with a greater number of patients.

References

Alter M (1966) Dermatoglyphic analysis as a diagnostic tool. Medicine 46: 1–12

Blanquet V, Goldgaber D, Turleau C, Creau-Golberg N, Delabar J, Sinet PM, Roudier M, de Grouchy J (1987) The amyloid protein (AD–AP) cDNA hybridizes in normal and Alzheimer individuals near the interface of 21q21 and q22.1. Ann Génét 30: 68–69

Boller F, Hecaen H (1979) L'évaluation des fonctions neuropsychologiques: examen standard de l'unité de recherches neuropsychologiques et neurolinguistiques. Rev Psychol Appl 29: 247–266

Boller F, Lopez OL, Moossy J (1988) Diagnosis of dementia: clinico-pathological correlations. Arch Neurol, in press

Cummins H, Midlo C (1943) Finger prints, palms and soles. Blakiston, Philadelphia

Delabar J, Lamour Y, Gegonne A, Davous P, Roudier M, Nicole A, Ceballos I. Amouyel P, Stehelin D, Sinet PM (1986) Rearrangement of chromosome 21 in Alzheimer's disease. Ann Génét 29: 226–228

Diagnostic and Statistical Manual of Mental Disorders (DSM III) (1980) 3rd edition. Washington, American Psychiatric Association, pp 107–112
Folstein MF, Folstein SE, McHugh PR (1975) "Mini mental state" a pratical method for grading cognitive state of patients for the clinician. J Psychiatr Res 12: 189–198
Fraser FC, Nora JJ (1986) Genetics of man, 2nd ed, Lea and Febiger Philadelphia, pp 233–240
Ghidoni E, Chiessi G, Dallari A, Pattacini F, Solime F (1987) Fingerprint patterns and genetic risk factors in Alzheimer's disease. Neuroscience (Suppl S) 22: 439
Holt SB (1968) The genetics of dermal ridges. Charles C Thomas, Springfield, Ill
Lafourcade J. Rethore MO (1967) Les dermatoglyphes. In: Journées parisiennes de pédiatrie, Flammarion, Paris, pp 87–111
Loeb C, Gandolfo C (1983) A Diagnostic evaluation of degenerative and vascular dementia. Stroke 14: 399–401
Luxenberg JS, Plato CC, Fox KM, Friedland RP, Rapoport SI (1987) Dermatoglyphics in dementia of the Alzheimer's type. Neurology [Suppl 1] 37: 333
McKhann G, Drachmann D, Folstein M, Katzman R, Price D, Stadlan E (1984) Clinical diagnosis of Alzheimer's disease: report of the NINCDS-ADRDA work group under the auspices of the Department of health and human services task force on Alzheimer's disease. Neurology 34: 939–944
Oliver C, Holland AJ (1986) Down's syndrome and Alzheimer's disease: a review. Psychol Med 16: 307–322
Plato CC, Cureghino JJ, Steinberg FS (1973) Palmar dermatoglyphics of Down's syndrome, revisited. Pediatr Res 7: 111–118
Podlisny MB, Lee G, Selkoe DJ (1987) Gene dosage of the β amyloid precursor protein in Alzheimer's disease. Science 238: 669–671
Roudier M, Marcie P, Davous P, Podrabinek N, Lamour Y (1986) Neuropsychological study of senile dementia of Alzheimer type. In: Bès A, Cahn J, Cahn R, Hoyer S, Marc-Vergnes JM, Wisniewski HM (eds), Senile dementia, early detection. Libbey Eurotext, Paris, pp 614–618
St George-Hyslop PH, Tanzi RE, Polinsky RJ, Neve RL, Pollen D, Drachman D, Growdon J, Cupples LA, Nee L, Myers R, O'Sullivan D, Watkins PC, Amos JA, Deutsch CK, Bodfish JW, Kinsbourne M, Feldman RG, Bruni A, Amaducci L, Foncin J-F, Gusella JF (1987) Absence of duplication of chromosome 21 genes in familial and sporadic Alzheimer's disease. Science 238: 664–666
Schaumann B, Alter M (1976) Dermatoglyphics in medical disorders. Springer, New York
Schwartz D (1963) Methodes statistiques à l'usage des médecins et biologistes. Flammarion, Paris
Seltzer B, Sherwin I (1986) Fingerprint pattern. Differences in early- and late-onset primary degenerative dementia. Arch Neurol 43: 665–668
Smith GF (1967) Correlation of dermal patterns on fingertips and toes in mongolism. In: CIBA Foundation Study Group (ed) Mongolism. Churchill, London, pp 35–40
Smith GF, Berg JM (1976) Down's Anomaly. Churchill Livingstone, New York
Tanzi RE, Bird ED, Latt SA, Neve RL (1987) The amyloid protein is not duplicated in brains from patients with Alzheimer's disease. Science 238: 666–669
Turpin R, Lejeune J (1959) Etude dermatoglyphique des paumes des mongoliens et de leurs parents et germains. Sem Hôp (Paris) 29: 3955–3967
Turpin R, Schutzenberger MP (1949) L'étude des dermatoglyphes. Sem Hôp (Paris) 25: 2553–2562
Walker NF (1957) The use of dermal configurations in the diagnosis of mongolism. J Pediatr 50: 19–26
Weinreb HJ (1985) Fingerprint patterns in Alzheimer's disease. Arch Neurol 42: 50–54
Weinreb HJ (1986) Dermatoglyphic patterns in Alzheimer's disease. J Neurogenet 3: 233–246

A Phylogenetic Hypothesis for Alzheimer's Disease

S. I. Rapoport

Summary

It is proposed that Alzheimer's disease is a human phylogenetic disease because of evidence that paired helical filaments, characteristic of the postmortem Alzheimer brain, are not found in brains of nonhuman primates; because of functional studies in life, and pathological studies postmortem, that the association neocortices and their connections are specifically involved throughout the course of the disease; and because of evidence that genes on chromosome 21 contribute to Alzheimer pathology in some families as well as in Down's syndrome. It is argued that the association necortices and their connections, which underwent integrated elaboration during recent hominid evolution, became vulnerable to Alzheimer pathology through the genomic processes that promoted their evolution. Some genes involved in integrated phylogeny of the association system, therefore, may contribute to the genetic liability for Alzheimer's disease in man.

Introduction

Alzheimer's disease, the fourth most common cause of death in the United States, is the major cause of dementia in the elderly (Katzman 1976). Yet its pathogenesis is poorly understood. None of the present hypotheses for its cause can explain most of the functional defects, pathology, or epidemiology of Alzheimer's disease (reviewed by Rapoport 1988b).

I have recently suggested (Rapoport 1988b) that Alzheimer's disease is a neurodegenerative disorder which is specific to man because of molecular genetic events which promoted rapid evolution of the hominid brain, and particularly of the association neocortices and nonneocortical regions to which they are connected. These regions underwent "integrated phylogeny" during recent hominid evolution.

In this paper, I reexamine the phylogenetic hypothesis for Alzheimer's disease. Concurrent evolution of association regions is described first, after which the molecular events that might have promoted their evolution are explored. Neuropathological and cerebral metabolic studies are presented that confirm that Alzheimer's disease selectively affects the association system. Similarities between Alzheimer's disease, Down's syndrome, and Pick's disease are evaluated. Finally, a polygenic model for Alzheimer's disease is presented, and is related to a similar model for evolution of the association neocortices in hominids.

Brain Evolution

The fossil record of early man (family Hominidae) extends backwards about 5 million years, when man and the great apes diverged genetically from the chimpanzee (King and Wilson 1975). Evolution of the hominid brain occurred through discontinuous steps of rapid growth and differentiation, separated by periods of relative stability (Fig. 1, Table 1). About 3.7 million years ago, endocranial volume equaled 400 cm^3 in *Australopithecus afarensis*, the first upright human ancestor. By 200000 years ago,

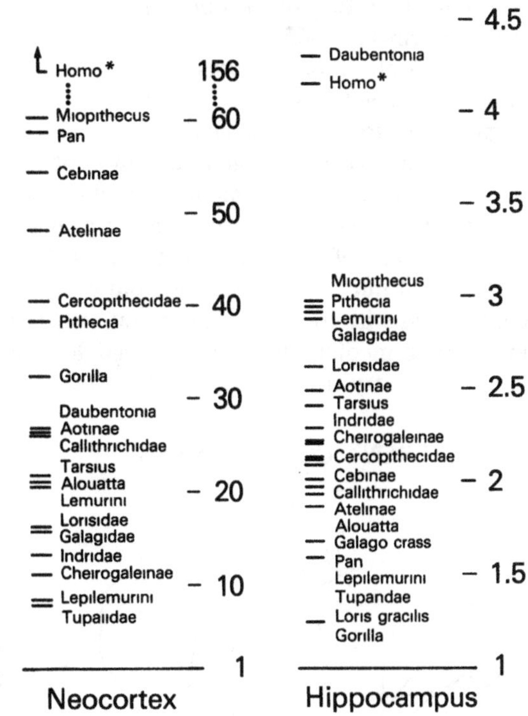

Fig. 1. Progression indices of neocortex and hippocampus in primates. Indices are numbers of times by which neocortex and hippocampus exceed respective value in a typical basal insectivore of equal body weight. (Adapted from Stephan and Andy 1970)

Table 1. Cranial capacity in primates. Data from Hofman (1983), Campbell (1985), and Cann (1987)

Species	Average (range) (cm^3)	Age (million years)
Lemur	(10–70)	58–65
Chimpanzee	383 (282–500)	25–5
Hominids		
Austropithecus afarensis[a]	440 (380–500)	4.0–2.3
A. africanus	450 (435–530)	3.0–2.0
A. robustus	500	2.0–1.5
A. bosei	515 (506–530)	2.5–1.2
Homo habilis	666 (660–752)	2.3–1.5
H. erectus	950 (775–1225)	1.3–0.4
H. sapiens recens	1330 (1000–2000)	0.2

[a] Ancestor of both *A. Africanus* and *Homo habilis*

endocranial volume had reached 1465 cm^3 in modern *Homo sapiens* (Hofman 1983; Campbell 1985; Cann 1987).

As it evolved, the hominid brain underwent reorganization and additions, particularly in the association neocortices. The frontal and occipital association areas occupy much larger fractions of the cerebral cortex in the human brain than in the brain of higher primates, and larger fractions in higher primates than in lower primates and other mammals (Holloway 1968). A postparietal gyrus, specific to the human brain, is found at the junction of projection areas for vision, somesthetic ability and hearing, and contributes to cerebral dominance and visual and auditory processing (Critchley 1953; Geschwind 1965).

Neocortical elaboration was accompanied by elaboration of phylogenetically older brain regions with which the neocortex established new connections. The posterior hippocampal formation expanded, particularly at the CA1 and subicular regions and the entorhinal cortex, while attenuation of the intrahemispheric hippocampal commissures allowed hippocampal connections with the ipsilateral association neocortices to promote hemispheric asymmetry (Fig. 1 and 2; Stephan and Andy 1970; Van Hoesen et al. 1979; Goldman-Rakic 1984; Demeter et al. 1985). The small cell corticobasal nuclei of the amygdaloid complex also expanded and established new connections with the medial temporal association neocortex, while phylogenetically unmodified medial and central amygdaloid nuclei receded and the nucleus of the lateral olfactory tract disappeared entirely (Fig. 3; Herzog and Van Hoesen 1976;

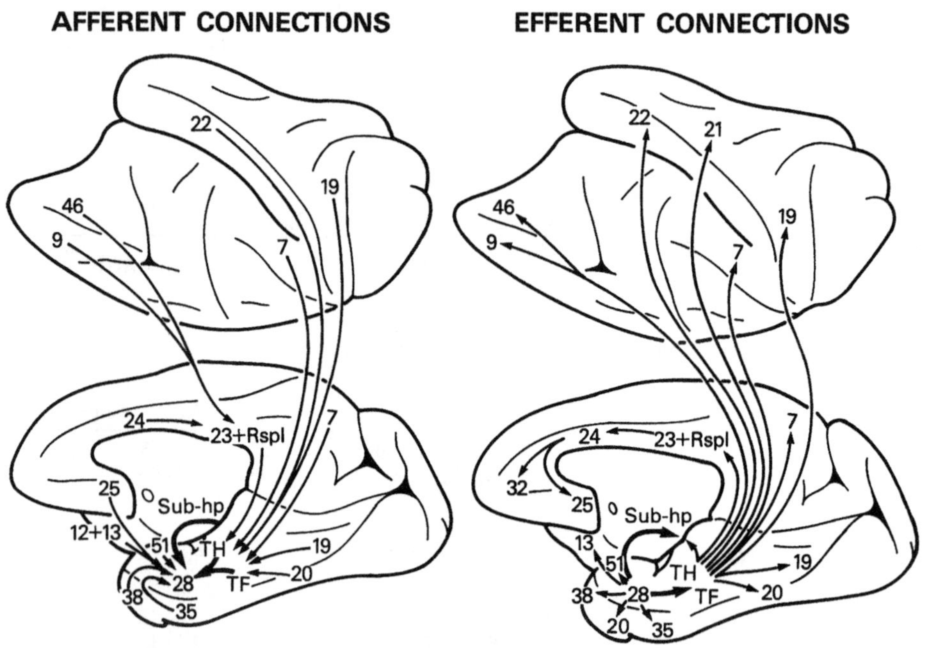

Fig. 2. Afferent and efferent cortical connections of parahippocampal gyrus in rhesus monkey, shown in lateral *(inverted)* and medial views of cerebral hemisphere. *Numbers* refer to cortical areas as described by Van Hoesen (1982). In addition to the above connections, temporal and parietal association areas are connected ipsilaterally with frontal association area; all also are connected to contralateral homologous association areas. (From Van Hoesen 1982)

Stephan and Andy 1977). The nucleus basalis of Meynert, which provides cholinergic projections to the entire neocortex, became condensed first in Carnivores, and later was elaborated in higher primates, particularly homo sapiens and *Cetacea* (Gorry 1963; Braak 1978).

The association system in primates is organized as follows (Fig. 2). Primary visual, somatosensory and auditory projection areas, as well as the primary motor area of the neocortex, are connected to association fields in the parietal, frontal, and temporal lobes. These fields in turn are connected reciprocally with the prefrontal cortex, and with paralimbic and limbic areas (including the hippocampus and parahippocampal gyrus), the latter connections investing information with emotional tone and placing it in long-term memory (Pandya and Seltzer 1982; Van Hoesen 1982). Ablation of either the hippocampus, prefrontal cortex, or amygdaloid body interferes somewhat with memory, whereas combined ablation of the hippocampus and amygdala, or of the hippocampus and prefrontal regions, produces striking memory deficits (Mishkin 1978; Milner and Petrides 1984). The prefrontal cortex, caudate nucleus, globus pallidus, substantia nigra, and thalamus also form a complex association loop which regulates "internal" initiation of movement in the absence of sensory guidance (Alexander et al. 1986).

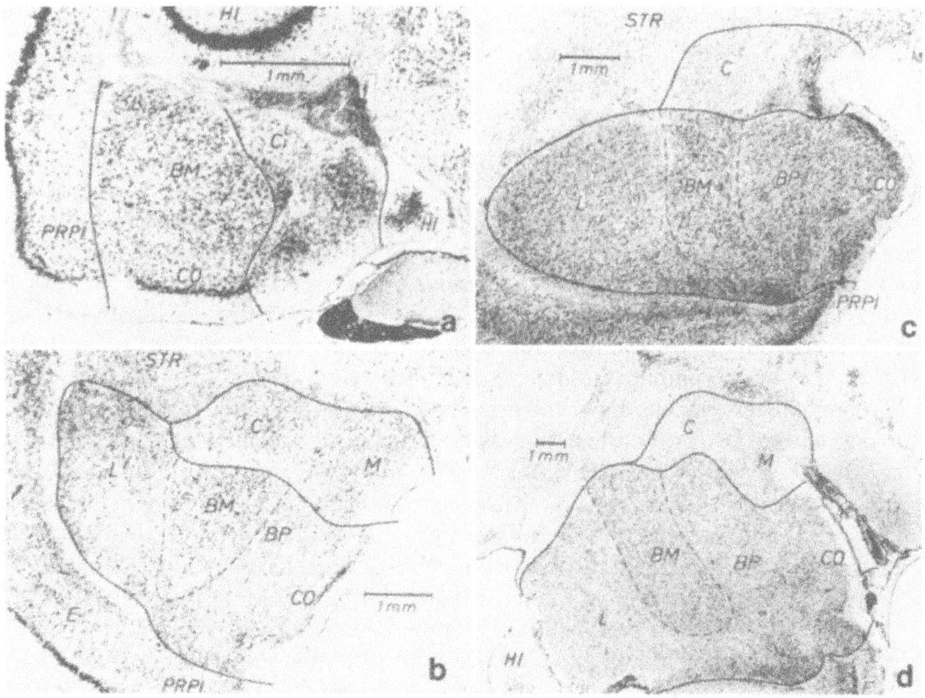

Fig. 3a–d. Frontal sections through the amygdaloid complex of a *Hemicentetes semispinosus* (an insectivore); **b** *Propithecus verreauxi* (a prosimian); **c** *Alouatta seniculus* (a simian); and **d** *Homo sapiens*. Note progressive expansion of small cell (parvocellular) basal-cortical nuclear complex. *BM*, basal nucleus magnocellular; *BP*, basal nucleus parvocellular; *HI*, hippocampus; *E*, entorhinal cortex; *CO*, cortical nucleus; *PRPI*, prepiriform cortex; *STR*, striatum; *C*, central nucleus; *M*, medial nucleus; *L*, lateral nucleus. (From Stephan and Andy 1977)

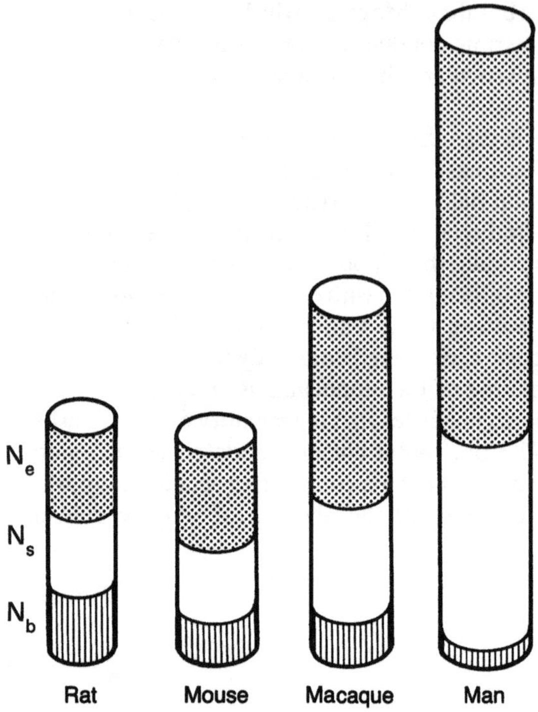

Fig. 4. Relative dimensions of neocortical columnar unit in four mammalian species. Although the diameters of each column are approximately the same, the proportions of secondary projection neurons (N_e), interneurons (N_s) and primary projection neurons (N_b) (represented by *subcylinders*), as well as columnar length, vary. (From Hofman 1985)

Pyramidal association neurons in the frontal cortex, which are found mainly in layer III, and less frequently in layers IV and V, are reciprocally connected with ipsilateral parietal association neurons, and via the corpus callosum with contralateral homologous association neurons that integrate right and left hemispheric activities. Ipsilateral and contralateral association fibers terminate in neocortical association areas in distinct, vertically oriented receptive fields, or columns. Terminal distributions of projections from the prefrontal cortex to the parahippocampal gyrus and presubicular cortices also are columnar (Goldman and Nauta 1977; Goldman-Rakic 1984).

Indeed, the cortical column is the organizational and operational building block of the mammalian cerebral cortex. Widths of cortical columns, between 300 μm to 700 μm, are similar in the rat, squirrel monkey, and rhesus monkey, although length varies with cortical thickness (Fig. 4; Hofman 1985). As the neocortex in the rhesus monkey is five times larger than in the squirrel monkey, and 20 times larger than in the rat, phylogenetic expansion of the cortical surface must have been accompanied by increased numbers of columns (Goldman-Rakic 1984; Sawaguchi and Kubota, 1986).

«En bloc» replication of functionally related groups of cortical columns during mammalian evolution may explain the multiple representations of visual, somatosensory, and auditory receptive areas in the primate neocortex (Fig. 5; Van Essen 1979; Kaas 1982). Multiple representations are infrequent in primitive mammals such as the hedgehog, which has no more than two visual and two somatosensory representations. However, cats have at least 13 visual areas, five somatosensory areas, and seven auditory areas, while the owl monkey has at least 10 visual areas, six somatosensory areas, four auditory areas and two more motor-somatic representations (Fig. 5).

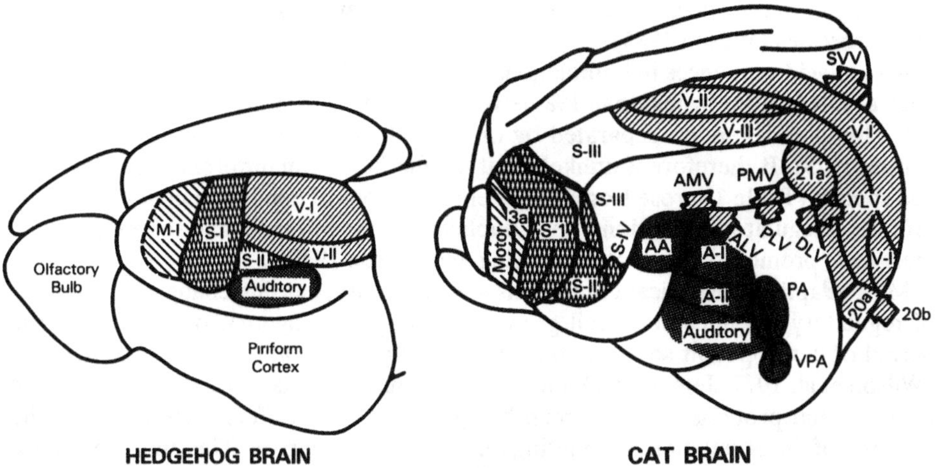

Fig. 5. Sensory and motor-sensory areas of cortex in a prototypical mammal, the hedgehog, and a moderately advanced mammal, the cat. The hedgehog has only a few areas; primary motor *(M-I)*, primary and secondary somatic (*S-I* and *S-II*), primary and secondary visual (*V-I* and *V-II*), and auditory *(A)* fields. The cat has acquired additional subdivisions including primary, secondary, and tertiary *(III)* fields, anterior auditory *(AAF)*, posterior auditory *(PFA)*, and splenial visual *(SVA)* fields. (Adapted from Kaas 1982)

Ontogeny

The temporal sequence of myelination in the human brain during development reflects the phylogenetic recency of the association neocortices (Yakovlev and Lecours 1967). Fiber tracts derived from association areas continue to myelinate up to at least the third decade of life, particularly in commissural and association fibers of the outermost layers of the cerebral hemispheres. Intracortical nerve fibers in frontal, parietal, and temporal association areas are myelinated into the fourth decade. The brain of the rhesus monkey also demonstrates later functional and biochemical maturation of the frontal and parietal association neocortices than of primary sensory and motor regions (Goldman-Rakic et al. 1987). Consistent with their evolutionary history, ontogeny of individual regions of the cerebellum and amygdaloid complex corresponds to recency of elaboration during neocortical evolution (Humphrey 1972; Sarnat and Netsky 1981).

Molecular Evolution

Mutations, Duplications, and Rearrangements

Molecular evolution of amino acid and nucleotide sequences occurs at fairly steady rates in all organisms, as frequently as 1% per 0.7 million years for immunoglobulins to 1% per 400 million years for H4 histones, which are genes considered to be structurally conserved (Wilson et al. 1977). However, evolution of phenotype varies markedly between species and illustrates the importance of environmental and cultural processes (Wilson 1985).

Amino acid sequences in homologous proteins, and electrophoretic differences in nuclear DNA differ by less than 1% between humans and chimpanzees, and indicate that Homo and Pan are separated by only 5 million years of evolution (King and Wilson 1975). It therefore is unlikely that the marked brain differences between the two species (Table 1) arose from infrequent mutations of genes coding for structural proteins. Regulatory mutations, gene duplications, or chromosomal rearrangements must have promoted this evolution (King and Wilson 1975).

Most adaptively significant mutations are regulatory, causing changes in activities of regulatory enzymes or of cell growth or recognition factors, or prolonging the period of development so as to allow continued production of postmitotic neurons (Wilson et al. 1977; Jerson, in Gould 1977). Because of mutations, about one-fifth of enzymes and proteins in any human being have a form different from that in the majority of the population, accounting for population diversity. This high prevalence of polymorphism is maintained because slightly deleterious mutations may be neutral or minimally disadvantageous for natural selection, and therefore can be fixed in the population genome (Harris and Hopkinson 1972).

Rapid phenotypic evolution also may follow gene duplication (Ohno 1970), which is introduced into the genome at sites of unequal crossover during the early prophase I stage of meiosis, or during unequal chromatid exchange during meiosis II or premeiotic stages, and is especially frequent at chromosomal sites of molecular instability (Donlon et al. 1986). Multiple copies of genes in the human genome frequently occur as clusters (families) of tandemly arranged repetitious genes, providing one solution to the problem of synthesizing additional amounts of gene products. Homogeneity in each family is maintained through unequal crossover, which allows repeated genes within a species to remain similar to one another as they diverge by "concerted evolution" in structure and number from repeated genes in other species (Hood et al. 1975; Zimmer et al. 1980).

Another factor that can initiate rapid phenotypic evolution is chromosomal rearrangement. The position of a gene on a chromosome, as well as its distance from heterochromatin (repetitive sequences that are not transcribed), are capable of modifying its expression (Lima-de-Faria 1983). Indeed, differences in rates of phenotypic evolution between mammals and frogs have been ascribed to differences in rates of chromosomal rearrangements (Wilson et al. 1974).

Although their expressed nuclear DNA does not differ by more than 1%, humans and chimpanzees differ distinctly with respect to chromosome rearrangements. Human chromosome 2 is a telomeric fusion of two acrocentric chimpanzee chromosomes. There are at least 9 pericentric inversions between chromosomes in the two species (breakage of the p and q arms in a chromosome and inversion around the centromere), multiple other rearrangements, and differences in amounts and locations of heterochromatin (De Grouchy et al. 1978; Yunis et al. 1980). For example, human satellite (III) heterochromatin is found only on human chromosome 9, whereas a homologous satellite heterochromatin is located on 10 different chimpanzee chromosomes (Jones et al. 1972).

Molecular Basis of Brain Evolution

There is little information as to how "integrated phylogeny" of the association neocortices and its connections in hominids was promoted by regulatory mutations, gene duplications, and chromosomal rearrangements. We can speculate that regulatory mutations or chromosomal rearrangements altered the regional intensities or sequences of expressions of genes coding for morphoregulatory cell-surface recognition or adhesion molecules (SAMs and CAMs; Edelman 1987), or for neurotrophic factors which promoted integrated phylogeny. For example, the trophic "nerve growth factor" influences the integrity of the septum-basal forebrain complex, together with its hippocampal and neocortical projection areas (Large et al. 1986; Kromer 1987). Other factors are known to regulate development of the limbic system and retina (Trisler 1982; Levitt and Cooper 1985). Altered expression of trophic factors could increase production of association neurons or reduce their programmed death during development (Cowan 1973).

It also has been argued that retardation of maturation – neoteny – contributed to phylogeny of the hominid brain (Gould 1977). Retardation would prolong mitotic activity of the primitive pseudostratified columnar cells on the ventricular surface of the developing neural tube, the progenitors of postmitotic, differentiated neurons that eventually migrate to the cortical surface (Boulder Committee 1970).

There is evidence that multiplication of columns during neocortical evolution (see above) occurred by interdigitation of new columns among the old in some cases, and by «en bloc» replication in others (Sawaguchi and Kubota 1986). The former process, which might have followed a chromosomal rearrangement or a regulatory mutation, may account for the different surface areas of the forelimb somatosensory cortices in two species of otter, corresponding to sensory discrimination capabilities of the forepaws in the two species (Radinsky 1968).

On the other hand, the multiple representations of visual, somatosensory, and auditory receptive areas in the neocortex of higher mammals (Fig. 5; Van Essen 1979; Kaas 1982) suggest «en bloc» replication following gene duplication. The complex association functions and structural relations of the new columns could have arisen from subsequent mutations of the duplicated genes, which were relatively free of selection pressures (Ohno 1970), or from local morphoregulatory modulation (Edelman 1987). Gene duplication during evolution probably caused duplicate A and A1 layers in the lateral geniculate nucleus of weasels, with no apparent difference between the two layers (Sanderson 1974).

Alzheimer's Disease: a Phylogenetic Disease of Association Neocortices and Their Connections

Criteria for Phylogenetic Neurological Disease

The above view of brain evolution suggests several criteria that a human neurological disease should satisfy if it is phylogenetic, that is, introduced or made more likely during hominid speciation. First, the fully manifest disease should be specifically human; in nonhuman primates, however, it might be partially manifest. As a corollary, a gene product characteristic of the disease, if present in the human brain, should be absent or in a lesser concentration in brains of nonhuman primates. A second criterion is that the disease be manifest mainly in association brain regions which evolved through "integrated phylogeny" during recent hominid evolution. It might first appear at puberty, when these regions rapidly mature (Feinberg 1982–1983), or in later life due to their selective degeneration. Third, the disease should have a substantial genetic cause, related to the genetic events that promoted evolution of the association system in hominids.

As shown below, many aspects of Alzheimer's disease are consistent with these criteria, suggesting that Alzheimer's disease is phylogenetic (Rapoport 1988b). First, Alzheimer's disease, as far as we know, has not been demonstrated in nonhuman primates; the neurofibrillary tangles and paired helical filaments, found in large quantities in the Alzheimer brain, are absent from the nonhuman brain, whereas the senile (neuritic) plaques in the Alzheimer brain are distinct from those in the brains of nonhuman primates because they contain paired helical filaments. Second, cognitive, pathological, and metabolic studies of Alzheimer's disease and Down's syndrome patients demonstrate selective degeneration of the frontal, parietal, and temporal association neocortices, and of the posterior hippocampus, entorhinal cortex, basocortical amygdaloid complex, and nucleus basalis of Meynert. Third, Alzheimer's disease is familial and inherited in some families, with chromosome 21 being implicated, and Alzheimer pathology occurs routinely in older subjects with trisomy 21. Altered expression of genes on chromosome 21, due to duplication (in Down's syndrome) or mutation (possibly in Alzheimer families), can be pathogenic in Alzheimer's disease.

Neuropathology

Pathological, metabolic, and cognitive studies indicate that Alzheimer's disease is a degenerative disease which preferentially involves the phylogenetically new association regions and their newly elaborated connections in the human brain (Rapoport et al. 1986; Rapoport 1988a). Its earliest and most prominent neuropsychological feature is recent memory impairment. The first cognitive deficits to appear that are related to neocortical dysfunction are impairments of attention, abstract reasoning, language, and visuospatial abilities (Haxby et al. 1985; Haxby et al. 1986).

The phosphorylation pattern in the Alzheimer brain appears altered, due possibly to increased protein kinase activity (Saitoh and Dobkins 1986). The postmortem Alzheimer brain contains an abnormally phosphorylated microtubular protein tau (an axonal protein) in neurofibrillary tangles and neuritic plaques (Wood et al. 1986); a 68000 dalton phosphorylated protein possibly related to tau (Wolozin et al. 1986); and an abnormally phosphorylated microtubular associated protein 2, MAP-2 (Kosik et al. 1984); the postmortem Alzheimer brain displays neuritic plaques – dystrophic nerve terminals that frequently accumulate amyloid protein; intracellular deposits of neurofibrillary tangles which contain paired helical filaments that probably are derived by phosphorylation of normal neurofilaments; and granulovacuolar degeneration and Hirano bodies (Terry 1978). Neuritic plaques in a given region represent the effect of degenerative processes in distant innervating neurons or their axons, whereas neurofibrillary tangles identify local degenerating neurons.

Neurofibrillary tangles with paired helical filaments are unique to man (Selkoe et al. 1987; Kemper 1984). They are found in CA1 pyramidal cells of the hippocampus, the glomerular formation of the hippocampal gyrus, association regions of the neocortex and in nuclei of the hypothalamus, substantia nigra, locus coeruleus, reticular formation of the brain stem, and amygdaloid complex (Wisniewski 1978; Terry 1978; Wisniewski et al. 1979; Kemper 1984). Tangles are not specific to Alzheimer's disease, and occur in other chronic neurological disorders (e.g., postencephalitic Parkinson's disease, amyotrophic lateral sclerosis, dementia pugilistica, and Down's syndrome), as well as in brains of healthy elderly people.

Neuritic plaques, which frequently contain paired helical filaments, are found in normal human brain and in Down's syndrome, as well as in slow viral infections in humans – kuru and Creutzfeldt-Jakob disease, and in animals – scrapie in mice (Wisniewski 1978). Neuritic plaques, but neither neurofibrillary tangles nor paired helical filaments, have been identified in brains of senescent subhuman primates, polar bears, and dogs (Terry and Wisniewski 1972; Selkoe et al. 1987). Plaques are not found in brains of old dogs with a proven health record (Ball et al. 1983). As viral encephalitis is common in nonbarrier-reared dogs (Fox 1970), plaques in these (or other) animals may reflect prior viral infection.

In Alzheimer's disease, neuropathology is less frequent in the primary somatosensory, auditory and visual cortices, or primary motor cortex, brain stem or cerebellum, than in the more recently evolved frontal, parietal, and temporal association neocortices (Fig. 6; Brun and Gustafson 1976; Terry 1978; Ball and Nuttal 1981; Pearson et al. 1985). Severe and progressive neuron loss is evidenced by ventricular dilatation, measured with quantitative computer assisted *X*-ray tomography (Creasey et al. 1986; Luxenberg et al. 1986).

There is additional evidence of pathology in recently evolved neocortical association structures. The thickness of the temporal association cortex is not reduced (Terry et al. 1981), whereas volume and length are lessened in relation to ante mortem severity of dementia (Duyckaerts et al. 1985), suggesting drop out of association columns. The predilection of neuritic plaques for layers III and V (to a lesser extent, layers II and VI) of the association cortices (Fig. 7; Pearson et al. 1985; Rogers and Morrison 1985) corresponds to the distribution of large pyramidal cells subserving associational inputs and outputs (Goldman and Nauta 1977), many of which are lost in Alzheimer's disease. Within the visual and auditory cortices, neurofibrillary tangles are found predominantly in layers II and V of the higher order association regions (Brodmann areas 20 and 22), but are rare in the primary sensory regions (Brodmann areas 17 and 18, Table 2; Lewis et al. 1986).

Alzheimer neuropathology within the hippocampal formation is found particularly in layers II and III of the entorhinal cortex, the subiculum, the CA1 region, and the outer two-thirds of the molecular layer of the dentate gyrus of the hippocampus (Fig. 8; Ball and Nuttal 1981; Hyman et al. 1984, 1986). These areas, elaborated during recent hominid evolution (see above), connect the hippocampal formation reciprocally, directly or indirectly, with the association neocortices, as well as with the basal forebrain, thalamus, and hypothalamus, and their involvement may functionally

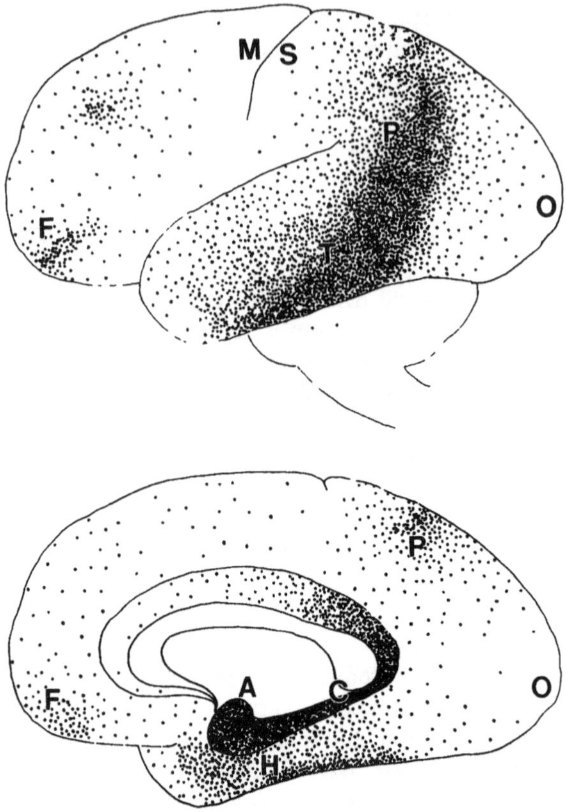

Fig. 6. Distribution and severity of senile (neuritic) plaques on lateral *(upper figure)* and medial *(lower figure)* aspects of brain in an average Alzheimer case. Association areas of parietal *(P)* and temporal (T) lobes and to some extent of frontal *(F)* cortex are affected. Amygdala *(A)*, parahippocampal gyrus *(H)*, and posterior cingulate *(C)* also are deeply affected. The occipital *(Q)*, somatosensory *(S)* and primary motor *(M)* cortices are spared. (Adapted from Brun and Gustafson 1976)

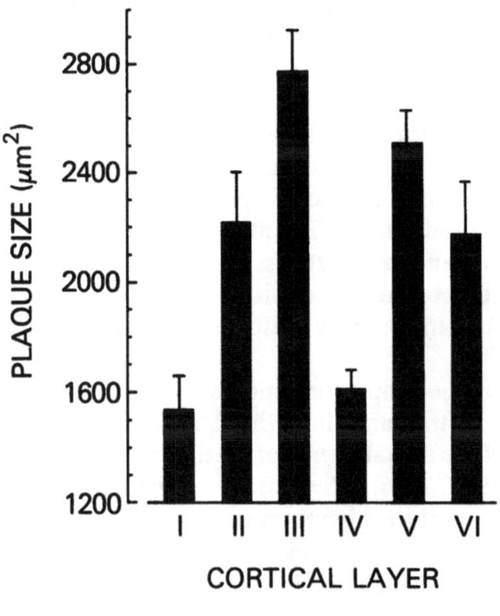

Fig. 7. Mean cross-sectional area of senile (neuritic) plaques in cortical lamina of association brain regions of Alzheimer patients. Plaques are most frequent in those layers which contain pyramidal association neurons (From Rogers and Morrison 1985)

Table 2. Neurofibrillary tangle counts in primary and secondary visual cortices from Alzheimer's disease patients. Tangles are more frequent in association (peristriate) than primary sensory (striate) areas. Data from Pearson et al. (1985)

Case no.	Tangles per field (n = 10)			
	Area 18 (peristriate)		Area 17 (striate)	
	Supragranular	Infragranular	Supragranular	Infragranlular
1	0.8 ± 2.1	0	0	0
2	0.8 ± 1.0	1.7 ± 1.2	0.1 ± 0.3	0
3	0.3 ± 0.9	0.2 ± 0.4	0	0
4	5.8 ± 3.1	4.1 ± 2.5	0.1 ± 0.3	0
5	11.3 ± 10.5	4.2 ± 2.4	0.5 ± 0.7	0.4 ± 0.9
6	11.2 ± 7.9	3.0 ± 2.3	5.3 ± 1.8	0.6 ± 0.8
7	12.4 ± 4.4	6.8 ± 2.7	1.8 ± 1.6	0.5 ± 0.7
8	24.6 ± 7.4	14.5 ± 5.6	6.7 ± 4.9	2.7 ± 2.5

Mean ± standard deviation

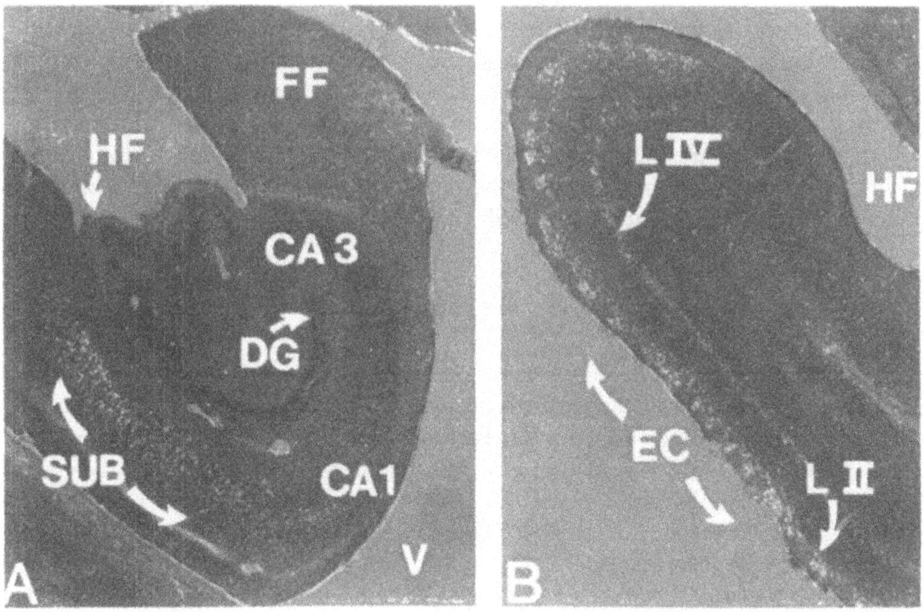

Fig. 8 A, B. Distribution of neurofibrillary tangles in the hippocampal formation in a patient with Alzheimer's disease. Congo red-stained sections in cross-polarized light show tangles as yellow red. **A** Subicular and CA1 fields contain numerous tangles that are, by comparison, sparse in adjacent CA3 and presubicular fields. **B** Tangles in laminar distribution in entorhinal cortex in layers II and IV. *CA*, cornu ammonis; *DG*, dentate gyrus; *EC*, entorhinal cortex; *FF*, fimbria-fornix; *HF*, hippocampal fissure; *L II* and *IV*, layers II and IV; *SUB*, subiculum; *V*, ventricle. Cells affected are those which regulate input and output between hippocampal formation and association and other nonhippocampal regions. (From Hyman et al. 1984)

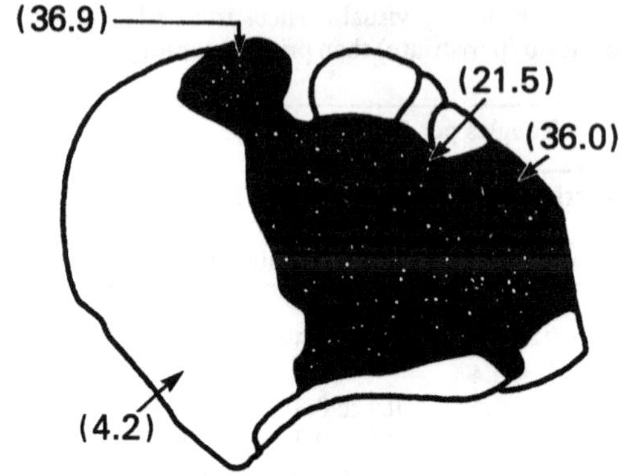

Fig. 9. Distribution of senile (neuritic) plaques in amygdaloid complex of Alzheimer patients. Numbers of plaques per square millimenter are given. Plaques are most frequent in recently elaborated basal and cortical nuclei (see Fig. 3). (From Kemper 1984)

remove the hippocampal formation from the cerebral association system (Hyman et al. 1984).

Although cell loss is greatest in the phylogenetically older medial and central nuclei of the amygdala (Herzog and Kemper 1980), neuritic plaques and neurofibrillary tangles are most plentiful in the recently elaborated small-cell basal-cortical nuclear complex, which communicates with the medial temporal association cortex (Figs 3 and 9; Jamada and Mehraein 1968; Stephan and Andy 1977; Kemper 1984). The amygdala also communicates with the nucleus basalis of Meynert, hippocampal complex, and locus coeruleus, all of which demonstrate Alzheimer neuropathology (Whitlock and Nauta 1956; Krettek and Price 1978; Kemper 1984). The nucleus basalis is depleted of large cholinergic neurons in Alzheimer's disease. These neurons normally project to the entire neocortex and to the dorsal hippocampus, and drop out asymmetrically in relation to the asymmetrical numbers of neuritic plaques in the left and right neocortices (Arendt et al. 1985; Whitehouse 1987).

Neurochemistry

The Alzheimer brain is defective in a large number of neurotransmitter markers: choline acetyltransferase (the synthesizing enzyme for acetylcholine), acetylcholinesterase (the enzyme which destroys free acetylcholine), noradrenaline, and neuropeptides (Yates et al. 1983). Receptors for nicotine, serotonin, glutamate, and somatostatin also are depleted (Whitehouse 1987). Some of the deficits can be related to the distribution of Alzheimer neuropathology.

For example, receptors for glutamate, the putative neurotransmitter in cortico-cortico association pathways and in pathways between the association neocortices and subcortical regions, are diminished in neocortical layers which contain dendrites of association neurons, and in the stratum moleculare and pyramidal cells of the CA1 region of the hippocampus and the subiculum (Fonnum et al. 1981; Greenamyre et al. 1987), regions which demonstrate Alzheimer pathology. Furthermore, reductions of acetylcholinesterase and choline acetyltransferase activities in all neocortical regions studied, primary sensory and motor as well as associative, reflect the profound loss of cholinergic neurons in the nucleus basalis of Meynert (see above; Davies 1979; Rossor et al. 1982). Somatostatin-like and neuropeptide Y immunoreactivities are depleted in most cortical regions, an exception being the postcentral primary somatosensory gyrus (Beal et al. 1986).

Metabolic Dysfunction of Association Neocortices

Metabolic and cognitive studies indicate that the association neocortices, which demonstrate neuropathology postmortem, are abnormal early and throughout the course of Alzheimer's disease. Although the brain makes up only 2% of body weight, it uses 20% of the glucose consumed by the body, primarily to maintain local electrical activity (Sokoloff 1981). Local glucose utilization can be measured in awake subjects with the method of positron emission tomography (PET).

PET studies performed on subjects at rest (eyes covered, ears plugged with cotton) demonstrate reduced glucose utilization in the parietal and temporal association cortices of mildly and moderately demented patients with Alzheimer's disease, as compared with controls, but no reductions in the sensorimotor and occipital (primary visual) regions; increased left-right metabolic differences (asymmetry) in the parietal, temporal and frontal association areas, but not the primary sensorimotor or visual areas; and fewer significant correlations, indicative of reduced coupling, between glucose metabolic rates in homologous association regions in the right and left

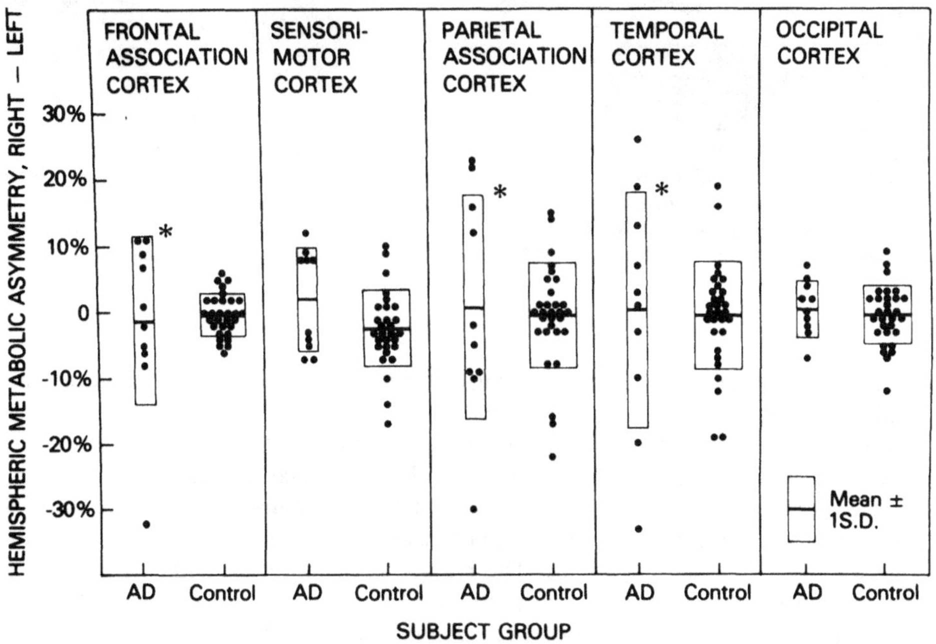

Fig. 10. Right-left differences in regional cerebral metabolic rates for glucose ($rCMR_{glc}$), normalized to mean, in five cortical regions from Alzheimer's disease (AD) patients and age-matched controls. $rCMR_{glc}$ was determined by positron emission tomography (PET). *Asterisks* indicate that variance was greater in AD patients than in controls ($P < 0.05$) in association but not in primary-sensory and motor cortices. (Data from Haxby et al. 1985)

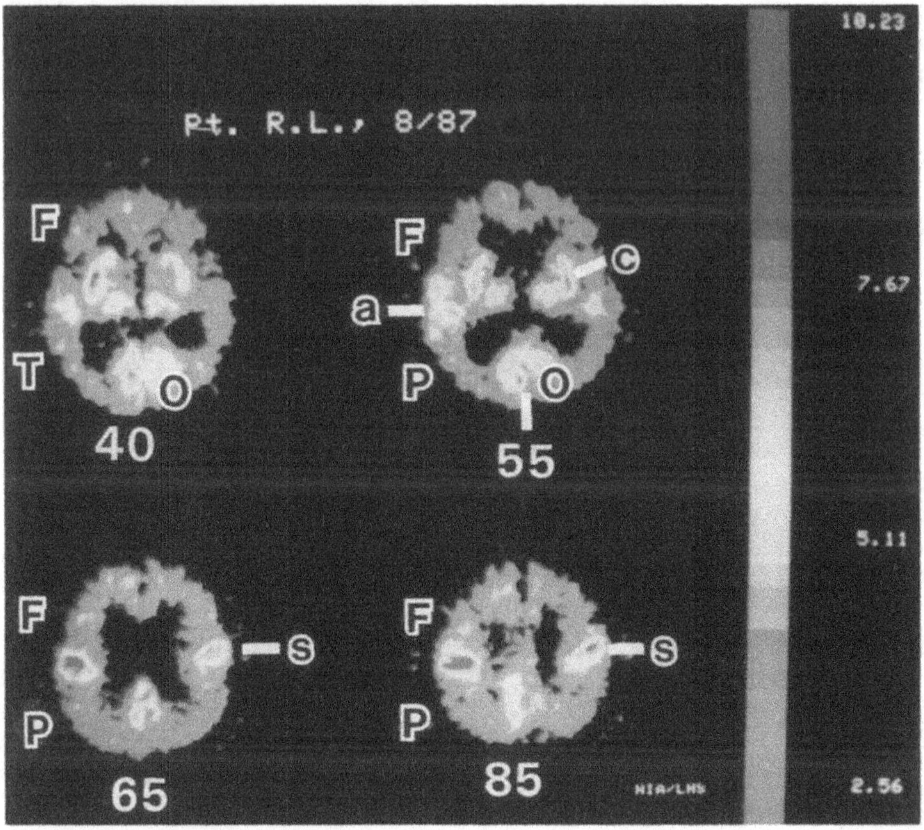

Fig. 11. Regional cerebral metabolic rates for glucose $rCMR_{glc}$, as determined with PET, in severely demented Alzheimer patient. A high metabolic rate is retained in the primary sensory-motor cortices *(s)*, the primary occipital cortex *(O)*, the auditory cortex *(a)*, and the caudate nucleus *(c)*, but is reduced elsewhere throughout the brain. *P*, parietal lobe; *F*, frontal lobe; *T*, temporal lobe; *O*, occipital lobe. (Courtesy of Laboratory of Neurosciences, National Institute on Aging)

cerebral hemispheres (Tables 3 and 4; Figs 10 and 11; Haxby et al. 1985; Duara et al. 1986; Rapoport et al. 1986; Rapoport 1988a; Horwitz et al. 1987).

Moderately demented Alzheimer patients with lower left than right hemispheric glucose metabolism have comparatively lower language than visuospatial test scores, and vice versa, as expected from the known location of language functions in association regions of the left hemisphere, and of visuospatial functions in the right hemisphere in right-handed individuals. The metabolic asymmetries and correlated language-visuospatial differences may correspond to asymmetrical and long-standing pathology of the association neocortices (Arendt et al. 1985).

Table 3. Relative metabolic rates in patients with Alzheimer's disease, in relation to severity. The metabolic ratio is the regional cerebral metabolic rate for glucose ($rCMR_{glc}$) in an association cortical region, to $rCMR_{glc}$ in a primary sensory or motor cortical region. Severity of dementia is given in terms of Folstein Minimental State Examination score – mild, 21–30; moderate, 11–20; severe, 0–10. Data from Haxby et al. (1985)

Metabolic ratio	Control (30)[a]	Mild AD (12)	Moderate AD (15)	Severe AD (8)
Parietal association / Sensorimotor	0.93 ± 0.05	0.83 ± 0.09[b]	0.85 ± 0.09[b]	0.72 ± 0.08[b]
Frontal association / Sensorimotor	0.97 ± 0.07	0.94 ± 0.06	0.92 ± 0.11	0.87 ± 0.18[b]
Lateral temporal association / Occipital	0.85 ± 0.08	0.76 ± 0.11[b]	0.77 ± 0.11[b]	0.66 ± 0.09[b]

[a] Number of subjects in parenthesis
[b] Mean ± S.D. differs from control by Bonferroni *t*-test ($P < 0.05$)
AD, Alzheimer's disease

Table 4. Significant differences in numbers of reliable partial correlations between pairs of regional cerebral metabolic rates for glucose, in mildly to moderately demented Alzheimer patients (DAT) as compared with age-matched controls. There are fewer correlations, indicative of less integrated neuronal activity, in Alzheimer patients in the parietal and frontal association areas, and between homologous left and right association areas. Data from Horwitz et al. (1987)

Brain regions	Total possible	Control	DAT
Frontal parietal	220	32	12[a]
Homologous (left-right)	28	22	14[a]

[a] Significantly different from control by χ^2 ($P < 0.05$)

Alzheimer Pathology in Down's Syndrome

Down's syndrome is a genetic disorder in which an extra portion of chromosome 21 leads to mental retardation, and frequently to dementia in middle age. Brains of Down subjects older than 40 years exhibit neuritic plaques, neurofibrillary tangles, and granulovacuolar degeneration, with the same density, chemical, and antigenic properties, and regional distributions as do brains of Alzheimer patients (Ball and Nuttal 1981; Mann et al. 1984). Layers II and III of the entorhinal cortex, and the CA1 pyramidal cell layer and subiculum of the hippocampus, are most affected, as are the association but not primary motor and sensory neocortices. As in Alzheimer's disease, cholinergic neurons are lost from the nucleus basalis of Meynert (Casanova et al. 1985). In addition, the Down brain displays decrements of the same neurotransmitter markers (choline acetyltransferase, acetylcholinesterase, somatostatin, and noradrenaline) as does the Alzheimer brain, as well as reduced dopamine (Yates et al. 1983).

Although all Down subjects older than 40 years have Alzheimer neuropathology, only about one-half of those over 40 are demented (Wisniewski et al. 1985). Quantita-

Table 5. Regional cerebral metabolic rates for glucose, measured with positron emission tomography, in association neocortices relative to primary sensorimotor regions in younger and older Down subjects and in age-matched controls. Metabolism reduced in parietal and temporal association cortices, compared with sensorimotor cortex. Data from Schapiro et al. (1986)

Metabolic ratio	*Healthy controls*		*Down syndrome*	
	< 35 YR (n = 24)	*35+ YR (n = 32)*	*< 35 YR (n = 15)*	*35+ YR (n = 7)*
Parietal/sensorimotor				
Right hemisphere	0.954 ± 0.010	0.971 ± 0.011	0.943 ± 0.009	0.868 ± 0.27[a]
Left hemisphere	0.959 ± 0.010	0.964 ± 0.010	0.930 ± 0.011	0.862 ± 0.040
Temporal/sensorimotor				
Right hemisphere	0.900 ± 0.022	0.844 ± 0.014	0.884 ± 0.023	0.787 ± 0.037
Left hemisphere	0.918 ± 0.021	0.859 ± 0.013	0.896 ± 0.020	0.766 ± 0.032[a]

Means ± S.E.
[a] Differs from mean in age-matched controls ($P < 0.05$), by Bonferroni statistics

tive computer-assisted tomography demonstrates progressive ventricular dilatation in these demented subjects over a period of about 1 year, as in older Alzheimer patients (M.B. Schapiro et al., in preparation).

PET shows abnormal glucose metabolism in the association but not sensory or motor neocortices of demented as well as nondemented middle-aged Down subjects, as in Alzheimer patients (Table 5; Schapiro et al. 1986). Right-left metabolic asymmetry is increased, and glucose utilization is reduced in the parietal and frontal association neocortices. The above observations indicate that Alzheimer-type degeneration is fundamentally the same in Down's syndrome and in Alzheimer's disease.

Pick's Disease and Alzheimer's Disease

Pick's disease, which has an age of onset between 50 and 60 years, has many clinical and pathological similarities to Alzheimer's disease (Wechsler et al. 1982; Constantinidis 1986). Like Alzheimer's disease, it occurs sporadically and within families. It is characterized by progressive dementia and aphasia, with restlessness and loss of normal inhibitions in the early stages, indicative of frontal lobe release. An initial PET study confirms metabolic dysfunction in the frontal lobes (Kamo et al. 1987).

In Pick's disease, there is dilatation of the lateral ventricles, accompanied by circumscribed atrophy of phylogenetically recent association frontal and temporal regions, but the primary motor and sensory gyri are spared, as in Alzheimer's disease (Tomlinson and Corsellis 1984). Pyramidal cells are lost from layers II, III and V of the temporal and frontal association cortices, and many remaining cells are swollen and denuded of dendritic spines, also as in Alzheimer's disease (Wechsler et al. 1982). Neuritic plaques (often without amyloid) and neurofibrillary tangles can be present (Wechsler et al. 1982). Argyrophilic Pick inclusion bodies are found in neurons of the association cerebral cortex, and within neurons of the CA1 layer of the hippocampus, of the adjacent subiculum and of the entorhinal cortex – regions also showing pathology in Alzheimer's disease (Ball 1979). These Pick bodies contain aggregates of 15 nm filaments which share antigenic determinants with abnormally phosphorylated microtubule-associated protein, tau, found also in the Alzheimer brain (Pollock et al. 1986). Together, these observations indicate that Pick's disease and Alzheimer's disease are remarkably similar in their clinical symptoms, their predilection for the association as compared with primary sensory and motor neocortices, and certain antigenic determinants.

Brain Evolution and Genomic Character Function for Alzheimer's Disease

In order to relate Alzheimer's disease to the molecular events that promoted rapid evolution of the hominid brain, let us consider genetic models that describe adaptation to a given environment by means of simultaneous adjustments of components of the species genome (Kimura 1983). The simplest of such models include a frequency distribution of individuals with a given character, which may, for example, be weight, and a "fitness" function which gives the phenotypic advantage of a numerical value for the character.

Let us define a genomic character function $B(x)$ of genes expressed in the association regions and their connections in the primate brain. Let $B(x)$ equal the sum of genes x_i, each multiplied by its number n_i in the genome, the extent of its expression e_i (between 0 and 1), and by environmental or other factors, a_i:

$$B(x) = a_1e_1n_1x_1 + a_2e_2n_2x_2 + \ldots a_ie_in_ix_i \ldots \quad (Eq.\ 1)$$

For a homozygous gene pair, $n_i = 2$. Different alleles, causing protein polymorphism, make the value of $B(x)$ distributed within a species. Because as yet many of the components of $(B(x)$ are unknown, $B(x)$ represents an additive model of gene interaction, rather than more complex nonadditive processes (Bishop 1983).

Figure 12 relates a hypothetical bimodal "fitness" function to the numerical value of $B(x)$, in chimpanzee and homo sapiens (Wilson et al. 1977); hominid evolution was accompanied by higher values of $(B(x)$. In each species, an optimal value of $B(x)$ exists which gives a maximum expected phenotypic advantage, on either side of which higher or lower values of $B(x)$ reduce "fitness." Advantage can be reduced by trisomy 21 or by gene deletions.

Liability to a phylogenetic neurological disease may appear following an evolutionary alteration in the genomic character function which determines the structure and function of brain regions in which the disease becomes manifest. To examine this liability, a "disease" function, rather than a "fitness" function, might more appropriately be related to a genomic character function.

Let us assume that liability for Alzheimer's disease is related to the value of a genomic character function $G(x)$, which depends on genes x_j multiplied by factors which were defined for Eq 1,

$$G(x) = a_1e_1n_1x_1 + a_2e_2n_2x_2 + \ldots a_je_jn_jx_j \ldots \quad (Eq.\ 2)$$

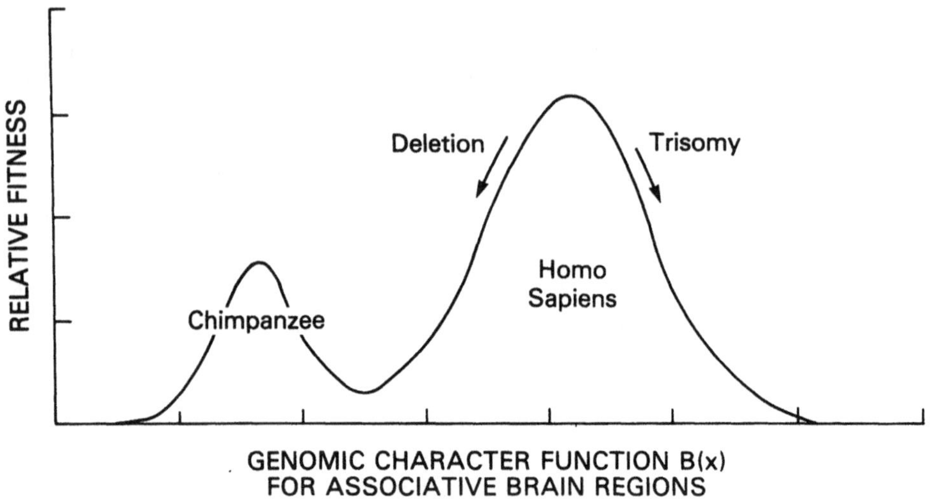

Fig. 12. Relative fitness (phenotypic competitive advantage) in relation to genomic function $B(x)$ for the association neocortices and their connections in chimpanzee and human brains. $B(x)$ given by Eq. 1 (in text), and shown in arbitrary units. (From Rapoport 1988b)

In the case of Down's syndrome, $n_j = 3$ if x_j is homozygous and is on the 21q22 region of chromosome 21 (Patterson et al. 1982). $G(x)$ probably includes some of the genes contributing to $B(x)$ in Eq. 1, in view of the specificity of Alzheimer pathology for newly evolved regions in the hominid brain. The environmental factors a_i in $G(x)$ are particularly important, as the concordance of Alzheimer's disease in homozygous twins is only about 40% (Bishop 1983; Nee et al. 1987).

Let the frequency distributions of $G(x)$ be represented by the normal probability functions illustrated in Fig. 13 (bottom), for each of five populations: I (chimpanzee), II (average human population, sporadic disease), III (humans with one first-degree relative who had Alzheimer's disease before the age of 70, familial disease), IV (humans with two first-degree relatives who had Alzheimer's disease before the age of 70, familial disease), and V (Down's syndrome subjects). As illustrated in Fig. 13 (top), the cumulative probability that subjects in each group will get Alzheimer's disease in their lifetime (up to age 90 for humans) increases in relation to the value of $G(x)$, and equals 0, 0.064, 0.23, 0.45, and 1.0 for groups I to V, respectively.

It is assumed that Alzheimer's disease does not occur in nonhuman primates, in view of the presence of neurofibrillary tangles with paired helical filaments only in the human brain (see above). The other probabilities are obtained from Heston et al. (1981), and Wiśniewski et al. (1985). In the general population, the risk of contracting Alzheimer's disease within a lifespan of 90 years is 6.4%. Having a first-degree relative (sibling or parent) who had the disease prior to age 70 increases the cumulative risk to 19%–23%. If both a sibling and parent had the disease prior to age 70, the cumulative risk becomes 45%, in the range of an autosomal dominant trait. In Down's syndrome, the risk of Alzheimer pathology is 100% after 40 years of age.

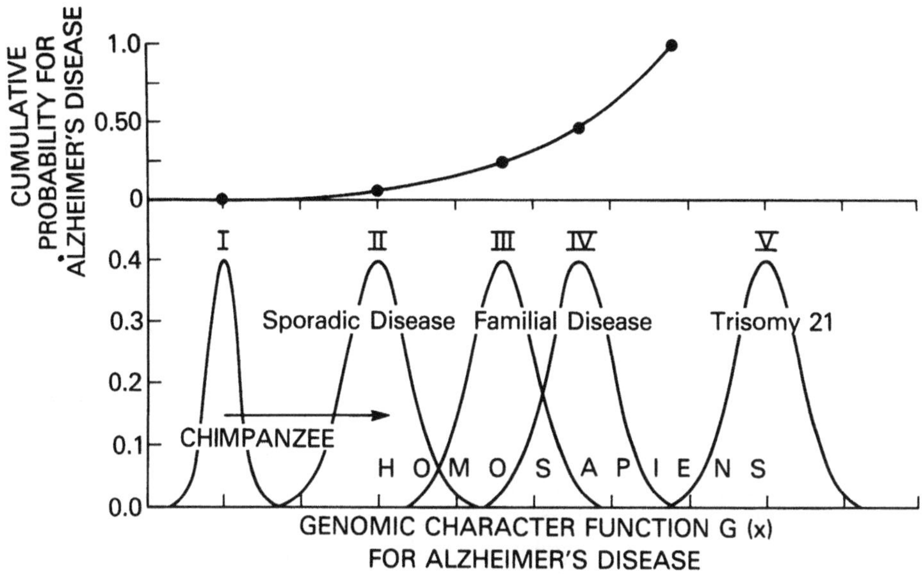

Fig. 13. Genomic character function $G(x)$ for Alzheimer's disease, in relation to hominid speciation and likelihood of developing disease in an individual lifetime. $G(x)$ (Eq. 2, text) is given in arbitrary units. *Bottom:* Normal distributions for $G(x)$ in selected species between primative chimpanzees and modern Homo sapiens. In the latter species, lower values of $G(x)$ are found in individuals likely to develop sporadic Alzheimer's disease, whereas higher values are found in individuals belonging to liable families, and highest values occur in subjects with trisomy 21. *Top:* Individual lifetime likelihoods for Alzheimer's disease as a function of $G(x)$, taken from Heston et al. (1981) (see text). Arrows indicate threshold value of $G(x)$ above which Alzheimer's disease has a finite likelihood in a lifetime.

The analysis asserts a common multifactorial pathogenesis for sporadic and familial Alzheimer's disease, and for Alzheimer pathology in Down's syndrome, related to the genomic character function $G(x)$. Evolution of the hominid brain was accompanied by an increase in the value of $G(x)$ and a finite vulnerability to Alzheimer's disease, as well as by an increased value of the genomic character function $B(x)$ for expression of newly evolved brain regions. The invariable appearance of Alzheimer pathology in adult Down's subjects suggests, furthermore, that $G(x)$ includes genes on chromosome 21. Increased expression of a gene in trisomy 21 may be similar to a regulatory mutation of the gene in early-onset Alzheimer's disease, in its effect on $G(x)$.

Additional evidence for involvement of chromosome 21 is abundant. Trisomy 21 is more frequent in families of Alzheimer probands than in the general population (Heston et al. 1981). Band 21q22 on chromosome 21, which must be trisomic for expression of the Down phenotype, contains only 50–100 genes (Patterson et al. 1982). However, a specific nucleotide sequence of DNA (restriction fragment length polymorphisms D21S1 and D21S11), located in the 21q11.2→21q21 region of chromosome 21, is linked to Alzheimer's disease in several families with mean ages of onset between 40 and 52 years (St George-Hyslop et al. 1987). This fragment is closer to the centromere of chromosome 21 than is the 21q22 fragment specific for the Down phenotype, indicating that the Alzheimer locus in Down's syndrome is distinct from the locus for retardation.

More recently, in families with mean ages of onset exceeding 60 years, linkage with the D21S1/D21S11 probes for chromosome 21 was excluded, whereas a family with an onset at 49 years demonstrated this linkage (Roses et al. 1988). Different loci for late and early onset Alzheimer's disease are consistent with a polygenic, multifactorial pathogenesis.

An amyloid polypeptide, identified in neuritic plaques and in the vasculature of the Alzheimer as well as the Down brain, has been suggested to be pathogenic in the Alzheimer process (Glenner and Wong 1984; Masters et al. 1985). The discovery that the gene coding for a brain protein which contains the 42 amino acid sequence of amyloid, as well as 57 additional amino acids, is localized at region 21q11.2→21q22.2 of chromosome 21 (Goldgaber et al. 1987; Tanzi et al. 1987), seemed to confirm the initiating role of this chromosome in Alzheimer's disease. More recently, however, it was shown that Alzheimer's disease is not tightly linked to the amyloid β-protein gene on chromosome 21, suggesting that abnormal expression of the amyloid gene is a posttranscriptional event regulated by other, more critical genes (Tanzi et al. 1987).

Conclusions

The hypothesis that Alzheimer's disease is a human phylogenetic disease is based on a number of factors. Pathological and immunological investigations show that paired helical filaments, characteristic of the disease in the postmortem brain, are not found in brains of nonhuman primates. Behavioral and functional studies in life, and pathological studies postmortem, reveal that the association system and its connections are specifically involved throughout the course of the disease, and there is evidence that genes on chromosome 21 contribute to Alzheimer pathology in some families as well as in patients with Down's syndrome.

It is argued that the association neocortices and their connections, which underwent concerted elaboration during recent hominid evolution, became vulnerable to Alzheimer pathology through the genomic processes that promoted this evolution – regulatory mutations, gene duplications, and chromosomal rearrangements. Therefore, some genes involved in brain evolution probably contribute to the genomic character function $G(x)$ for Alzheimer's disease, which increased during neocorticalization. Accordingly a better understanding of the genomic events that promoted this evolution should provide insight into the genetic basis of Alzheimer's disease, which might be related to withdrawal or abnormal transport of the morphogenetic and trophic factors which promoted "integrated phylogeny" of the association regions (Appel 1981; Creasey and Rapoport 1985).

Conversely, if Alzheimer's disease is phylogenetic, information about its genetic causes, derived perhaps with restriction fragment length polymorphisms, might elucidate the molecular basis of brain evolution. In a similar vein, Bishop (1983) has suggested that the study of retroviruses would reveal both the basis of carcinogenesis and clues to the control of normal development.

Several approaches can test the hypothesis that genes pathogenic in Alzheimer's disease were involved in the evolution of association regions in the hominid brain. Differences in gene expression, using subtraction hybridization, for example, could be looked at between association cortical regions, on the one hand, and primary sensory and motor regions, on the other; or between newly expanded and relatively static parts of the hippocampal formation or amygdaloid formation in brains from healthy subjects as well as from Alzheimer patients. To narrow the field, the 1% differences in nuclear DNA and protein amino acids between man and chimpanzee (King and Wilson 1975) might first be examined in relation to brain differences between the two species. Comparative anatomic studies might help to identify critical trophic or morphogenetic factors which changed during evolution of brain regions at risk for disease, and thereby focus the search for the factors whose withdrawal might contribute to pathology. Comparative biochemistry could elucidate differences in gene expression in the brain regions of various mammalian species, regions which display Alzheimer pathology only in man.

Having identified differences in gene expression, we then must understand how these differences account for modified brain structure and function, and vulnerability to Alzheimer's disease. We must discover how these genes interact with each other and the environment so as to produce disease only in later life.

References

Alexander GE, DeLong MR, Strick PL (1986) Parallel organization of functionally segregated circuits linking basal ganglia and cortex. Annu Rev Neurosci 9: 357–381

Appel SH (1981) A unifying hypothesis for the cause of amyotrophic lateral sclerosis, parkinsonism and Alzheimer disease. Ann Neurol 10: 499–505

Arendt T, Bigl V, Tennstedt A, Arendt A (1985) Neuronal loss in different parts of the nucleus basalis is related to neuritic plaque formation in cortical target areas in Alzheimer's disease. Neuroscience 14: 1–14

Ball MJ (1979) Topography of Pick inclusion bodies in hippocampi of demented patients. A quantitative study. J Neuropathol Exp Neurol 38: 614–620

Ball MJ, MacGregor J, Fyfe IM, Rapoport SI, London ED (1983) Paucity of morphological changes in the brains of aging Beagle dogs: further evidence that Alzheimer lesions are unique for primate central nervous system. Neurobiol Aging 4: 127–131

Ball MJ, Nuttal K (1981) Topography of neurofibrillary tangles and granulovacuoles in hippocampi of patients with Down's syndrome: quantitative comparison with normal ageing and Alzheimer's disease. Neuropathol Appl Neurobiol 7: 13–20

Beal MF, Mazurek MF, Svendsen CN, Bird ED, Martin JB (1986) Widespread reduction of somatostatin-like immunoreactivity in the cerebral cortex in Alzheimer's disease. Ann Neurol 20: 489–495

Bishop DT (1983) Multifactorial inheritance. In: Emery AEH, Rimoin DL (eds), Principles and practice of medical genetics, vol 1. Churchill Livingstone, Edinburgh, pp 111–119

Boulder Committee (1970) Embryonic vertebrate central nervous system: revised terminology. Anat Rec 166: 257–262

Braak H (1978) Pigment architecture of the human telencephalic cortex. III. Regio praesubicularis. Cell Tissue Res 190: 509–523

Brun A, Gustafson L (1976) Distribution of cerebral degeneration in Alzheimer's disease. A clinico-pathological study. Arch Psychiatr Nervenkrankh 223: 15–33

Campbell BG (1985) Humankind emerging, 4th edn. Van Nostrand Reinhold, New York

Cann RL (1987) In search of Eve. A DNA trail leads to a single African woman, 200,000 years old. Sciences Sept/Oct: 30–37

Casanova MF, Walker LC, Whitehouse PJ, Price DL (1985) Abnormalities of the nucleus basalis in Down's syndrome. Ann Neurol 18: 310–313
Constantinidis J (1986) Heredity and dementia. Gerontology 32 [Suppl 1]: 73–79
Cowan WM (1973) Neuronal death as a regulative mechanism in the control of cell number in the nervous system. In: Rockstein M (ed), Development and aging in the nervous system. Academic, New York, pp 19–41
Creasey H, Rapoport SI (1985) The aging human brain. Ann Neurol 17: 2–10
Creasey H, Schwartz M, Frederickson H, Haxby JV, Rapoport SI (1986) Quantitative computed tomography in dementia of the Alzheimer type. Neurology 36: 1563–1568
Critchley M (1953) The parietal lobes. Arnold, London
Davies P (1979) Neurotransmitter-related enzymes in senile dementia of the Alzheimer type. Brain Res 171: 319–327
De Grouchy J, Turleau C, Finaz C (1978) Chromosomal phylogeny of the primates. Annu Rev Genet 12: 289–328
Demeter S, Rosene DL, Van Hoesen GW (1985) Interhemispheric pathways of the hippocampal formation, presubiculum, and entorhinal and posterior parahippocampal cortices in the rhesus monkey: the structure and organization of the hippocampal commissures. J Comp Neurol 233: 30–47
Dolon TA, Lalande M, Wyman A, Bruns G, Latt SA (1986) Isolation of molecular probes associated with the chromosome 15 instability in the Prader-Willi syndrome. Proc Nat Acad Sci USA 83: 4408–4412
Duara R, Grady CL, Haxby J, Sundaram M, Cutler NR, Heston L, Moore A, Schlageter N, Larson S, Rapoport SI (1986) Positron emission tomography in Alzheimer's disease. Neurology 36: 879–887
Duyckaerts C, Hauw JJ, Piette F, Rainsard C, Poulain V, Berthaux P, Escourolle R (1985) Cortical atrophy in senile dementia of the Alzheimer type is mainly due to a decrease in cortical length. Acta Neuropathol (Berl) 66: 72–74
Edelman GM (1987) Neural darwinism. The theory of neuronal group selection. Basic, New York
Eldredge N, Gould J (1972) Punctuated equilibria: an alternative to phyletic gradualism. In: Schopf TJM (ed) Models in paleobiology. Freeman Cooper, San Francisco pp 82–115
Feinberg I (1982–1983) Schizophrenia: caused by a fault in programmed synaptic elimination during adolescence? J Psychiatr Res 17: 319–334
Fonnum F, Soreide A, Kvale I, Walker J, Walaas I (1981) Glutamate in cortical fibers. Adv Biochem Psychopharmacol 27: 29–41
Fox MW (1970) Central nervous system. In: Andersen AC (ed) The beagle as an experimental dog. Iowa State University Press, Ames, pp 350–373
Geschwind N (1965) Disconnexion syndromes in animals and man. Brain 88: 237–294
Glenner GG, Wong CW (1984) Alzheimer's disease and Down's syndrome: sharing of a unique cerebrovascular amyloid fibril protein. Biochem Biophys Res Comm 122: 1131–1135
Goldgaber D, Lerman MI, McBride OW, Saffiotti U, Gajdusek DC (1987) Characterization and chromosomal localization of cDNA encoding brain amyloid of Alzheimer's disease. Science 235: 877–880
Goldman PS, Nauta WJH (1977) Columnar distribution of cortico-cortical fibers in the frontal association, limbic, and motor cortex of the developing Rhesus monkey. Brain Res 122: 393–413
Goldman-Rakic PS (1984) Modular organization of prefrontal cortex. Trends Neurosc 7: 419–424
Goldman-Rakic PS, Isseroff A, Schwartz ML, Bugbee NM (1987) The neurobiology of cognitive development. In: Mussen PH (ed) Handbook of child psychology, 4th edn, vol 2. Infancy and developmental psychobiology. Wiley, New York, pp 281–344
Gorry JD (1963) Studies on the comparative anatomy of the ganglion basale of Meynert. Acta Anat 55: 51–104
Gould SJ (1977) Ontogeny and phylogeny. Harvard University Press, Cambridge
Greenamyre JT, Penney JB, D'Amato CJ, Young AB (1987) Dementia of the Alzheimer's type: changes in hippocampal L-[^{3}H] glutamate binding. J Neurochem 48: 543–551
Harris H, Hopkinson DA (1972) Average heterozygosity per locus in man: an estimate based on the incidence of enzyme polymorphisms. Ann Hum Genet 36: 9–20
Haxby JV, Duara R, Grady CL, Cutler NR, Rapoport SI (1985)Relations between neuropsychological and cerebral metabolic asymmetries in early Alzheimer's disease. J Cereb Blood Flow Metab 5: 193–200

Haxby JV, Grady CL, Duara R, Schlageter N, Berg G, Rapoport SI (1986) Neocortical metabolic abnormalities precede nonmemory cognitive deficits in early Alzheimer's-type dementia. Arch Neurol 43: 882–885

Herzog AG, Kemper TL (1980) Amygdaloid changes in aging and dementia. Arch Neurol 37: 625–629

Herzog AG, Van Hoesen G (1976) Temporal neocortical afferent connections to the amygdala in the rhesus monkey. Brain Res 115: 57–69

Heston LL, Mastri AR, Anderson VE, White J (1981) Dementia of the Alzheimer type. Clinical genetics, natural history, and associated conditions. Arch Gen Psychiatry 38: 1085–1090

Hofman MA (1983) Encephalization in hominids: evidence for the model of punctuationalism. Brain Behav Evol 22: 102–117

Hofman MA (1985) Neuronal correlates of corticalization in mammals: a theory. J Theoret Biol 112: 77–95

Holloway RL Jr (1968) Evolution of the primate brain: some aspects of quantitative relations. Brain Res 7: 121–172

Hood L, Campbell JH, Elgin SCR (1975) The organization, expression, and evolution of antibody genes and other multigene families. Annu Rev Genet 9: 305–353

Horwitz B, Grady CL, Schlageter NL, Duara R, Rapoport SI (1987) Intercorrelations of regional cerebral glucose metabolic rates in Alzheimer's disease. Brain Res 407: 294–306

Humphrey T (1972) The development of the human amygdaloid complex. In: Eleftheriou BE (ed) The neurobiology of the amygdala. Plenum Press, New York, pp 21–82

Hyman BT, Van Hoesen GW, Damasio AR, Barns CL (1984) Alzheimer's disease: cell specific pathology isolates the hippocampal formation. Science 225: 1168–1170

Hyman BT, Van Hoesen GW, Kromer LJ, Damasio AR (1986) Perforant pathway changes and the memory impairment of Alzheimer's disease. Ann Neurol 20: 472–481

Jamada M, Mehraein P (1968) Verteilungsmuster der senilen Veränderungen im Gehirn. Die Beteiligung des limbischen Systems bei hirnatrophischen Prozessen des Seniums und bei Morbus Alzheimer. Arch Psychiatr Nervenkrankh 211: 308–324

Jones KW, Prosser J, Corneo G, Ginelli E, Borrow M (1972) Satellite DNA, constitutive heterochromatin, and human evolution. In: Modern aspects of cytogenetics: constitutive heterochromatin in man. Symposia Medic Hoechst 6: 45–74

Kaas JH (1982) The segregation of function in the nervous system: why do sensory systems have so many subdivisions? Contrib Sensory Physiol 7: 201–240

Kamo H, McGeer PL, Harrop R, McGeer E, Calne DB, Martin WRW, Pate BD (1987) Positron emission tomography and histopathology in Pick's disease. Neurology 37: 439–445

Katzman R (1976) The prevalence and malignancy of Alzheimer disease: a major killer. Arch Neurol 33: 217–218

Kemper T (1984) Neuroanatomical and neuropathological changes in normal aging and in dementia. In: Albert ML (ed) Clinical neurology of aging. Oxford University Press, Oxford, pp 9–52

Kimura M (1983) The neutral theory of molecular evolution. Cambridge University Press, Cambridge

King MC, Wilson AC (1975) Evolution at two levels in humans and chimpanzees. Science 188: 107–116

Kosik KS, Duffy LK, Dowling MM, Abraham C, McCluskey A, Selkoe DJ (1984) Microtubule-associated protein 2: monoclonal antibodies demonstrate the selective incorporation of certain epitopes in Alzheimer neurofibrillary tangles. Proc Nat Acad Sci USA 81: 7941–7945

Krettek JE, Price JL (1978) A description of the amygdaloid complex in the rat and cat with observations on intra-amygdaloid axonal connections. J Comp Neurol 178: 255–280

Kromer LF (1987) Nerve growth factor treatment after brain injury prevents neuronal death. Science 235: 214–216

Large TH, Bodary SC, Clegg DO, Weskamp G, Otten U, Reichardt LF (1986) Nerve growth factor expression in the developing rat brain. Science 234: 352–355

Levitt P, Cooper V (1985) Cell surface localization of the limbic antigen: an ultrastructural immunocytochemical analysis. Soc Neurosci Abstracts 11: 1106

Lewis DA, Campell MJ, Huntley GW, Benson DL, Terry RD, Morrison JH (1986) Laminar and regional specificity of tangle and plaque distribution in Alzheimer's disease (AD): a quantitative study of visual and auditory cortices. Soc Neurosci Abstracts 12: 943

Lima-De-Faria A (1983) Molecular evolution and organization of the chromosome. Elsevier, Amsterdam
Luxenberg J, Creasey H, Haxby J, Sundaram M, Rapoport SI (1986) The rate of ventricular enlargement in dementia of the Alzheimer type (DAT) correlates with rate of neuropsychological deterioration. J Nucl Med 27: 1024
Mann DMA, Yates PO, Marchyniuk B (1984) Alzheimer's presenile dementia, senile dementia of Alzheimer type and Down's syndrome in middle age form an age related continuum of pathological changes. Neuropathol Appl Neurobiol 10: 185–207
Masters CL, Simms G, Weinmann NA, Multhaup G, McDonald BL, Beyreuther K (1985) Amyloid plaque core protein in Alzheimer disease and Down syndrome. Proc Natl Acad Sci USA 82: 4245–4259
Milner B, Petrides M (1984) Behavioural effects of frontal-lobe lesions in man. Trends Neurosci 7: 403–407
Mishkin M (1978) Memory in monkeys severely impaired by combined but not by separate removal of amygdala and hippocampus. Nature 273: 297–298
Nee LE, Eldridge R, Sunderland T, Thomas CB, Katz D, Thompson KE, Weingartner H, Weiss H, Julian C, Cohen R (1987) Dementia of the Alzheimer type: clinical and family study of 22 twin pairs. Neurology 37: 359–363
Ohno S (1970) Evolution by gene duplication. Springer, Berlin Heidelberg New York
Pandya DN, Seltzer B (1982) Association areas of the cerebral cortex. Trends Neurosci 5: 386–390
Patterson D, Jones C, Scoggin C, Miller YE, Graw S (1982) Somatic cell genetic approaches to Down's syndrome. Ann NY Acad Sci 396: 69–91
Pearson RCA, Esiri MM, Hiorns RW, Wilcock GK, Powell TPS (1985) Anatomical correlates of the distribution of the pathological changes in the neocortex in Alzheimer's disease. Proc Natl Acad Sci USA 82: 4531–4534
Pollock NJ, Mirra SS, Binder LI, Hansen LA, Wood G (1986) Filamentous aggregates in Pick's disease, progressive supranuclear palsy, and Alzheimer's disease share antigenic determinants with microtubule-associated protein, tau. Lancet II: 1211
Radinsky LB (1968) Evolution of somatic sensory specialization in otter brains. J Comp Neurol 134: 495–506
Rapoport SI (1988a) Alzheimer's disease: phylogenetic vulnerability of associative neocortex and its connections. Cold Spring Harbor, Banbury Report. Cold Spring Harbor Laboratory, New York, in press
Rapoport SI (1988b) Brain evolution and Alzheimer's disease. Rev Neurol 144: 79–90
Rapoport SI, Horwitz B, Haxby JV, Grady CL (1986) Alzheimer's disease: metabolic uncoupling of associative brain regions. Can J Neurol Sci 13: 540–545
Rogers J, Morrison JH (1985) Quantitative morphology and regional and laminar distributions of senile plaques in Alzheimer's disease. J Neurosci 5: 2801–2808
Roses AD, Pericak-Vance MA, Haynes CS, Haines JL, Gaskell PA, Yamaoka L, Hung WY, Heyman AL, Clark CM (1988) Linkage analysis in late onset familial Alzheimer's disease (AD). Ninth International Workshop on Human Gene Mapping, in press
Rossor MN, Emson PC, Iverson LL, Mountjoy CQ, Roth M, Fahrenkrug J, Rehfeld JF (1982) Neuropeptides and neurotransmitters in cerebral cortex in Alzheimer's disease. In: Corkin S, Davis KL, Growdon JH, Usdin E, Wurtman RJ (eds) Alzheimer's disease: a report of progress in research. Aging, vol 19. Raven, New York, pp 15–24
Saitoh T, Dobkins KR (1986) Increased in vitro phosphorylation of a M_r 60,000 protein in brain from patients with Alzheimer disease. Proc Natl Acad Sci USA 83: 9764–9767
Sanderson KJ (1974) Lamination of the dorsal lateral geniculate nucleus in carnivores of the weasel *(Mustelidae)*, raccoon *(Procynoidae)* and fox *(Canidae)* families. J Comp Neurol 153: 239–266
Sarnat HB, Netsky MG (1981) Evolution of the nervous system, 2nd edn. Oxford University Press, Oxford
Sawaguchi T, Kubota K (1986) A hypothesis on the primate neocortex evolution: column-multiplication hypothesis. Int J Neurosci 30: 57–64
Schapiro MB, Haxby JV, Grady CL, Rapoport SI (1986) Cerebral glucose utilization, quantitative tomography, and cognitive function in adult Down syndrome. In: Epstein CJ (ed), The neurobiology of Down syndrome. Raven, New York, pp 89–108

Selkoe DJ, Bell DS, Podlisny MB, Price DL, Cork LC (1987) Conservation of brain amyloid proteins in aged mammals and humans with Alzheimer's disease. Science 235: 873–877
Sokoloff L (1981) Localization of functional activity in the central nervous system by measurement of glucose utilization with radioactive deoxyglucose. J Cereb Blood Flow Metab 1: 7–36
Stephan H, Andy OJ (1970) The allocortex in primates. In: Noback CR, Montagna W, (eds) The primate brain, advances in primatology, vol 1. Appleton-Century-Crofts, New York, pp 109–135
Stephan H, Andy OJ (1977) Quantitative comparison of the amygdala in insectivores and primates. Acta Anat 98: 130–153
St George-Hyslop PH, Tanzi RE, Polinsky RJ, Haines JL, Nee L, Watkins PC, Myers RH, Feldman RG, Pollen D, Drachman D, Growdon J, Bruni A, Foncin J-F, Salmon D, Frommelt P, Amaducci L, Sorbi S, Piacentini S, Stewart GD, Hobbs WJ, Conneally PM, Gusella JF (1987) The genetic defect causing familial Alzheimer's disease maps on chromosome 21. Science 216: 885–890
Tanzi RE, Gusella JF, Watkins PC, Bruns GAP, St George-Hyslop P, Van Keuren ML, Patterson D, Pagan S, Kurnit DM, Neve RL (1987) Amyloid β protein gene: cDNA, mRNA distribution, and genetic linkage near the Alzheimer locus. Science 235: 880–884
Tanzi RE, St George-Hyslop PH, Haines JL, Polinsky RJ, Nee L, Foncin J-F, Neve RL, McClatchey AI, Conneally PM, Gusella JF (1987) The genetic defect in familial Alzheimer's disease is not tightly linked to the amyloid β-protein gene. Nature 329: 156–157
Terry RD (1978) Ultrastructural alterations in senile dementia. In: Katzman R, Terry RD, Bick KL, (eds) Alzheimer's disease: senile dementia and related disorders. Aging, vol 7. Raven, New York, pp 375–382
Terry RD, Peck A, Deteresa R, Schechter R, Horoupian DS (1981) Some morphometric aspects of the brain in senile dementia of the Alzheimer type. Ann Neurol 10: 184–192
Terry RD, Wisniewski HM (1972) Ultrastructure of senile dementia and of experimental analogs. In: Gaitz CM (ed) Advances in behavioral biology, vol 3. Aging and the brain. Plenum, New York
Tomlinson BE, Corsellis JAN (1984) Ageing and the dementias. In: Adams JH, Corsellis JAN, Duchen LW (eds) Greenfield's Neuropathology 4th edn. Wiley, New York, pp 950–1025
Trisler D (1982) Are molecular markers of cell position involved in the formation of neural circuits? Trends Neurosci 5: 306–310
Van Essen DC (1979) Visual areas of the mammalian cerebral cortex. Annu Rev Neurosci 2: 227–263
Van Hoesen GW (1982) The parahippocampal gyrus. New observations regarding its cortical connections in the monkey. Trends Neurosci 5: 345–350
Van Hoesen GW, Rosene DL, Mesulam M-M (1979) Subicular input from temporal cortex in the rhesus monkey. Science 205: 608–610
Wechsler AF, Verity MA, Rosenschein S, Fried I, Scheibel AB (1982) Pick's disease. A clinical, computed tomographic, and histological study with Golgi impregnation observations. Arch Neurol 39: 287–289
Whitehouse PJ (1987) Neurotransmitter receptor alterations in Alzheimer disease: a review. Alzh Dis Assoc Disord 1: 9–18
Whitlock DG, Nauta WJH (1956) Subcortical projections from the temporal neocortex in *Macaca mulatta*. J Comp Neurol 106: 183–212
Wilson AC (1985) The molecular basis of evolution. Sci Am 253: 164–173
Wilson AC, Carlson SS, White TJ (1977) Biochemical evolution. Annu Rev Biochem 46: 573–639
Wilson AC, Sarich VM, Maxson LA (1974) The importance of gene rearrangement in evolution: evidence from studies of rates of chromosomal, protein, and anatomical evolution. Proc Natl Acad Sci USA 71: 3028–3030
Wisniewski HM (1978) Possible viral etiology of neurofibrillary changes and neuritic plaques. In: Katzman R, Terry RD, Bick KL (eds) Alzheimer's disease: senile dementia and related disorders. Aging, vol 7. Raven, New York, pp 555–557
Wisniewski K, Jervis GA, Moretz RC, Wisniewski HM (1979) Alzheimer neurofibrillary tangles in diseases other than senile and presenile dementia. Ann Neurol 5: 288–294
Wísniewski KE, Wísniewski HM, Wen GY (1985) Occurrence of neuropathological changes and dementia of Alzheimer's disease in Down's syndrome. Ann Neurol 17: 278–282
Wolozin BL, Pruchnicki A, Dickson DW, Davies P (1986) A neuronal antigen in the brains of Alzheimer patients. Science 232: 648–650

Wood JB, Mirra SS, Pollock NJ, Binder LI (1986) Neurofibrillary tangles of Alzheimer's disease share antigenic determinants with the axonal microtubule-associated protein tau (τ). Proc Nat Acad Sci USA 83: 4040–4043
Yakovlev PI, Lecours A-R (1967) The myelogenetic cycles of regional maturation of the brain. In: Minkowski A (ed) Regional development of the brain in early life. Davis, Philadelphia, pp 3–70
Yates CM, Simpson J, Gordon A, Maloney AFJ, Allison Y, Ritchie IM, Urquhart A (1983) Catecholamines and cholinergic enzymes in pre-senile and senile Alzheimer-type dementia and Down's syndrome. Brain Res 280: 119–126
Yunis JJ, Sawyer JR, Dunham K (1980) The striking resemblance of high-resolution G-banded chromosomes in man and chimpanzee. Science 208: 1145–1148
Zimmer EA, Martin SL, Beverley SM, Kan Y, Wilson AC (1980) Rapid duplication and loss of genes coding for the α chains of hemoglobin. Proc Natl Acad Sci USA 77: 2158–2162

Chromosome 21, Trisomy 21, and Alzheimer's Disease

P.-M. Sinet, Z. Rahmani, J.-L. Blouin, A. Nicole, I. Ceballos, N. Creau-Goldberg, C. Turleau, J. de Grouchy, J.-L. Huret, M. Poissonnier, and *J.-M. Delabar*

Summary

Down's syndrome is defined by a characteristic phenotype, mental retardation and associated pathological manifestations such as rapid aging and Alzheimer's disease. In most cases, Down's syndrome results from the presence of an extra chromosome 21 in all cells. Genes which in triplicate participate in Down's syndrome pathology have yet to be found. Studies of partial trisomies have shown that they are in the distal part (21q21→q22) of chromosome 21. We are currently investigating several patients with most of the features of Down's syndrome but an apparently normal karyotype. Enzymes coded by chromosome 21, namely superoxide dismutase (SOD) and cystathionine beta synthase, have been assessed, as well as gene copy number for the amyloid protein precursor, the protooncogene ETS2 and various anonymous DNA sequences. Results indicate that duplication of two regions might be important in Down's syndrome pathogeny: one containing the SOD gene, the other the protooncogene ETS2.

Introduction

Down's syndrome is the most common of the congenital defects, as it afflicts one of every 700 babies. This condition is associated with phenotypic abnormalities, mental retardation, a high frequency of visceral malformations (mainly cardiopathies), cancers, and leukemia, a shortened life expectancy with premature aging, and the constant occurrence after the age of 30 of brain lesions similar to those observed in Alzheimer's disease (for review, see Sinex and Merril 1982). In most cases, Down's syndrome results from the presence in all cells of an extra chromosome 21. The consequence of chromosome 21 excess is an overexpression of the proteins which are coded by genes on chromosome 21. So far, a gene-dosage effect has been confirmed for all the proteins whose genes are on chromosome 21 (Fig. 1). One can infer from these observations that the overexpression of one (or a few) chromosome 21 gene(s) is at the root of Alzheimer's type brain pathology in Down's syndrome.

The search for genetic cause(s) of Alzheimer's disease has become the subject of intensive investigations. In early-onset (before age 60) familial forms of the disease, there is evidence that a genetic defect lies on the proximal part of the long arm of chromosome 21 (St. George-Hyslop et al. 1987). In late-onset familial Alzheimer's disease, the genetic defect does not appear to be at the same locus (see Pericak-

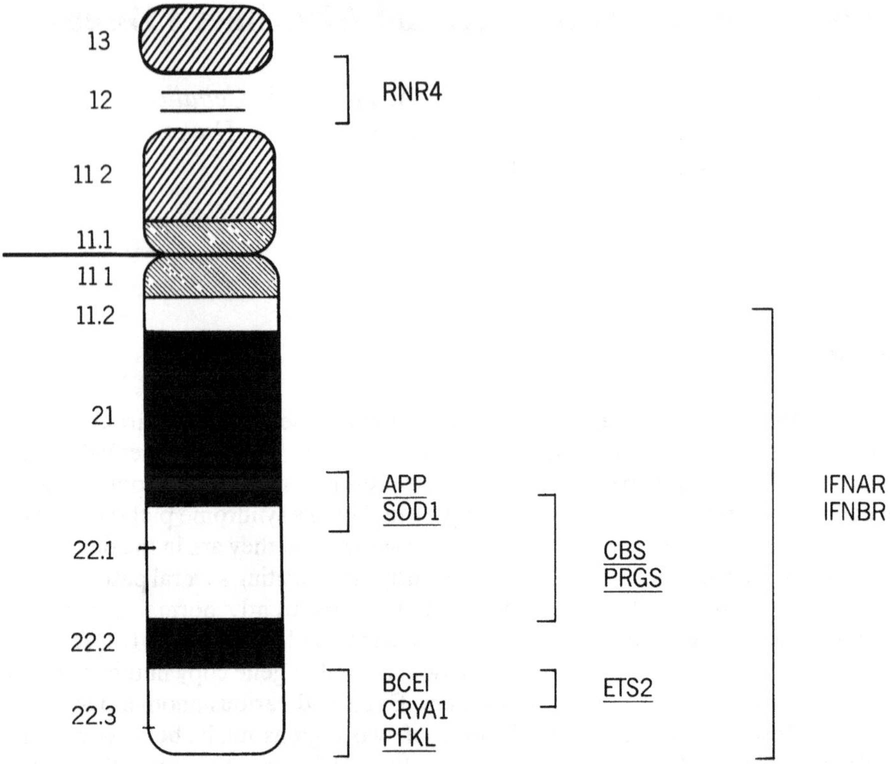

Fig. 1. Genes on chromosome 21. APP, amyloid beta (A4) precursor protein; BCEI, estrogen-inducible sequence, expressed in breast cancer; CRYA 1, crystallin, alpha A1 polypeptide; ETS2, avian erythroblastosis virus E26 (v-ets) oncogene homolog 2; INFAR, interferon-alpha, receptor for; IFNBR, interferon-beta, receptor for; PFKL, phosphofructokinase, liver type; PRGS, phosphoribosylglycinamide synthetase; RNR4, RNA, ribosomal 4; SOD1, superoxide dismutase 1, soluble

Vance, this volume). Thus, there is already some evidence that various genetic defects, i.e., different genes, might lead to brain lesions associated with Alzheimer's disease. Identifying the gene(s) involved in the pathogenesis of the Alzheimer's type brain lesions in Down's syndrome would be potentially very helpful to our understanding of Alzheimer's disease in general.

To attain this goal at least two complementary approaches are conceivable.

The first approach is to test possible pathogenic effects resulting from the overexpression of known chromosome 21 genes after their introduction in cells or animals (transgenic mice). Such an approach is presently applied with superoxide dismutase-1 (SOD-1). It has been proposed that high SOD-1 levels might harm trisomy 21 cells by causing an increased production of hydrogen peroxide H_2O_2 (Sinet 1982). Hydrogen peroxide may exert toxic actions by oxidizing sulfhydryl groups and initiating the peroxidation of unsaturated lipids. Glutathione peroxidase activity (GSHPx) that protects cells by removing peroxides is increased in red cells, fibroblasts (Sinet et al.

1979) and lymphocytes (Anneren and Epstein 1986) of Down's syndrome patients. As the gene coding for GSHPx is not on chromosome 21 but on chromosome 3, this increase might result from a regulatory response to oxidative challenges secondary to SOD-1 excess. The possibility of a relationship between SOD-1 and GSHPx increases has been investigated in cell and animal models such as transgenic mice in which extra copies of the human SOD-1 gene have been introduced. Mouse cells overexpressing the transfected human SOD-1 gene show an induction of GSHPx activity (Ceballos et al. 1988) and an enhancement of lipid peroxidation (Elroy-Stein et al. 1986), whereas transgenic mice for the same gene do not show the same phenomenon (see Epstein, this volume). This discordance between cell and transgenic mouse models requires further investigation. Enhanced lipid peroxidation is also observed in rat PC 12 cells (Elroy-Stein and Groner 1988) overexpressing human SOD-1. These SOD-1 transfected cells exhibit an impaired neurotransmitter uptake which is associated with a modification of the membrane composition of chromaffin granules. Thus, enhanced SOD-1 levels within cells might well be a cause of oxidative damage and functional impairments.

We can predict that the principle of manufacturing cell and animal models mimicking the overexpression of chromosome 21 genes will very likely provide answers to many questions regarding the pathogeny of Down's syndrome.

A second approach is to attain better knowledge of the genetic content and organization of chromosome 21 through the study of those rare patients who present clinical features of Down's syndrome without an extra chromosome 21.

The Down's syndrome phenotype has been observed in patients with partial trisomies of chromosome 21, resulting from unbalanced translocations or de novo duplications evidenced by cytogenetic analysis. From these observations, it was concluded that only the distal half of the long arm of chromosome 21, i.e., band 21q22, is involved in the pathogenesis of Down's syndrome (Aula et al. 1973; Couturier et al. 1979; Crippa et al. 1984; Habedank and Rodewald 1982; Jenkins et al. 1983; Mattei et al. 1981; Niebuhr 1974; Pfeiffer et al. 1977; Poissonnier et al. 1976; Sinet et al. 1976; Taysi et al. 1982; Williams et al. 1975).

Recent observations of patients with clinical features of Down's syndrome but no visible anomaly of the karotype suggest that duplication(s) of (a) short segment(s) of chromosome 21 might be sufficient to induce Down's syndrome phenotype (Delabar et al. 1987; Huret et al. 1987). Molecular studies on these patients should help define the size and genetic content of such duplication(s). We present here results of the study of four Down's syndrome patients with 46 chromosomes: some of these results have been previously published (Delabar et al. 1987; Huret et al. 1987).

Patients

F. G. is a patient with a visible rearrangement of one chromosome 21 that is a de novo duplication of chromosome 21 from 21q21 to 21q22.2 (Poissonnier et al. 1976). S.P. (Huret et al. 1987), E.D. (Delabar et al. 1987), and S.B. (J. de Grouchy and C. Turleau, personal observation) are patients with an apparently normal karyotype.

Enzymatic activities

Superoxide dismutase (SOD-1) and cystathionine beta synthase (CBS) are encoded by sequences located on chromosome 21 (Fig. 1) and have been shown to present a 50% increase in trisomy 21 patients (Sinet et al. 1976; Chadefaux et al. 1985). SOD-1 and CBS activity were assayed on erythrocytes and fibroblasts, respectively. When compared to normal controls SOD-1 activity was found to have increased by 40% in S. P., 40% in F. G., and 25% in E. D. CBS assay revealed an increased activity in E. D. and F. G., but no increase in S. P. The most likely explanation of these results is that three copies of the CBS gene are present in the genomes of E. D. and F. G. and that three copies of the SOD-1 gene are present in S. P., E. D., and F. G. We have tested this latter hypothesis by estimating the gene copy number for SOD-1 in the DNA of these patients. Other sequences were also quantified to further explore the possibility of microrearrangements of chromosome 21.

Gene dosage analysis

Quantification of the copy number of five chromosome 21 sequences was carried out as described previously (Delabar et al. 1987; Huret et al. 1987). Probes were human cDNAs corresponding to the amyloid beta precursor protein (APP) (Goldgaber et al. 1987), SOD-1 (Lieman-Hurwitz et al. 1982), the proto-oncogene ETS-2 (gift from D. Stehelin), the phosphofructokinase liver type (PFKL; gift from Y. Groner), and a breast cancer inducible protein BCEI (Prudhomme et al. 1985). DNA was purified from blood and fibroblasts by standard techniques, digested by Eco RI, subjected to electrophoresis in 0.8% agarose gels, blotted and successively hybridized with the different chromosome 21 probes and three reference probes encoding collagen genes COLIAI, COLIA2, COL5A2, located on chromosomes 17, 7, and 2, respectively (gift from F. Ramirez). Quantification of the DNA specific for each probe was carried out by densitometry, and the ratio between each chromosome 21 probe and reference probes provided estimates of the corresponding gene copy number. Table 1 presents the results of this analysis. APP gene copy number showed a 50% increase in patients F. G., S. B. and E. D.; the same was observed for SOD-1 and ETS-2 in S. P., E. D. and F. G. Neither PFKL nor BCEI (F. G. and S. B. not determined) was found increased in any case.

Table 1. Enzyme activities and DNA gene dosage: comparison between normal controls and Down's syndrome patients with partial duplication

	Enzyme activity				Gene dosage			
Genes	S.P.	E.D.	F.G.	S.B.	S.P.	E.D.	F.G.	S.B.
APP					=	+	+	+
SOD1	+	+	+	n.d.	+	+	+	n.d.
ETS2					+	+	+	=
CBS	=	+	+	n.d.				
PFKL	n.d.	n.d.	=	n.d.	=	=	=	=
BCEI					=	=	n.d.	n.d.

n.d., not determined; +, increase; =, no change

Discussion

Enzymatic and gene-dosage analysis of these four Down's syndrome patients without extra chromosome 21 suggest two interesting features. First, the increased SOD-1 activity found in F. G., S. P., and E. D. is compatible with a gene-dosage effect, since it is associated with three copies of the SOD-1 gene. Second, three genes are found duplicated in most cases: SOD-1, APP, and ETS2. These genes are normally located on two regions of chromosome 21 which are physically distant from each other.

In situ hybridization experiments on metaphasic chromosomes localize APP and SOD-1 at the interface between 21q21 and 21q22.1 (Delabar et al. 1987; Blanquet et al. 1987), whereas ETS2 is more distal on 21q22.2–21q22.3 (Watson et al. 1986; Blanquet et al. 1988). Moreover, linkage analysis (Watkins et al. 1987) indicates a relatively large genetic distance (20 CM) between SOD-1 and ETS2. In F. G. the duplication of APP, SOD-1, and ETS2 is compatible with the reported cytogenetic anomaly, that is a duplication of 21q21→21q22.2. In the three other patients, there are also three copies of SOD-1 and ETS2 but no modification of the karyotype. The duplication of a single fragment in which the distance between these two genes would be preserved should have been visible by cytogenetic analysis, as in F. G. The structure of the chromosome anomaly in these patients is, therefore, different from that in F. G. One can imagine that a complex rearrangement has brought together and duplicated the SOD-1 and ETS2 regions. Another possibility is that these two physically distant regions have been separately duplicated, the size of these duplications being too small to be visible by cytogenetic analysis.

In conclusion, two regions of chromosome 21 seem to have a special importance in the pathogeny of Down's syndrome: one at the interface between 21q21 and 21q22.1, where the APP and SOD-1 genes are located, and the other in 21q22.2→21q22.3, close to the ETS2 proto-oncogene. These observations also indicate that inframicroscopic duplications of chromosome 21 may cause profound developmental anomalies. Analysis of the genetic content of these duplications might enlighten our understanding of Down's syndrome and, possibly, its association with Alzheimer's disease.

References

Anneren KG, Epstein CJ (1986) Lipid peroxidation, superoxide dismutase-1 and glutathione peroxidase activities in trisomy 16 fetal mice and human trisomy 21 fibroblasts. Pediatr Res 21: 88–92

Aula P, Leisti J, Von Koskull H (1973) Patrial trisomy 21. Clin Genet 4: 241–251

Blanquet V, Goldgaber D, Turleau C, Creau-Goldberg N, Delabar J, Sinet P-M, Roudier M, de Grouchy J (1987) The β amyloid protein (AD-AP) cDNA hybridizes in normal and Alzheimer individuals near the interface of 21q21 and q22.1. Ann Genet 30: 68–69

Blanquet V, Turleau C, Stehelin D, Créau-Goldberg N, Delabar J-M, Sinet P-M, Davous P, de Grouchy J (1988) Regional mapping of ETS2 on chromosome 21 is different in a normal individual and in an Alzheimer disease patient. Human Gene Mapping 9, Paris, 1987. Cytogenet Cell Genet 46: 583

Ceballos I, Delabar JM, Nicole A, Lynch RE, Hallewell RA, Kamoun P, Sinet PM (1988) Expression of transfected human CuZn superoxide dismutase gene in mouse L cells and NS20Y neuroblastoma cells induces enhancement of glutathione peroxidase activity. Biochem Biophys Acta 949: 58–64

Chadefaux B, Rethore MO, Raoul O, Ceballos I, Poissonnier M, Gilgenkranz S, Allard D (1985) Cystathionine beta synthase: gene dosage effect in trisomy 21. Biochem Biophys Res Commun 128: 40–44

Couturier J, Dutrillaux B, Garber P, Raoul O, Croquette MF, Fourlinnie JF, Maillard E (1979) Evidence for a correlation between late replication and autosomal gene inactivation in a familial translocation t (x:21). Hum Genet 49: 319–326

Crippa L, Ballaman J, Engel E (1984) Trisomie partielle pour le segment 21 (q11→qter) résultant d'une translocation de novo entre les chromosomes 5 et 21. Ann Genet (Paris) 27: 190–193

Delabar J-M, Sinet P-M, Chadefaux B, Nicole A, Gegonne A, Stehelin D, Creau-Goldberg N, Turleau C, de Grouchy J (1987) Submicroscopic duplication of chromosome 21 and trisomy 21 phenotype (Down's syndrome), Hum Genet 76: 225–229

Elroy-Stein O, Bernstein Y, Groner Y (1986) Overproduction of human CuZn-superoxide dismutase in transfected cells: extenuation of paraquat-mediated cytotoxicity and enhancement of lipid peroxidation. EMBO J 5: 615–622

Elroy-Stein O, Groner Y (1988) Impaired neuro-transmitter uptake in PC12 cells overexpressing human CuZn-superoxide dismutase. Implication for gene dosage effects in Down's syndrome. Cell 52: 259–267

Goldgaber D, Lerman MI, McBride OW, Saffiotti U, Gajdusek DC (1987) Characterization and chromosomal localization of a cDNA encoding brain amyoid of Alzheimer's disease. Science 235: 877–880

Habedank M, Rodewald A (1982) Moderate Down's syndrome in three siblings having partial trisomy 21q22→21qter and therefore no SOD-1 excess. Hum Genet 60: 74–77

Huret J-L, Delabar J-M, Marlhens F, Aurias A, Nicole A, Berthier M, Tanzer J, Sinet P-M (1987) Down syndrome with duplication of a region of chromosome 21 containing the CuZn superoxide dismutase gene without detectable karyotypic abnormality. Hum Genet 75: 251–257

Jenkins EC, Duncan CJ, Wright CE, Giordano FM, Wilbur L, Wisniewski K, Sklower SL, French JH, Jones C, Brown WT (1983) Atypical Down syndrome and partial trisomy 21. Clin Genet 24: 97–102

Lieman-Hurwitz J, Dafni N, Lavie V, Groner Y (1982) Human cytoplasmic superoxide dismutase cDNA clone: a probe for studying the molecular biology of Down Syndrome. Proc Natl Acad Sci USA 79: 2808–2811

Mattei JR, Mattei MG, Baeteman MA, Giraud F (1981) Trisomy 21 for the region 21q223: identification by high-resolution R banding pattern. Hum Genet 56: 409–411

Niebuhr E (1974) Down's syndrome. The possibility of a pathogenetic segment on chromosome n°21. Humangenetik 21: 99–101

Pfeiffer RA, Kessel EK, Soer KH (1977) Partial trisomies of chromosome 21 in man. Two new observations due to translocations 19:21 and 4:21. Clin Genet 11: 207–213

Poissonnier M, Saint Paul B, Dutrillaux B, Chassaigne M, Gruyer P, Blignieres-Strouk G (1976) Trisomie 21 partielle (21q21→21q22.2). Ann Genet (Paris) 19: 69–73

Prud'homme JF, Fridlansky F, Le Cunff M, Atger M, Mercier-Bodart C, Pichon MF, Milgrom E (1985) Cloning of a gene expressed in human breast cancer and regulated by estrogen in MCF-7 cells. DNA 4: 11–21

Sinet P-M (1982) Metabolism of oxygen derivatives in Down syndrome. Ann NY Acad Sci 396: 83–94

Sinet P-M, Allard D, Lejeune J, Jerome H (1976) Trisomie 21 et superoxide dismutase-1 (IPO-A). Exp Cell Res 97: 47–55

Sinet P-M, Lejeune J, Jerome H (1979) Trisomy 21 (Down's syndrome) glutathione peroxidase, hexose monophosphate shunt and I. Q. Life Sci 24: 29–34

Sinex EM, Merril CR (1982) (eds) Alzheimer's disease, Down's syndrome and aging. Ann NY Acad Sci, Vol 396

St George-Hyslop PH, Tanzi RE, Polinsky RJ, Haines JL, Nee L, Watkins PC, Myers RH, Feldman RG, Pollen D, Drachman D, Growdon J, Bruni A, Foncin J-F, Salmon D, Frommelt P, Amaducci L, Sorbi S, Piacentini S, Stewart GD, Hobbs WJ, Conneally PM, Gusella JF (1987) The genetic defect causing familial Alzheimer's disease maps on chromosome 21. Science 235: 885–890

Taysi K, Sparkes RS, O'Brien TJ, Dengler DR (1982) Down's syndrome phenotypes and autosomal gene inactivation in a child with presumed (X:21) de novo translocation. J Med Genet 19: 144–148

Watkins P, Stewart G, Tanzi RE (1987) Personnal communication

Watson DK, McWilliams-Smith MJ, Kozack C, Reeves R, Gearhart J, Nunn MF, Nash W, Fowle JR 3d, Duesberg P, Papas TS (1986) Conserved chromosomal positions of dual domains of the ets protooncogene in cats, mice and humans. Proc Natl Acad Sci USA 83: 1792–1796

Williams JD, Summut RL, Martens PR, Kimbrell RA (1975) Familial Down's syndrome due to t(10:21) translocation: evidence that the Down phenotype is related to trisomy of a specific segment of chromosome 21. Am J Hum Genet 27: 478–485

Trisomic and Transgenic Mice in the Study of the Pathogenesis of Alzheimer's Disease and Down's Syndrome

C. J. Epstein

Summary

Morphological, chemical, and metabolic data indicate that the pathological process occurring in the brains of adults with Down's syndrome (DS) is very similar to, if not indistinguishable from, that which occurs in the brains of individuals with Alzheimer's disease (AD). However, discrepancies in the frequency of dementia and possibly in the numbers and distributions of lesions suggest that the pathogenetic mechanisms operative in the two conditions are not necessarily or even likely to be identical. The critical fact that must be kept in mind when considering the effects of trisomy 21 in the causation of DS and of its phenotypic features, including AD, is that the basic problem stems from the presence of an *extra* but *normal* chromosome. Several mechanisms have been proposed to explain the relationship of this increased dosage of chromosome 21 genes to the development of AD. These mechanisms include direct injury to the nervous system as the result of increased activity of one or a few genes, as well as indirect effects brought about by abnormalities in the development of the trisomic nervous system or by increased susceptibility to injurious agents. Several model systems for studying these mechanisms have been developed: the trisomy 16 mouse, the trisomy 16 ↔ 2n mouse chimera, and, most recently, transgenic mice carrying the human CuZn-superoxide dismutase (SOD) gene. In the brains of the transgenic mice, total CuZn-SOD is increased 1.6- to 1.9-fold, but glutathione peroxidase activity and endogenous lipid peroxidation are not increased. It therefore appears that, in a normal environment, an increase in CuZn-SOD activity to the range found in DS does not by itself produce demonstrable alterations in spontaneous lipid peroxidation or in an enzyme system associated with oxygen radical metabolism.

Relationship of Alzheimer's Disease to Down's Syndrome

Since the time that a pathological relationship between Down's syndrome (DS) and Alzheimer's disease (AD) was first suspected (Struwe 1929), a large body of evidence has been accumulated to support the existence of this relationship. These data have been extensively reviewed and discussed elsewhere (Epstein 1983, 1986, 1987; Oliver and Holland 1986) and are summarized in Table 1. Taken together, the morphological, chemical, and metabolic data indicate that the pathological process occurring in the brains of adults with DS is very similar to, if not indistinguishable from, that which occurs in the brains of individuals with AD.

Table 1. Similarities between adults with Down's syndrome and individuals with Alzheimer's disease. (Modified from Epstein 1987)

Neuropathology	
	Similar qualitative and quantitative appearance and geographical distribution of granulovascular changes, senile plaques, neurofibrillary tangles, and neuronal loss (Ellis et al. 1974; Whalley and Buckton 1979; Ball and Nuttall 1980, 1981; Mann et al. 1984, 1987a, b; Wisniewski et al. 1985a, b; Ball et al. 1986; Williams and Matthysse 1986)
Neurochemistry	
	Enzymes: decreased choline acetyltransferase and acetylcholinesterase (Yates et al. 1980; Godridge et al. 1987)
	Monoamines: decreased norepinephrine, dopamine, and serotonin (5-HT) (Yates et al. 1981; Nyberg et al. 1982; Godridge et al. 1987)
	Similar/identical structure(s) of β_2 protein cerebrovascular amyloid fibrils and of amyloid plaque core proteins (Masters et al. 1985; Wong et al. 1985)
	Elevation in concentration of Alz-50 (67K) protein antigen (Wolozin et al. 1986)
Cerebral metabolism	
	Reduction in cerebral glucose metabolism from premorbid levels (de Leon et al. 1983; Foster et al. 1984; Schapiro et al. 1987)
Neuropsychology	
	Dementia in ≥ 25% of DS adults; gradual loss of intellectual functions in most or all DS adults (Thase et al. 1982, 1984; Wisniewski et al. 1985b; Schapiro et al. 1987)

The pathological lesions of AD may appear as early as the second or third decades of life in DS (Wisniewski et al. 1985b) and are virtually invariant by the fourth and fifth decades (Malamud 1972; Whalley and Buckton 1979; Wisniewski et al. 1985b). What has been perplexing and controversial, however, is the relationship between these abnormalities and the psychological and behavioral changes that take place in older individuals with DS. Although there does appear to be a gradual loss of a variety of intellectual functions in later decades, irrespective of whether dementia is actually diagnosed (Thase et al. 1982, 1984; Schapiro et al. 1987), frank dementia – as manifested by loss of skills of daily living and of vocational skills, impaired abstract thinking or judgment, disturbances of higher cortical function, and personality changes – seems to occur in only about 25% of the affected individuals with DS (Wisniewski et al. 1985b). Wisniewski and Rabe (1986) reject the notion that the absence of dementia in the majority of DS individuals with the pathology of AD indicates that the pathology and the development of psychological and behavioral changes are unrelated. Rather, they believe that the appearance of dementia, both in AD that occurs in the non-DS population and in adults with DS, is dependent on the pathological abnormalities (as measured by numbers of plaques and tangles) exceeding some threshold value, a value which, they suggest, is higher in DS than in non-DS individuals. In support of this idea, they present data, taken from the studies of Wisniewski et al. (1985b) on DS and of Blessed et al. (1968) and Wilcock and Esiri (1982) for non-DS AD, which show that demented individuals in both groups have higher densities of plaques and tangles than do nondemented individuals. These data, which are really not directly comparable, suggest that the putative threshold density of plaques and tangles for dementia is higher in DS than in the non-DS group (Wisniewski and Rabe 1986). This hypothesis would provide a convenient explanation for why only a fraction of adults with DS are clinically demented and thereby have both the pathological and clinical characteristics of AD, but why it should be so is not obvious. In fact, just the opposite might have been suspected – that a brain which is already functionally compromised should have a lower, rather than a higher, threshold for the development of dementia.

Another possible explanation for the discrepancy between the pathology and appearance of dementia may reside in the geographic location and intensity of the lesions. Similar patterns of nerve-cell loss were found to be present in DS and AD by Mann et al. (1984) and by Ball et al. (1986). In the latter study it was found that the rank order for tangles and granulovacuoles in various parts of the hippocampi of individuals with DS closely resembled the rank order in brains of individuals with AD. However, Mann et al. (1987b) have observed that, while all areas of the brain damaged in AD were also damaged in DS, the reductions in relative nerve-cell number and mean nucleolar volume were significantly less in many areas in DS. Similarly, the number of plaques in the temporal cortex was less in DS than in AD. Thus, it may still turn out that geographical distributions of lesions (at least in temporal terms) in AD and DS are not identical and that there are certain groups of neurons which are of particular importance in the development of dementia and are more affected in non-DS AD than in DS.

The reason for dwelling on the matter of the frequency of dementia in DS is that it points to what may be an important difference in pathogenesis between sporadic and familial AD, on the one hand, and the AD associated with DS, on the other. While it seems quite reasonable, particularly in light of the genetic data mentioned below, to operate from the premise that the pathogenetic mechanisms are related in the two situations, it would appear that they are probably not identical (see also Glenner 1988). Although it might even be questioned whether the term AD should actually be used with reference to DS, I think that the data summarized in Table 1 are sufficient to make this terminology legitimate.

Possible Mechanisms for the Development of Alzheimer's Disease in Down's Syndrome

The critical fact that must be kept in mind when considering the effects of trisomy 21 in the causation of DS and its phenotypic features, including AD, is that the basic problem stems from the presence of an *extra* but *normal* chromosome. Therefore, the abnormalities must be related to the presence of an extra set of normal genes rather than to genes that are in some way abnormal (Epstein 1983, 1986, 1988). A trisomy is, therefore, a disorder of gene dosage, and all available evidence indicates, not only for genes on human chromosome 21 but also for the more than 40 other human and mouse genes that have been examined, that the presence of three rather than two copies of a gene results in the synthesis of 150% of the normal amount of the gene product (Epstein 1986).

For loci on chromosome 21 gene-dosage effects have been confirmed for superoxide dismutase-1, the interferon-α/β receptor, cystathionine β-synthase, phosphofructokinase (liver type), phosphoribosylglycinamide synthetase, and leukocyte functional antigen LFA-1 – the β subunit of which is coded for by a locus on chromosome 21 (Epstein 1986; Taylor 1987).

Two major difficulties prevent us from being able to reason from knowledge of the genetic structure of chromosome 21 to an understanding of its role in the pathogenesis of AD in DS. The first is that we know the identities of only relatively few of the loci carried by chromosome 21. Moreover, we do not have sufficient information to implicate any particular region of the chromosome, and it is not even known whether the AD component of the phenotype of trisomy 21 actually resides in the chromosomal region implicated in producing the somatic phenotype of DS. In this regard it is of interest that the brain of a 73-year-old man with "typical" DS but a normal karyotype did not show any of the changes of AD (Williams and Matthysse 1986). The second major difficulty in understanding the role of trisomy 21 is that we have virtually no understanding of the pathogenesis of any feature of AD. It is hard to think of mechanisms for a process the nature of which is not really understood.

Genes on Chromosome 21

Despite these difficulties, we do know certain things about chromosome 21 that may be relevant. Perhaps of greatest interest is that two genes related to the development of AD have recently been shown to actually be present on this chromosome: FAD, a gene of unknown identity that is considered to be the cause of dominantly inherited familial Alzheimer's disease; and APP, the gene for a large putative transmembrane protein (amyloid precursor protein) which contains within its sequence the small 4200 dalton polypeptide that constitutes the β-fibrils of cerebrovascular amyloid. Although it was initially hoped that these two loci might actually be the same, it is now known that they are quite distant from one another (Van Broeckhoven et al. 1987; Tanzi et al. 1987b). Still, it is not inconceivable that they are somehow related.

Putting these two loci aside for the moment, it is possible to consider two classes of pathogenetic relationships between DS and AD (Epstein 1983; Epstein et al. 1988). The first is that the genetic imbalance in trisomy 21 (DS) directly causes AD. This could occur if increased dosage of one or more loci results in increased activities of certain gene products which, in turn, result in injury to the brain (Sinet 1982). A related proposition is that AD (unrelated to DS) is itself the result of a microduplication of chromosome 21 (Schweber 1985, 1986; Zemlan et al. 1986). The second possibility is that the genetic imbalance in trisomy 21 (DS) indirectly causes AD by enhancing susceptibility to exogenous agents that cause AD or by causing the nervous system to be intrinsically defective from early in life and therefore predisposed to degenerative changes. Although it has been suggested, I regard another proposal in this class, that DS leads to AD by causing premature aging, as being without foundation (Epstein 1983, 1986, 1987).

Microduplication of Chromosome 21

The notion that AD might be the result of a microduplication of chromosome 21 was initially strengthened by the mapping of FAD and APP to chromosome 21 and by the early reports of increased gene copy numbers for APP, SOD 1, and ETS 2 (a proto-oncogene) in the cells of individuals with AD (Delabar et al. 1987; Schweber et al. 1987). However, other investigators have been unable to confirm increased copy numbers for either APP or SOD 1 (St George-Hyslop et al. 1987; Tanzi et al. 1987a; Podlisny et al. 1987), although Schweber (1988) has presented evidence that a probe for exon V of the SOD 1 gene does detect an extra copy of this region in AD DNA. Another reason for questioning the microduplication hypothesis is that it might be expected, were such a duplication actually present in familial AD, that the time of appearance of the disease in such families, both pathologically and clinically, would resemble that found in DS. But this does not appear to be the case. For example, in the very large pedigree studied by Nee et al. (1983), the age of clinical onset ranged from 47 to 59 years – later than the onset of pathology in DS but with a much higher frequency of dementia. In fact, the dissociation between pathology and dementia in DS in itself argues against attributing AD simply to a microduplication or partial trisomy of chromosome 21. Nevertheless, all theoretical arguments aside, the claims of Schweber (1988) certainly deserve to be critically tested.

Superoxide Dismutase

Although a microduplication of chromosome 21 has not been proven to exist in AD, this does not necessarily mean that the presence of an extra copy of one or a few genes in trisomy 21 does not cause the AD associated with DS. In this regard, much has been written about the increased concentration of superoxide dismutase-1 (CuZn-superoxide dismutase, SOD-1) in trisomic cells and tissues and its potential role in the pathogenesis of both the mental retardation and AD associated with DS (Sinet 1982; Sinet et al. 1979). SOD-1 catalyzes the conversion (dismutation) of O_2- (superoxide) radicals to H_2O_2 and O_2, and H_2O_2 and O_2 can further react to form the highly reactive and injurious hydroxyl radical (OH·). Direct evidence for functional alterations in the metabolism of oxygen as a result of increased SOD-1 activity is quite limited. However, Elroy-Stein et al. (1986) have found that cells overexpressing SOD-1 by 2- to 6-fold after transfection with a cloned human SOD-1 gene are more resistant to the lethal effects of paraquat, an agent which leads to the generation of superoxide radicals. Similarly, the transfection of rat PC12 cells with the same gene has led to the appearance of transformed cells with 1.5 to 2 times normal SOD-1 activity and a reduced uptake of dopamine and norepinephrine (Elroy-Stein and Groner 1988). The latter has been attributed to a diminished pH gradient across the membranes of the chromaffin granules which is postulated to result from impairment of H^+-ATPase activity by some type of peroxidation reaction.

If increased activity of SOD-1 is injurious to the brain, it would be expected that this would manifest itself as an increase in lipid peroxidation. And, in fact, Brooksbank and Balazs (1984) did observe such an increase in brains of fetuses with trisomy 21. However, those investigators also found significant alterations in the composition of polyunsaturated fatty acids in the trisomic brains which could explain, in whole or in part, the increase in lipid peroxidation (Brooksbank et al. 1985). In studies of an animal model system, the trisomy 16 mouse fetus (see below), no increase in lipid peroxidation was found in fetal brains in which SOD-1 activity was increased 1.5-fold (Anneren and Epstein 1986). It must be concluded, therefore, that a relation between increased SOD-1 activity and the pathogenesis of AD in DS remains to be demonstrated.

Another locus certainly worthy of consideration as a candidate for being "the" causal locus of AD in DS is APP. However, at this time one can only speculate on how the presence of an extra copy of this gene could lead either to the deposition of cerebrovascular amyloid alone or to the full-blown pathology of AD.

Intrinsic Defects in the DS Nervous System

Turning to a more indirect relationship between trisomy 21 and the development of AD, one possibility worthy of further consideration is that the neurons of individuals with DS are intrinsically defective and predisposed to degenerative changes from the beginning of life. That the nervous system in DS is abnormal from early in life is obvious from the neonatal hypotonia and early onset of developmental delay and mental retardation. But is there anything different about the nervous system in DS that distinguishes it from other causes of mental retardation which are not associated with the development of AD later in life? Recent investigations have focused on decreases in neuronal density and synaptogenesis and on abnormalities of dendrites in the brains of infants and children with DS (Sylvester 1983; Ross et al. 1984; McGeer et al. 1985; Becker et al. 1986). The most detailed studies of neuronal density and synaptogenesis in the early DS brain have been carried out by Wisniewski et al. (1986). They studied 73 DS brains from individuals between birth and 14 years of age and found neuronal densities to be decreased by 10% to 50% in several areas, including the visual, parahippocampal, and visual cortices. On the basis of their observations, they concluded that there is an arrest of prenatal neurogenesis and of prenatal and postnatal synaptogenesis in DS.

None of the observations just cited proves that abnormalities of the early development of the DS brain predispose it to the degenerative changes of AD later in life. Unless accompanied by chemical or functional alterations that could compromise neuronal integrity, deficiencies in cell number should not, in themselves, lead to premature cell degeneration. However, examples of chemical and functional abnormalities in the DS nervous system have already been mentioned – for example, altered composition of polyunsaturated fatty acids in fetal DS membranes (Brooksbank et al. 1985) and abnormal electrical properties in cultured fetal DS dorsal root ganglion cells (Scott 1986, Nieminen and Rapoport 1986) – thus, it is conceivable that these derangements, superimposed on an existing deficiency of neurons, could well play a role in the development of AD.

Enhanced Susceptibility of Trisomy 16 Chimeras to Scrapie

Another possible suggestion of an indirect effect, that DS enhances the susceptibility of the brain to some exogenous agent that causes AD, suffers from the difficulty that no such exogenous agent has ever been related to the pathogenesis of AD. Nevertheless, it is of interest that trisomy 16 ↔ diploid (Ts16 ↔ 2n) mouse chimeras, which constitute an animal model for human trisomy 21/diploid mosaics (mouse chromosome 16 carrying many genes present on human chromosome 21; Cox et al. 1984), show an accelerated course in the development of scrapie (Epstein et al. 1988). When inoculated intracerebrally as weanlings with the scrapie prion, the time between inoculation and appearance of the first symptoms of scrapie was reduced by about 17 days (11%) in the Ts16 ↔ 2n chimeras. The disease then proceeded with a fulminant course, so that death occurred within 3 to 4 days, rather than in about 15 days as in the controls. Overall, therefore, the time between inoculation and death was reduced by about 30 days (18%). The Ts16 ↔ 2n chimeras do not carry any known mutations. Rather, they possess a population of brain cells, probably of the order of 40% as estimated from earlier work (Cox et al. 1984), that differs from a similar population in the control chimeras only in the presence of an extra chromosome 16. How this extra chromosome might be acting is presently a matter for conjecture, but it could be through any of a number of mechanisms involving altered neurochemical (Coyle et al. 1986), neurodevelopmental (Oster-Granite et al. 1986), or neurophysiological (Orozco et al. 1987, 1988) properties of the trisomic neurons.

Experimental Systems

The use of animal models to study the pathogenesis of AD is not a new concept, and such models have been used to investigate both toxic and infectious etiologies (Dickinson et al. 1979; Committee on Animal Models for Research on Aging 1981; Crapper-McLachlan and De Boni 1982). However, the use of an animal model to study the pathogenesis of DS is a relatively new approach, and it is worth considering whether both conditions could be studied simultaneously in a model system.

Mouse Trisomy 16

The development of trisomic mouse models for DS is based on the premise that it should be possible to study the effects of increased doses of particular human chromosome 21 genes, or sets of such genes, by using mice that are trisomic for the particular mouse chromosome or chromosomes that carry the human chromosome 21 homologous loci. Of the limited number of identified loci now known to be present on human chromosome 21, five (superoxide dismutase-1, SOD1; phosphoribosylglycinamide synthetase, PRGS; the interferon-α/β receptor, IFNRA; ETS2; and APP) have been mapped to mouse chromosome 16 (Cox et al. 1980; Francke and Taggart 1979; Lin et al. 1980; Lovett et al. 1987; Watson et al. 1986; Fig. 1). These results strongly suggest that a human chromosome 21 region of significant size has been evolutionarily conserved between man and mouse. This region is the same one to which the

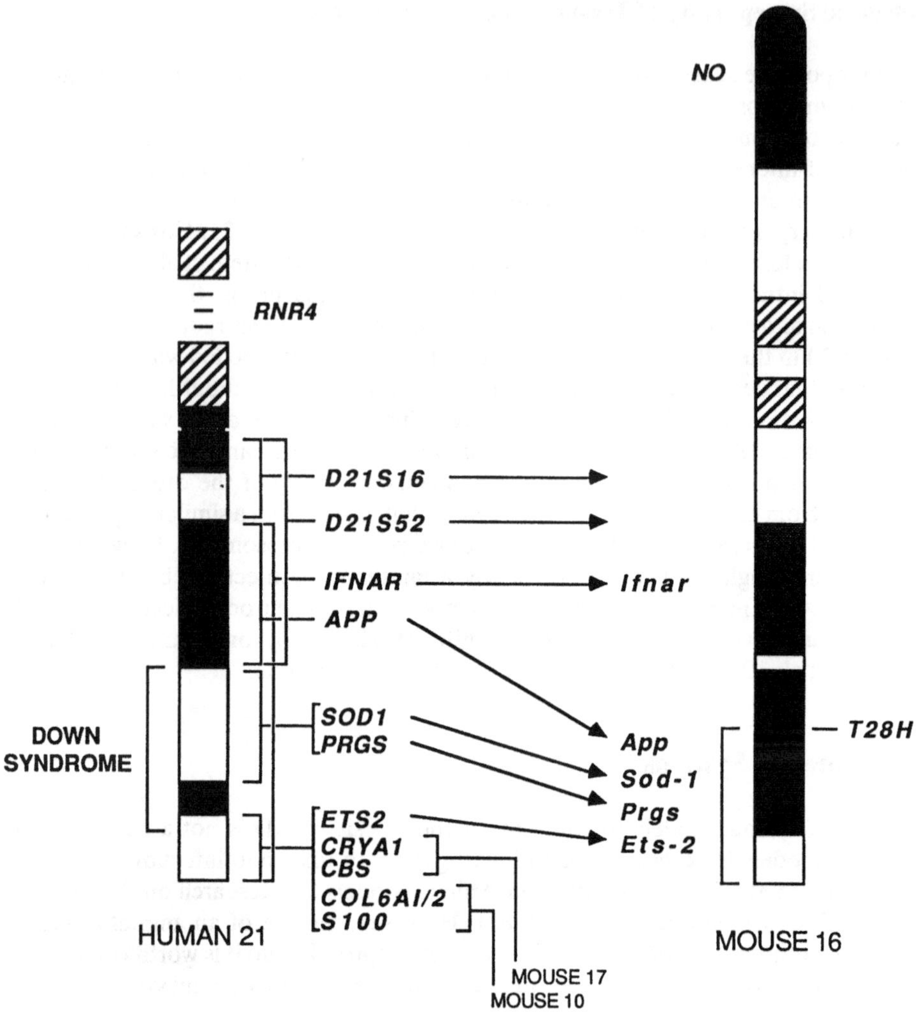

Fig. 1. Location of human chromosome 21 genes in the mouse genome

phenotype of Down's syndrome (DS) has been localized (Fig. 1). In addition, two anonymous DNA sequences, D21S16 and D21S52, which are proximal to 21q22.1, have also been mapped to mouse chromosome 16 (Cheng et al. 1987). It seems reasonable to infer that other homologous loci and sequences are also present on the two chromosomes in question and that we are dealing with many more than just the genes mapped to date.

However, not all loci in the distal part of human chromosome 21 map to mouse 16. In particular, several genes found in the distal 21q22.3 band have been found in the mouse to be on chromosome 17 (α-crystallin, CRYA1; breast cancer estrogen-inducible sequence, BCEI; cystathionine β-synthase, CBS), or on chromosome 10 (collagen α1(VI) and α2(VI), COL6A1 and COL6A2; the β subunit of brain protein S100) (Cox et al. in preparation; Cheng et al. 1987; Allore et al. 1988; Münke et al. 1988).

Neuroanatomical and neurochemical findings in mouse Ts16 are indicative of retarded brain development which leads to a reduced cortical surface, permanent deficiency of cortical neurons, and arrested development of the neurons within certain neurotransmitter systems (for review, see Coyle et al. 1986; Oster-Granite et al. 1986). Cultured dorsal root ganglion (DRG) neurons from fetal Ts16 mice have, as was noted above, a variety of specific changes in electrophysiological properties (Orozco et al. 1987, 1988) which are similar to those found in cultured human trisomy 21 fetal DRG neurons (Nieminen and Rapoport 1986).

When the brains of Ts16 mouse fetuses were assayed for SOD-1 and glutathione peroxidase (GSHPx) activities and for lipid peroxidation, the expected 1.5-fold increase in SOD-1 activity was observed. However, unlike what had been observed in human trisomic erythrocytes and lymphocytes (Sinet et al. 1975; Annerén et al. 1985) but similar to what was found in DS fetal brain (Brooksbank and Balazs 1984), GSHPx activity was not increased in trisomy 16 mouse brain. Furthermore, unlike what was observed in human fetal DS brains, in which there was a 50% increase in lipid peroxidation as measured by malonaldehyde production (Brooksbank and Balazs 1984), the level of lipid peroxidation was actually decreased in the Ts16 mouse brain. Whatever the explanation for the differences in lipid peroxidation, these results indicate that under the relatively short time span of these experiments, which are necessarily limited by the need to work with fetal animals (since Ts16 mice do not survive after birth), a 1.5-fold increase in SOD-1 activity in brain is not necessarily accompanied by either an elevation in GSHPx or by an increase in lipid peroxidation.

Transgenic Mice

In 1966, Lederberg (1966) predicted the construction of mice carrying genes from human chromosome 21, and this has been achieved through the techniques of making transgenic mice. There were two reasons for wanting to make such animals. First, as was noted with regard to the work on Ts16 mouse fetuses, the animals only live to term, a period that may be too short for observing long-term effects on the brain or other organs. Second, whether one is using Ts16 mice or Ts16 ↔ 2n chimeras, a large number of genes are unbalanced simultaneously, and it is therefore impossible to attribute definitively a particular phenotypic effect to a specific gene or set of genes. Both objections can be overcome by making transgenic animals in which the dosage of individual genes of interest is increased to the level found in the usual trisomic state.

As a model system for testing this approach and to further our studies of the effects of increased SOD-1 activity, we have prepared, in collaboration with Yoram Groner of the Weizmann Institute, Israel, transgenic mice carrying the gene for human SOD-1. This is the same cloned gene that was used for the successful in vitro transfection studies mentioned earlier (Elroy-Stein et al. 1986) and that has recently been used for the transfection of rat PC12 pheochromocytoma cells (Elroy-Stein and Groner 1988).

To date, five lines of transgenic mice carrying between 1 and 12 copies of the human SOD-1 gene have been developed in San Francisco (Epstein et al. 1987), and their properties are shown in Table 2. (An additional four lines have been prepared in

Table 2. Properties of human SOD-1 (Cu/Zn-SOD) transgenic mice

Transgenic strain	Integrated copies of SOD-1 gene (n)	Ratio (transgenic/control) of specific activities of total SOD-1	
		Brain	Erythrocytes
TgHS/SF-155	1	1.6	1.7
TgHS/SF-218	8	1.8	1.7
TgHS/SF-229	12	1.9	2.0
TgHS/SF-242	3		(1.1)[a]
TgHS/SF-287	1		(1.2)[a]

[a] Single sets of assays

Israel.) All strains of transgenics are phenotypically normal, and the founders have lived to over 1 year of age without developing any obvious neurological problems. It is apparent from the data in Table 2 that expression of the human enzyme is not proportional to gene copy number in either brain or erythrocytes. Furthermore, when several other tissues are examined, the relative expressions of the transgene(s) and the endogenous mouse SOD-1 gene are not constant. In general, expression of the transgene is highest in brain and erythrocytes, and it tends to be lowest in the liver.

As was the case in the Ts16 mice, the elevation of SOD-1 activity in the transgenic animals does not appear to cause a significant increase in the activity of GSHPx in red cells and brain. Similarly, endogenous lipid peroxidation does not appear to be increased. These results, combined with those on Ts16 mouse fetuses cited earlier, indicate that increased GSHPx activity found in human Ts21 cells may not necessarily be a direct consequence of increased SOD-1 activity. The same may also be the case for lipid peroxidation, although it should be noted that Elroy-Stein and Groner (1988) did observe a 1.65-fold increase in lipid peroxidation in their transformed PC12 cells.

Preliminary investigations using paraquat in vivo to induce the intracellular generation of superoxide radicals have not revealed any differences in response between transgenic and control animals insofar as SOD-1 and GSHPx activities and lipid peroxide concentrations are concerned. However, since paraquat probably does not cross the blood-brain barrier, no effects would be expected to occur in brain. Experiments examining the effects of hypoxia and hyperoxia in vivo on the brain and other tissues of transgenic mice are currently in progress.

The transgenic approach to making models for human DS is, of course, applicable to any gene of interest that has been cloned. Insofar as specific human chromosome 21 loci are concerned, work to date has concentrated on SOD-1, since this is the first human chromosome 21 gene that has been fully cloned and hypotheses concerning the potential effects of elevated SOD-1 activity already existed. However, there is no compelling reason to believe at this time that SOD-1 is necessarily involved in the pathogenesis of AD, and it will therefore be of interest to develop and examine strains of transgenic mice incorporating other known human chromosome 21 genes, such as that for the amyloid β-protein, or even larger genomic segments. Accordingly, work is now being carried out in several laboratories to make transgenic animals carrying extra copies of the gene, APP, for the amyloid β-protein precursor. In this work the questions are, of course, whether the presence of increased amounts of the amyloid precursor is in itself sufficient to lead to the deposition of cerebrovascular amyloid and, if so, whether this deposition results in the other pathological changes characteristic of AD. And, if excess APP itself is not sufficient to cause AD, what about increased APP and SOD-1?

The search may be a long one, but ultimately it should be possible, by increasing the expression in the mouse of the appropriate regions of human chromosome 21 (or of the homologous mouse chromosome[s]), to simulate the pathogenesis of AD in a model system. If that can be accomplished, then the question of how to prevent it can then be posed.

Acknowledgment. This work was supported by grand HD-17001 from the National Institute of Child Health and Human Development, grants from the Hurd Foundation and the Weingart Foundation, and a gift from Clipped Wings (United Airlines Stewardess Alumnae)

References

Allore R, O'Hanlon D, Price R, Neilson K, Willard HF, Cox DR, Marks A, Dunn RJ (1988) Gene encoding the β subunit of S100 protein is on chromosome 21: implications for Down syndrome. Science 239: 1311–1313

Annerén KG, Epstein CJ (1986) Lipid peroxidation and superoxide dismutase-1 and glutathione peroxidase activities in trisomy 16 fetal mice and human trisomy 21 fibroblasts. Pediatr Res 21: 88–92

Annerén G, Edgvist LE, Gebre-Medhin M, Gustavson KH (1985) Glutathione peroxidase activity in erythrocytes in Down's syndrome. Abnormal variation in relation to age and sex through childhood and adolescence. Trisomy 21 1: 9–17

Ball MJ, Nuttall K (1980) Neurofibrillary tangles, granulovacuolar degeneration, and neuron loss in Down syndrome: quantitative comparison with Alzheimer dementia. Ann Neurol 7: 462–465

Ball MJ, Nuttall K (1981) Topography of neurofibrillary tangles and granulovacuoles in hippocampi of patients with Down's syndrome: quantitative comparison with normal aging and Alzheimer's disease. Neuropathol Appl Neurobiol 7: 13–20

Ball MJ, Schapiro MB, Rapoport SI (1986) Neuropathological relationships between Down syndrome and senile dementia Alzheimer type. In: Epstein CJ (ed), The neurobiology of Down syndrome. Raven, New York, pp 45–58

Becker LE, Armstrong DL, Chan F (1986) Dendritic atrophy in children with Down's syndrome. Ann Neurol 20: 520–526

Blessed G, Tomlinson BE, Roth M (1968) The association between quantitative measures of dementia and senile changes in the cerebral grey matter of elderly subjects. Br J Psychiatry 114: 797–817

Brooksbank BWL, Balazs R (1984) Superoxide dismutase, glutathione peroxidase and lipoperoxidation in Down's syndrome fetal brain. Dev Brain Res 16: 37–44

Brooksbank BWL, Martinez M, Balacz R (1985) Altered composition of polyunsaturated fatty acyl groups in phosphoglycerides of Down's syndrome fetal brain. J Neurochem 44: 869–874

Cheng SV, Nadeau JH, Tanzi RE, Watkins PC, Sacchi N, Neve RL, Gusella JF (1987) Synteny in man and mouse of DNA markers from the chromosomal region linked to familial Alzheimer's disease and Down syndrome. Am J Hum Genet 41: A161

Committee on Animal Models for Research on Aging (1981) Mammalian models for research on aging. National Academy Press, Washington DC, pp 291–307

Cox DR, Epstein LB, Epstein CJ (1980) Genes coding for sensitivity to interferon *(IfRec)* and soluble superoxide dismutase *(SOD-1)* are linked in mouse and man and map to chromosome 16. Proc Natl Acad Sci USA 77: 2168–2172

Cox DR, Smith SA, Epstein LB, Epstein CJ (1984) Mouse trisomy 16 as an animal model of human trisomy 21 (Down syndrome): formation of viable trisomy 16 ↔ diploid mouse chimeras. Dev Biol 101: 416–424

Coyle JT, Gearhart JD, Oster-Granite ML, Singer HS, Moran TH (1986) Brain neurotransmitters: implications for Down syndrome from studies of mouse trisomy 16. In Epstein CJ (ed), The neurobiology of Down syndrome. Raven, New York, pp 153–169

Crapper-McLachlan DR, DeBoni U (1982) Models for the study of pathological neural aging. Aging 18: 61–71

Delabar J-M, Goldgaber D, Lamour Y, Nicole A, Huret J-L, de Grouchy J, Brown P, Gadjusek DC, Sinet P.-M (1987) β Amyloid gene duplication in Alzheimer's disease and karyotypically normal Down syndrome. Science 235: 1390–1392

de Leon MJ, Ferris SH, George AE, Reisberg B, Christman DR, Kricheff II, Wolf AP (1983) Computed tomography and positron emission transaxial tomography evaluations of normal aging and Alzheimer's disease. J Cereb Blood Flow Metab 3: 391–394

Dickinson AG, Fraser H, Bruce M (1979) Animal models for the dementias. In: Glen AIM, Whalley LJ (eds) Alzheimer's disease. Early recognition of potentially reversible deficits. Churchill Livingstone, Edinburgh, pp 42–45

Ellis WG, McCulloch JR, Corley CL (1974) Presenile dementia in Down's syndrome. Ultrastructural identity with Alzheimer's disease. Neurology 24: 101–106

Elroy-Stein O, Groner Y (1988) Impaired neurotransmitter uptake in PC12 cells overexpressing human Cu/Zn-superoxide dismutase – implication for gene dosage effects in Down syndrome. Cell 52: 259–267

Elroy-Stein O, Bernstein Y, Groner Y (1986) Overproduction of human Cu/Zn-superoxide dismutase in transfected cells: extenuation of paraquat-mediated cytotoxicity and enhancement of lipid peroxidation. EMBO J 5: 615–622

Epstein CJ (1983) Down's syndrome and Alzheimer's disease, implications and approaches. In: Katzman R (ed) Banbury report 15, Biological aspects of Alzheimer's disease. Cold Spring Harbor Laboratory, Cold Spring Harbor, pp 169–182

Epstein CJ (1986) Consequences of chromosome imbalance. Principles, mechanisms, and models. Cambridge University Press, New York

Epstein CJ (1987) Down syndrome and Alzheimer disease. What is the relationship? In: Glenner GG, Wurtman RJ (eds) Advancing frontiers in Alzheimer's disease research. University of Texas Press, Austin, pp 155–173

Epstein CJ (1988) Mechanisms of the effects of aneuploidy in mammals. Annu Rev Genet (in press)

Epstein CJ, Avraham KB, Lovett M, Smith S, Elroy-Stein O, Rotman G, Bry C, Groner Y (1987) Transgenic mice with increased Cu/Zn-superoxide dismutase activity: animal model of dosage effects in Down syndrome. Proc Natl Acad Sci USA 84: 8044–8048

Epstein CJ, Anneren KG, Foster D, Groner Y, Prusiner SB, Smith SA (1988) Pathogenetic relationships between Down syndrome and Alzheimer disease: studies with animal models. In: Banbury report 27: Molecular neuropathology of aging. Cold Spring Harbor Laboratory, Cold Spring Harbor, pp 339–355

Foster NL, Chase TN, Mansi L, Brooks R, Fedio P, Patronas NJ, DiChiro G (1984) Cortical abnormalities in Alzheimer's disease. Ann Neurol 16: 649–654

Francke U, Taggart RT (1979) Assignment of the gene for cytoplasmic superoxide dismutase (SOD-1) to a region of the chromosome 16 and of Hprt to a region of the X chromosome in the mouse. Proc Natl Acad Sci USA 76: 5230–5233

Glenner GG (1988) Alzheimer's disease, its proteins and genes. Cell 52: 307–308

Godridge H, Reynolds GP, Czudek C, Calcutt NA, Benton M (1987) Alzheimer-like neurotransmitter deficits in adult Down's syndrome brain tissue. J Neurol Neurosurg Psychiatry 50: 775–778

Lederberg J (1966) Experimental genetics and human evolution. Bull Atomic Sci 22 (8): 4–11

Lin P-F, Slate DL, Lawyer FC, Ruddle FH (1980) Assignment of the murine interferon sensitivity and cytoplasmic superoxide dismutase genes to chromosome 16. Science 209: 285–287

Lovett M, Goldgaber D, Ashley P, Cox DR, Gajdusek DC, Epstein CJ (1987) The mouse homolog of the human amyloid β protein (AD–AP) gene is located on the distal end of mouse chromosome 16: further extension of the homology between human chromosome 21 and mouse chromosome 16. Biochem Biophys Res Commun 144: 1069–1075

Malamud N (1972) Neuropathology of organic brain syndromes associated with aging. In: Gaitz CM (ed) Aging and the brain. Plenum, New York, pp 63–87

Mann DMA, Yates PO, Marcyniuk B (1984) Alzheimer's presenile dementia, senile dementia of Alzheimer type and Down's syndrome in middle age form: an age related continuum of pathologic changes. Neuropathol Appl Neurobiol 10: 185–207

Mann DMA, Yates PO, Marcyniuk B (1987a) Dopaminergic neurotransmitter systems in Alzheimer's disease and in Down's syndrome at middle age. J Neurol Neurosurg Psychiatry 50: 341–344

Mann DMA, Yater PO, Marcyniuk B, Ravindra CR (1987b) Loss of neurons from cortical and subcortical areas in Down's syndrome patients at middle age. Quantitative comparisons with younger Down's patients and patients with Alzheimer's disease. J Neurol Sci 80: 79–89

Masters CL, Sims G, Weinman NA, Multhaup G, McDonald BL, Beyreuther K (1985) Amyloid plaque core protein in Alzheimer disease and Down syndrome. Proc Natl Acad Sci USA 82: 4245–4249

McGeer EG, Norman M, Boyes B, O'Kusky J, Suzuki J, McGeer PL (1985) Acetylcholine and aromatic amine systems in postmortem brain of an infant with Down's syndrome. Exp Neurol 87: 557–570

Münke M, Kraus JP, Ohura T, Francke U (1988) The gene for cystathionine β-synthase *(CBS)* maps to the subtelomeric region on human chromosome 21q and to proximal mouse chromosome 17. Am J Hum Genet 42: 550–559

Nee LE, Polinsky RJ, Eldridge R, Weingartner H, Smallberg S, Ebert M (1983) A family with histologically confirmed Alzheimer's disease. Arch Neurol 40: 203–208

Nieminen K, Rapoport SI (1986) Electrical membrane properties of cultured fetal dorsal root ganglia neurons from normal human and Down's syndrome. Soc Neurosci Abstracts 12: 1360

Nyberg P, Carlsson A, Winblad B (1982) Brain monoamines in cases with Down's syndrome with and without dementia. J Neural Transm 55: 289–299

Oliver C, Holland AJ (1986) Down's syndrome and Alzheimer's disease: a review. Psychol Med 16: 307–322

Orozco CB, Smith SA, Epstein CJ, Rapoport SI (1987) Electrophysiological properties of cultured dorsal root ganglion and spinal cord neurons of normal and trisomy 16 fetal mice. Dev Brain Res 32: 111–122

Orozco CB, Epstein CJ, Rapoport SI (1988) Voltage-activated sodium conductances in cultured normal and trisomy 16 dorsal root ganglion neurons from the fetal mouse. Dev Brain Res 38: 265–274

Oster-Granite ML, Gearhart JD, Reeves RH (1986) Neurobiological consequences of trisomy 16 in mice. In: Epstein CJ (ed) The neurobiology of Down syndrome. Raven, New York, pp 137–151

Podlisny MB, Lee G, Selkoe DJ (1987) Gene dosage of the amyloid β precursor protein in Alzheimer's disease. Science 238: 669–671

Ross MH, Galaburda AM, Kemper TL (1984) Down's syndrome: is there a decreased population of neurons? Neurology 34: 909–916

Schapiro MB, Haxby JV, Grady CL, Duara R, Schlageter NL, White B, Moore A, Sundaram M, Larson SM, Rapoport SI (1987) Decline in cerebral glucose utilization and cognitive function with aging in Down's syndrome. J Neurol Neurosurg Psychiatry 50: 766–774

Schweber M (1985) A possible unitary genetic hypothesis for Alzheimer's disease and Down syndrome. Ann NY Acad Sci 450: 223–238

Schweber M (1986) Unitary genetic hypothesis for Down syndrome and Alzheimer's disease. Am J Hum Genet 39: A100

Schweber M (1988) Down syndrome and the measurement of chromosome 21 DNA amounts in Alzheimer's disease. In: Blass J, Miner G, Miner L, Richter R, Valentine J (eds) Familial Alzheimer's disease: molecular genetics, clinical prospects and societal issues. Dekker, New York

Schweber M, Tuson C, Shiloh R, Ben-Neriah Z (1987) Triplication of chromosome 21 material in Alzheimer's disease. Neurology [Suppl 1] 37: 222

Scott BS (1986) Electrophysiological studies of Down syndrome nervous tissue in vitro. In: Epstein CJ (ed) The neurobiology of Down syndrome. Raven, New York, pp 121–135

Sinet P-M (1982) Metabolism of oxygen derivatives in Down syndrome. Ann NY Acad Sci 396: 83–94

Sinet P-M, Lejeune J, Jerome H (1979) Trisomy 21 (Down syndrome). Glutathione peroxidase, hexosemonophosphate shunt and IQ. Life Sci 24: 29–34

Sinet P-M, Michelson AM, Bazin A, Lejeune J, Jerome H (1975) Increase in glutathione peroxidase activity in erythrocytes from trisomy 21 subjects. Biochem Biophys Res Comm 67: 910–915

St George-Hyslop PH, Tanzi RE, Polinsky RJ, Neve RL, Pollen D, Drachman D, Growdon J, Cupples LA, Nee L, Myers RH, O'Sullivan D, Watkins PC, Amos JA, Deutsch CK, Bodfish JW, Kinsbourne M, Feldman RG, Bruni A, Amaducci L, Foncin J-F, Gusella JF (1987) Absence of duplication of chromosome 21 genes in familial and sporadic Alzheimer's disease. Science 238: 664–666

Struwe F (1929) Histopathologische Untersuchungen über Entstehung und Wesen der Senilen Plaques. Z Neurol Psychiatr 122: 291–307

Sylvester PE (1983) The hippocampus in Down's syndrome. J Ment Defic Res 27: 227–236

Tanzi RE, Bird ED, Latt SA, Neve RL (1987 a) The amyloid β protein gene is not duplicated in brains from patients with Alzheimer's disease. Science 238: 666–669

Tanzi RE, St George-Hyslop PH, Haines JL, Polinsky RJ, Nee L, Foncin J-F, Neve RL, McClatchey AJ, Conneally PM, Gusella JF (1987 b) The genetic defect in familial Alzheimer's disease is not tightly linked to the amyloid β-protein gene. Nature 329: 156–157

Taylor GM (1987) Altered expression of lymphocyte functional antigen in Down syndrome. Immunol Today 8: 366–369

Thase ME, Liss L, Smeltzer D, Maloon J (1982) Clinical evaluation of dementia in Down's syndrome. J Ment Defic Res 26: 239–244

Thase ME, Tigner R, Smeltzer DJ, Liss L (1984) Age-related neuropsychological deficits in Down's syndrome. Biol Psychiatr 19: 571–585

Van Broeckhoven C, Genthe AM, Vandenberghe A, Horstheinke B, Backhovens H, Raeymaekers P, Van Hul W, Wehnert A, Gheuens J, Cras P, Bruyland M, Martin JJ, Salbaum M, Multhaup G, Masters CL, Beyreuther K, Gurling, HMD, Mullan MJ, Holland A, Barton A, Irving N, Williamson R, Richards SJ, Hardy JA (1987) Failure of familial Alzheimer's disease to segregate with A4-amyloid gene in several European families. Nature 329: 153–155

Watson DK, McWilliams-Smith MJ, Kozak C, Reeves R, Gearhart J, Nunn MF, Nash W, Fowle JR, III, Duesberg P, Pappas TS, O'Brien SJ (1986) Conserved chromosomal positions of dual domains of the *ets* protooncogene in cats, mice, and humans. Proc Natl Acad Sci USA 83: 1792–1796

Whalley LB, Buckton KE (1979) Genetic factors in Alzheimer's disease. In: Glen AIM and Whalley LJ (eds) Alzheimer's disease. Early recognition of potentially reversible defects. Churchill Livingstone, Edinburgh, pp 36–41

Wilcock GK, Esiri MM (1982) Plaques, tangles, and dementia. A quantitative study. J Neurol Sci 56: 343–356

Williams RS, Matthysse S (1986) Age-related changes in Down syndrome brain and the cellular pathology of Alzheimer disease. Prog Brain Res 70: 49–67

Wisniewski HM, Rabe A (1986) Discrepancy between Alzheimer-type neuropathology and dementia in people with Down syndrome. Ann NY Acad Sci 477: 247–260

Wisniewski KE, Dalton AJ, Crapper McLachlan DR, Wen GY, Wisniewski HM (1985 a) Alzheimer's disease in Down's syndrome: clinicopathologic studies. Neurology 35: 957–961

Wisniewski KE, Wisniewski HM, Wen GY (1985 b) Occurrence of neuropathological changes and dementia of Alzheimer's disease in Down's syndrome. Ann Neurol 17: 278–282

Wisniewski K, Laure-Kamionowska M, Connell F, Wen GY (1986) Neuronal density and synaptogenesis in the postnatal stage of brain maturation in Down syndrome. In: Epstein CJ (ed) The neurobiology of Down syndrome. Raven, New York, pp 29–44

Wolozin BL, Pruchnicki A, Dickson DW, Davies P (1986) A neuronal antigen in the brains of Alzheimer's patients. Science 232: 648–650

Wong CW, Quaranta V, Glenner GG (1985) Neuritic plaques and cerebrovascular amyloid in Alzheimer disease are antigenically related. Proc Natl Acad Sci USA 82: 8729–8732

Yates CM, Simpson J, Maloney AJF, Gordon A, Reid AH (1980) Alzheimer-like cholinergic deficiency in Down syndrome. Lancet II: 979

Yates CM, Ritchie IM, Simpson J, Maloney AJ, Gordon A (1981) Noradrenaline in Alzheimer-type dementia and Down syndrome. Lancet II: 39–40

Zemlan FP, Thienhaus OJ, Bosmann HB (1986) Increased chromosome 21q22.1 marker in Alzheimer's disease and Down's syndrome. Soc Neurosci Abstr 12: 1314

Molecular Genetic Strategies in Familial Alzheimer's Disease: Theoretical and Practical Considerations

P. H. St George-Hyslop, L. Farrer, J. Haines, R. Myers, R. Polinsky, L. Nee, A. Bruni, S. Scorbi, S. Piacentini, L. Amaducci, J.-F. Foncin, R. G. Feldman, P. Frommelt, P. Watkins, R. Tanzi, J. Aalbo, J. Growdon, D. Drachman, D. Pollen, P. M. Conneally, and *J. Gusella*

Summary

Genetic linkage studies have provided evidence to indicate that there is a defective gene on chromosome 21 which causes the autosomal dominant form of Alzheimer's disease (AD), at least in the four large pedigrees examined. Further studies have indicated that the β-amyloid gene and the superoxide dismutase-1 gene are not the site of the familial AD (FAD) mutation, and that duplication of large regions of chromosome 21 is not the pathogenetic mechanism in either FAD or sporadic AD. Additional studies are currently under way to more precisely map the location of the FAD gene in order to expedite the ultimate goal of isolating and characterizing the actual FAD gene.

Introduction

The primary cause of Alzheimer's disease (AD) remains unknown. However, several epidemiological studies have reported that first-degree relatives of patients with AD have an increased risk of this disorder (Breitner et al. 1988; Fitch et al. 1988; Heston et al. 1981; Rocca et al. 1986). It is extremely important to note that such familial clustering of AD does not prove a genetic etiology. However, several extended pedigrees have been described in which the disease phenotype can be clearly followed through multiple generations (Foncin et al. 1985; Goudsmit et al. 1981; Nee et al. 1983). In these pedigrees at least, the familial form of AD (FAD) clearly results from a dominantly inherited defect in an autosomal gene. Apart from the obvious pattern of inheritance, and a somewhat younger age of onset, cases with *typical* FAD are phenotypically indistinguishable from those with the "sporadic" form of the disease (Davies 1986). Consequently, identification of the primary defect could provide powerful insights into the biochemical pathophysiology of FAD, and possibly also that of the non-familial form of the disease.

An initial step towards the eventual goal of isolating the FAD gene defect is to identify which of the 22 pairs of autosomal chromosomes carries this gene. The existence of large pedigrees with FAD suggests that the chromosomal location of the causative gene defect could be discovered by identifying a polymorphic genetic marker co-segregating with the disorder. The discovery of the chromosomal location of the FAD gene using this strategy will allow subsequent attempts to clone the disease gene based simply upon a knowledge of its chromosomal location. In the absence of unambiguous clues as to the likely identity of the FAD gene, this approach avoids the necessity of making any a priori assumptions as to the nature of the FAD gene defect.

Classical genetic linkage studies using polymorphic expressed protein markers, such as the blood group antigens, have been previously attempted in FAD without success (Feldman et al. 1963; Spence et al. 1986). However, in recent years the power of this genetic linkage strategy has been dramatically increased by the discovery of large numbers of DNA markers which detect restriction fragment length polymorphisms (RFLPs) in human genomic DNA. We have applied the strategy of genetic linkage analysis with DNA markers to four large kindreds with pathologically proven FAD.

Localization of the FAD Gene

A priori the FAD gene could have been located on any of the 22 autosomal chromosomes. However, it has been known for several years that the brains of elderly individuals with trisomy 21 almost invariably harbour the neuropathological changes of AD (Oliver and Holland 1986). Furthermore, it seems clear that at least some elderly Down's syndrome (DS) individuals also develop cognitive impairment in late life consistent with AD. These observations suggested that genes on chromosome 21 may have a special role in the pathogenesis of FAD, and prompted an intensive investigation of the molecular genetics of this autosome.

Several DNA markers from the obligate DS region of chromosome 21 (21q22-21qter) were tested for linkage to FAD. Contrary to initial expectations, all markers from this region gave negative LOD scores, allowing this region of chromosome 21 to be excluded as the site of the FAD mutation. However, two DNA markers (D21S1/D21S11 and D21S16) from the more proximal regions of chromosome 21 gave positive LOD scores. Initially the 2-point linkage analysis LOD scores generated independently at each of these loci were less than the +3 conventionally required to prove linkage. However, the more statistically efficient method of multipoint linkage analysis (LINKAGE ver 3.5) generated LOD scores greater than +4.0 for chromosomal locations in the vicinity of these markers, proving that a defective gene located on the proximal long arm of chromosome 21 is the cause of the autosomal dominant form of FAD at least in the four pedigrees examined (St George-Hyslop et al. 1987).

Localization of the gene coding for the precursor of the β-amyloid peptide (AAP gene) to the proximal long arm of chromosome 21 near to the markers D21S1/D21S11 and D21S16 has led to the suggestion that this gene may be the site of the FAD mutation (Goldgaber et al. 1987; Kang et al. 1987; Robakis et al. 1987; Kang et al. 1987). This possibility received tentative support from preliminary observations suggesting that regions of chromosome 21 which carry the AAP gene and/or the superoxide dismutase gene (SOD1) may be duplicated in genomic DNA from individuals with AD (Delabar et al. 1987; Schweber et al. 1987). However, we and several other groups were able to show that the FAD mutation was not tightly linked to either the AAP gene or the SOD1 gene. Furthermore, we were unable to document any association between the presence of particular RFLPs in either of these genes and the occurrence of sporadic AD. Finally, we were unable to discover chromosomal duplication at any locus on chromosome 21 in the genomic DNA extracted from a variety of tissues of individuals with either sporadic or familial AD. These results, taken together, imply that the FAD mutation probably does not reside in any of the presently known genes on chromosome 21 (St George-Hyslop et al. 1987). Consequently, the identity of the actual FAD gene will have to be pursued using the more laborious techniques of molecular genetics (e.g., chromosome walking, PFG mapping, etc.) which are also being applied to several other inherited diseases.

In order to clone the FAD gene using standard molecular genetic strategies it will be necessary to first achieve a better localization of this gene. Better localization of the gene with respect to a set of close flanking markers can be gained by the examination of additional markers and additional FAD pedigrees. Another critical question which will also need to be addressed in order to facilitate the isolation of the FAD gene is the issue of heterogeneity in AD. Obviously, if there are pedigrees with FAD due to a gene defect at another chromosomal locus, their inclusion in the analysis of pedigrees with a defect on chromosome 21 will cause confusion. Likewise, if kindreds with multiple affected members due to a very common environmentally induced illness (i.e., phenocopies) are included in the analysis (under the mistaken impression that they represent an incompletely penetrant dominant gene defect) a similar disruption of the analysis will occur. Consequently, we have set out below a number of issues which must be very critically addressed when genetic linkage studies and tests of heterogeneity are performed on FAD pedigrees.

Linkage Strategies

Genetic linkage strategies, in the crudest terms, attempt to show that the proportion of informative meiotic events in which the disease phenotype and a particular allele of the genetic marker co-segregate is greater than would be expected by chance alone for a given genetic distance (recombination frequency θ) between the marker and the disease gene. A number of parameters, such as the frequency of the disease gene in the population, the age-dependent risk of the disease for currently asymptomatic members (age of onset correction), other penetrance functions, mutation rates, etc., must be incorporated into the analysis. The validity of these parameters is obviously critical both to the correctness of the analyses and to the interpretation of the results of these analyses.

Estimates of both the overall maximum penetrance of the FAD gene and of the age-dependent penetrance of this gene are necessary in order to analyse the genetic data contributed by currently asymptomatic members of the pedigrees under study. If the penetrance of the AD gene is determined by age *and* by other genetic and/or environmental factors, some elderly individuals may in fact be asymptomatic gene carriers. Unless this possibility is accounted for, the analysis will consider these asymptomatic gene carriers as nongene carriers concordant for the linked allele of the marker (i.e., recombinants), thereby contributing towards negative LOD scores. Studies of monozygotic twins (MZ) showing incomplete (40%) concordance, and wide differences in age of onset of AD even in the concordant MZ twins, together with several published pedigrees showing occasional skipped generations, are quite compatible with, but do not prove, the possibility that penetrance is affected by factors other than age (Nee et al. 1987). In the large pedigrees which we have previously analysed, very accurate estimates of penetrance and age-dependent risk can be readily generated from the extensive multigeneration family history data. However, these factors must be specifically addressed by careful epidemiologic studies if smaller pedigrees are to be incorporated into the analysis.

The frequency of the disease gene in the general population is another significant parameter in the linkage analysis. Differences in the estimated frequency of the disease gene in the general population can significantly alter the interpretation of recombination events in some pedigrees. For instance, a high gene frequency would allow for the occasional acquisition of the disease from a "presymptomatic" married-in parent. On the other hand, a very low gene frequency would force the analysis to consider that the disease was always acquired from the parent in direct descent in the family. In the latter paradigm, all individuals discordant at the marker locus would be considered as obligate recombinants. However, if autosomal dominant FAD is in fact a very common disease with incomplete penetrance due to age or other factors, an appreciable proportion of "recombinant" individuals could simply reflect acquisition of the disease from the "presymptomatic" married-in parent rather than true recombination events. Unfortunately, the true frequency of the autosomal dominant FAD gene in the general population is unknown. Some epidemiologic surveys which have nonrandomly assessed the incidence of AD amongst first-degree relatives of AD patients have shown a 50% age-dependent cumulative risk of AD among these relatives (Breitner et al. 1988). These results would imply that autosomal dominant FAD may be very common. Conversely, some case-controlled epidemiologic surveys have failed to observe increased familial aggregation of AD, particularly in late onset cases (Chandra et al. 1987). Additionally, several studies of twins have shown similar concordance rates between monozygotic and dizygotic twins (Nee et al. 1987). These studies would seem to suggest that not all AD is due to a genetic defect. The possibility that a significant proportion of AD may have a non-genetic etiology requires consideration of an additional argument. If an appreciable proportion of AD in fact results from a non-genetic etiology, then some instances of "recombination" in FAD pedigrees could simply represent chance occurrence of the nongenetic (phenocopy) form of the disease in one member of the FAD pedigree. Resolution of the relative incidences of the sporadic and the true autosomal dominant forms of AD, and estimation of the true FAD gene frequency, will again require careful analysis of the incidence and inheritance of AD in family members of *randomly* or *sequentially* assessed AD patients.

Finally, the traditional maximum likelihood methods of genetic linkage analysis require that the mode of genetic transmission be identified. In the large FAD pedigrees which we have previously studied, the mode of genetic transmission is unambiguously that of an autosomal dominant trait. However, in many smaller pedigrees, the mode of transmission often cannot be unequivocally identified. It could be argued that many of these small pedigrees do not reflect genetic transmission, but rather reflect familial clusters of a very common nongenetic disease. Obviously, the inclusion of such "multiplex" kindreds with a non-genetic or multifactorial (gene plus environment) etiology will confound the analysis, and could lead to spurious conclusions both about gene location and about genetic heterogeneity in autosomal dominant FAD.

Practical Problems in Studying the FAD Gene

In addition to the problems associated with the genetic model used in the linkage analysis, there are several practical problems which arise in the study of disorders of late onset where the antemortem diagnosis depends largely on clinical evaluation. First, the pedigree structure of most late-onset multiplex FAD kindreds makes them a poor source of genetic information. In many multiplex FAD pedigrees the disease cannot be traced beyond the nuclear family, only a limited number of affected individuals are alive and available for study at any given time, and neither of the parents of the affected individuals is alive. Consequently, most of the genetic information contributed by these pedigrees is not definitive even when the marker and the disease gene are closely linked. Indeed, the most definitive information contributed by these pedigrees is the presence of an obligate recombination event when affected members of the pedigree are discordant at the marker locus. However, the significance of a recombination event in small nuclear pedigrees is often difficult to interpret. Such a recombination event could simply reflect the fact that the marker is not precisely at the disease gene. On the other hand, such a recombination event could equally well reflect etiologic heterogeneity (nongenetic or second gene etiology), diagnostic errors, acquisition of the disease from the married-in parent as discussed earlier, or even a case of nonpaternity. Indeed, one of the difficulties of late-onset pedigrees is that since neither parent is alive, suspected cases of non-paternity can almost never be proven. Consequently, most small multiplex pedigrees represent a poor source of genetic information. Modelling of typical nuclear FAD pedigrees (N. Wexler and J. Ott, personal communication) indicates that more than 50% of such pedigrees would give a LOD score more negative than 0.00 at 10 cM using a standard genetic marker 10 cM from the actual disease gene. These limitations, therefore, frustrate attempts to detect genetic linkage in small pedigrees using markers more than a few centiMorgans from the disease gene, and complicate the discovery of heterogeneity.

The second practical problem encountered in the study of FAD is the issue of diagnosis. Current criteria for the diagnosis of AD are reported to have a diagnostic error rate of approximately 10%. The diagnostic accuracy is probably much better in the large, early-onset pedigrees where the diagnosis has been established neuropathologically in multiple members, and where the differential diagnosis is more limited. In small, late-onset pedigrees, neuropathologic confirmation in other members is often lacking, and the clinical diagnosis may be less certain because other disorders such as multi-infarct dementia are a relatively more common cause of dementia in the elderly than in the young. Consequently, such diagnostic uncertainties represent additional limitations upon the analysis of small, late-onset kindreds with familial clustering of AD. In summary, genetic linkage studies have provided evidence to indicate that there is a defective gene on chromosome 21 which causes the autosomal dominant form of AD at least in the four large pedigrees examined. Further studies have indicated that the β-amyloid gene and the SOD1 gene are not the site of the FAD mutation, and that duplication of large regions of chromosome 21 is not the pathogenetic mechanism in either FAD or sporadic AD. Additional studies are currently underway to more precisely map the location of the FAD gene in order to expedite the ultimate goal of isolating and characterizing the actual FAD gene. A number of potential problems have been identified which may confound the analysis and which will require very careful consideration during the interpretation of linkage data, particularly when small, late-onset pedigrees are examined.

References

Breitner JCS, Silverman JM, Mohs RC, Davis KL (1988) Familial aggregation of Alzheimer's disease: comparison of risk among relatives of early- and late-onset cases, and among male and female relatives in successive generations. Neurology 38: 207–212

Chandra V, Philipose V, Bell PA, Lazaroff A, Schoenberg BS (1987) Case-controlled study of late onset "probable Alzheimer's disease." Neurology 37: 1295–1300

Davies P (1986) The genetics of Alzheimer's disease: a review and a discussion of the implications. Neurobiol Aging 7: 459–466

Delabar J-M, Goldgaber D, Lamour Y, Nicole A, Huret J-L, de Grouchy J, Brown P, Gajdusek DC, Sinet P-M (1987) β-amyloid gene duplication in Alzheimer's disease and karyotypically normal Down syndrome. Science 235: 1390–1392

Feldman RG, Chandler KA, Levy LL, Glaser GH (1963) Familial Alzheimer's disease. Neurology 13: 811–823

Fitch N, Becker R, Heller A (1988) The inheritance of Alzheimer's disease: a new interpretation. Ann Neurol 23: 14–19

Foncin J-F, Salmon D, Supino-Viterbo V, Feldman RG, Macchi G, Mariotti P, Scoppetta C, Caruso G, Bruni AC (1985) Demence presenile d'Alzheimer transmise dans une famille etendue. Rev Neurol (Paris) 141: 194–202

Goldgaber D, Lerman MI, McBride OW, Saffiotti U, Gadjusek DC (1987) Characterization and chromosomal localization of a cDNA encoding brain amyloid of Alzheimer's disease. Science 235: 877–880

Goudsmit J, White BJ, Weitkamp LR, Keats JB, Morrow CH, Gajdusek DC (1981) Familial Alzheimer's disease in two kindreds of the same geographic and ethnic origin. J Neurol Sci 49: 79–89

Heston LL, Mastri AR, Anderson VE, White J (1981) Dementia of the Alzheimer type: clinical genetics, natural history, and associated conditions. Arch Gen Psychiatry 38: 1085–1090

Kang J, Lemaire H-G, Unterbeck A, Salbaum JM, Masters CL, Grzeschik KH, Multhaup G, Beyreuther K, Muller-Hill B (1987) The precursor of the Alzheimer's disease amyloid A4 protein resembles a cell-surface receptor. Nature 325: 733–736

Nee L, Eldridge R, Sunderland T, Thomas CB, Katz D, Thompson KE, Weingartner H, Weiss H, Julian C, Cohen R (1987) Dementia of the Alzheimer type: clinical and family study of 22 twin pairs. Neurology 37: 359–363

Nee L, Polinsky RJ, Eldridge R, Weingartner H, Smallberg S, Ebert M (1983) A family with histologically confirmed Alzheimer disease. Arch Neurol 40: 203–208

Oliver C, Holland AJ (1986) Down's Syndrome and Alzheimer's disease: a review. Psychol Med 16: 307–322

Robakis NK, Wisniewski HM, Jenkins EC, Devine-Gage EA, Houck GE, Yao XL, Ramakrishna N, Wolfe G, Silverman WP, Brown WT (1987) Chromosome 21q21 sublocalization of gene encoding β-amyloid peptide in cerebral vessels and neuritic (senile) plaques of people with Alzheimer disease and Down syndrome. Lancet I: 384–385

Rocca WA, Amaducci LA, Schoenberg BS (1986) Epidemiology of clinically diagnosed Alzheimer disease. Ann Neurol 19: 415–424

Schweber M, Tuson C, Shiloh R, Ben-Neriah Z (1987) Triplication of chromosome 21 material in Alzheimer's disease. Neurology 37: 222

Spence MA, Heyman A, Marazita ML, Sparkes RS, Weinberg T (1986) Genetic linkage analysis in Alzheimer's disease. Neurology 36: 581–583

St George-Hyslop PH, Tanzi R, Polinsky R, Haines JL, Nee L, Watkins PC, Myers R, Feldman RG, Pollen D, Drachman D, Growdon J, Bruni A, Foncin J-F, Salmon D, Frommelt P, Amaducci L,

Sorbi S, Piacentini S, Stewart GD, Hobbs WJ, Conneally PM, Gusella JF (1987a) The genetic defect causing familial Alzheimer's disease maps on chromosome 21. Science 235: 885–890

St George-Hyslop PH, Tanzi RE, Polinsky RJ, Neve RL, Pollen D, Drachman D, Growdon J, Cupples LA, Nee L, Myers R, O'Sullivan D, Watkins PC, Amos JA, Deutsch CK, Bodfish JW, Kinsbourne M, Feldman RG, Bruni A, Amaducci L, Foncin J-F, Gusella JF (1987b) Absence of duplication of genes on chromosome 21 in familial and sporadic Alzheimer disease. Science 238: 664–666

Tanzi RE, Gusella JF, Watkins PC, Bruns GAP, St George-Hyslop PH, Van Keuren ML, Patterson D, Pagan S, Kurnit DM, Neve RL (1987) Amyloid β protein gene: cDNA, mRNA distribution, and genetic linkage near the Alzheimer locus. Science 235: 880–884

Genetic Linkage Studies in Late-Onset Alzheimer's Disease Families

M.A. Pericak-Vance, L.H. Yamaoka, C.S. Haynes, J.L. Haines, P.C. Gaskell, W.-Y. Hung, C.M. Clark, A.L. Heyman, J.A. Trofatter, J.P. Eisenmenger, J.R. Gilbert, J.E. Lee, M.J. Alberts, M.C. Speer, D.V. Dawson, R.J. Bartlett, N.L. Earl, T. Siddique, and *A.D. Roses*

Summary

Alzheimer's disease (AD) is a devastating neurological disorder and the leading cause of dementia among the elderly. Recent studies have localized the gene for familial AD to chromosome 21 in a series of early-onset AD families (EOAD; mean age-of-onset, < 60). Familial late-onset AD (LOAD; mean age-of-onset, > 60) is a more common clinical form of the disorder. Linkage studies undertaken to test the localization of LOAD families to chromosome 21 failed to establish linkage and excluded linkage from a portion of the region where the EOAD gene was localized. These findings suggest that more than one etiology may exist for familial Alzheimer's disease and indicate the need for continued screening of the genome in LOAD families.

Introduction

Alzheimer's disease (AD) is a catastrophic neurodegenerative disorder that affects millions of individuals of all races and ethnic backgrounds. The economic cost alone in nursing home, medical, and ancillary care is greater than $ 40 billion annually (US Congress, April 1987); no one can estimate the cost to families and society. There is no successful treatment or cure for AD. The age-of-onset is variable and has been reported from the fourth to the ninth decade of life, with the majority of cases occurring in later life.

The etiology of AD remains unclear. A genetic component has long been implicated in AD due to the familial clustering of AD cases (Folstein and Powell 1984; Breitner and Folstein 1984). Even though nongenetic cases may occur, it is unlikely that the aggregation of affected persons in families can be explained by chance alone (Lander and Botstein 1986). Autosomal dominant inheritance with age-dependent penetrance has been suggested to explain this aggregation. Recent epidemiological studies support this hypothesis, finding a cumulative incidence of approximately 50% probable AD by the ninth decade among relatives of AD probands (Mohs et al. 1987; Breitner et al. 1988). In addition, large multigenerational pedigrees with the rare, early onset AD (EOAD) have been described in which approximately 50% of relatives are affected in several generations (Nee et al. 1983). Inherent ascertainment biases in the data make it difficult to accept with confidence the results of segregation analysis aimed at determining the mode of inheritance. Formal segregation analyses in the past have proven troublesome (Weitkamp et al. 1983), and despite the numerous advances in segregation analysis in recent years, it is sometimes impossible to make definitive statements regarding inheritance patterns. Linkage analysis is one approach to establishing the existence of a genetic component in the expression of a particular trait. It is inherently more difficult for a nongenetic mechanism to mimic linkage than segregation.

Chromosome 21 had long been considered a possible site for the AD gene due to the reported association between AD and Down's syndrome (Heyman et al. 1984). In 1987, linkage of familial Alzheimer's disease (FAD) was reported to two probes on chromosome 21, D21S16 and D21S1/D21S11 (St George-Hyslop et al. 1987). D21S16 gave $\hat{\theta}$ (maximum recombination fraction) = 0.0 $\hat{z}$ (maximum *LOD* score) = 2.32 and D21S1/D21S11 gave $\hat{\theta}$ = 0.08 with $\hat{z}$ = 2.37. Maximizing the linkage information in a multipoint analysis resulted in a peak *LOD* score of 4.25, confirming the location of FAD on chromosome 21 in the four families analyzed. The mean ages-of-onset (M) in the families were 52, 48.7, 49.8, and 39.9 years.

Thirteen FAD Families

Diagnosis

We have examined and obtained blood for DNA and paternity studies from 106 members (32 affected) of 13 FAD (familial Alzheimer's disease) families each with multiple affected family members (Fig. 1). The total number of affected persons, living and deceased, in these families is 49. Five of the families have autopsy-confirmed AD. Nine of the 13 families have three or more family members affected with AD and four families have two AD-affected family members. The majority of the affected relatives were first-degree relatives. Sampled individuals from the 13 families were evaluated by a neurologist and associated diagnostic personnel of the Duke Alzheimer Disease Research Center (ADRC) and the clinical diagnosis of probable AD was made as formerly described (Pericak-Vance et al. 1986). Previously unpublished data from our center show confirmation of the clinical diagnosis of AD by pathological findings at autopsy in eight of eight independent individuals from families with multiple affected members.

Of the 49 affected family members included in the present study, only 12 were not examined by ADRC personnel. Most of these were deceased family members (i.e., parents of living affected persons). Of those individuals not available for examination, medical records were obtained and reviewed by a neurologist before clinical status was assigned. In making the diagnosis of AD, care was taken to exclude confounding causes of dementia such as depression and multiple infarct disease.

Chromosome 21 Probes as Markers

The mode of inheritance in these families is consistent with autosomal dominance with age-dependent penetrance. In 11 families *M* ranged from 60 to 80+ years. Two families (#317 and #208) have *M* = 56 and *M* = 54 years, respectively, and one family (#372) has exceptionally early age-of-onset (*M* = 49), which is similar to the EOAD

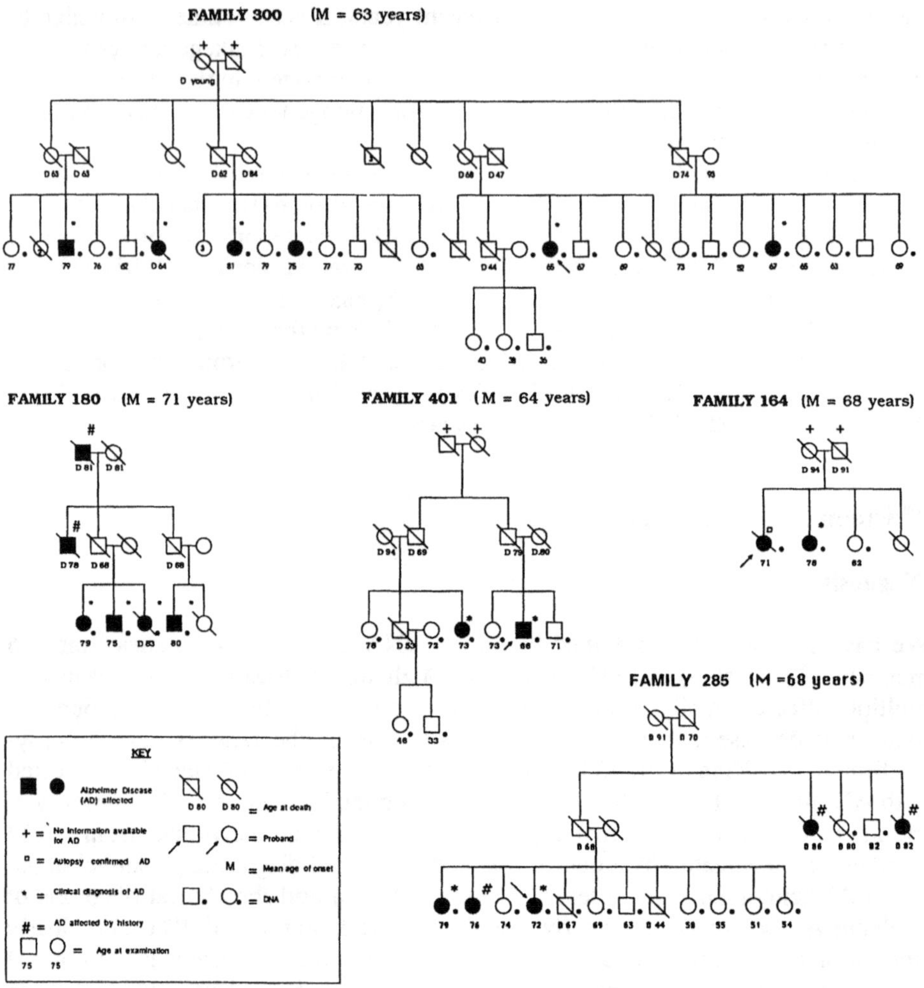

Fig. 1. The 13 Alzheimer's disease families used in the linkage analysis. DNA from each member within the pedigree was isolated from blood or from EBV-transformed lymphoblast cell lines. This genomic DNA was digested with the appropriate restriction enzyme and the resultant fragments were size-separated by submarine, agarose gel electrophoresis in TAE buffer (40 m*M* tris-acetate, 2 m*M* EDTA). The DNA fragments were transferred from the gel to a nylon filter support (Gene Screen Plus, NEN) by capillary action using the alkaline transfer procedure (Chomczynski and Quasba 1985). DNA probes were labelled with α-^{32}P-deoxycytidine triphosphate (NEN) by random oligonucleotide priming (Amersham). Labelled probes were hybridized to the filters for 18–24 h at 42° C in 50% formamide, 10% dextran sulphate, 1% SDS, 1 *M* NaCl; 20 m*M* sodium phosphate buffer, pH 7.0, 5X Denhardts; and 100 µg/ml salmon sperm DNA. The filters were washed twice in 2 X SSC at room temperature, then twice in 2 X SSC-1% SDS at 65° C. The filters were exposed to X-ray film (Kodak XAR-5) with a Dupont Cronex intensifying screen at −80° C for 24–72 h

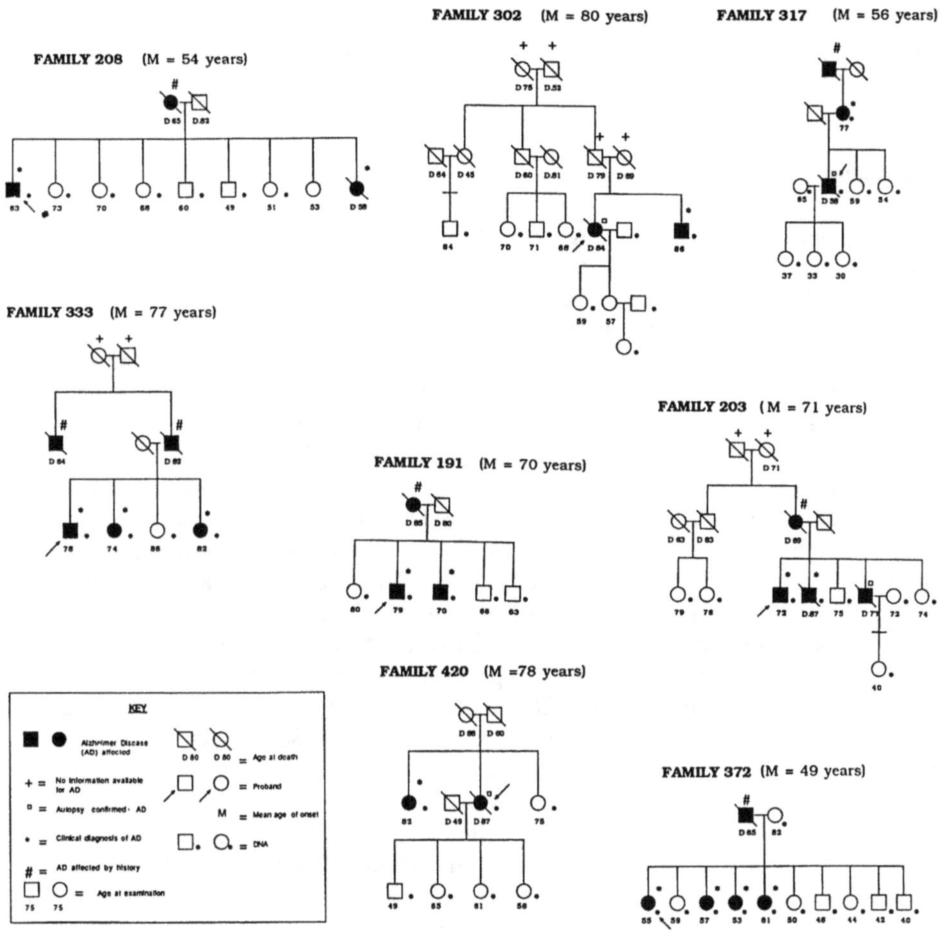

Fig. 1

families reported elsewhere (St George-Hyslop et al. 1987). As the majority of the families in our study are of the late-onset type (LOAD), the most common clinical form of the disease, we were interested in testing the EOAD chromosome 21 linked probes (St George-Hyslop et al. 1987) for linkage in our data set. Linkage of LOAD to these above probes is of critical significance in determining the overall etiology of AD. Exclusion of linkage of LOAD to this region of chromosome 21 would necessitate the further screening of other chromosome regions for linkage to identify the gene(s) involved in LOAD, and thus confirm the existence of a genetic component in this clinical entity.

The markers included in the analysis were the chromosome 21 probes, D21S1/D21S11 and D21S16, previously shown to be linked to AD in the EOAD families (St George-Hyslop et al. 1987). High molecular weight genomic DNA was prepared from lymphocytes as previously described (Pericak-Vance et al. 1986b; Bartlett et al. 1987). The restriction endonuclease digestion, agarose gel electrophoresis, Southern blotting, DNA probe labelling and hybridization were as outlined previously (St George-Hyslop et al. 1987; Pericak-Vance et al. 1986b). Genotypes were assigned accordingly.

Discussion

The data were analyzed for linkage using both the LIPED and LINKAGE computer programs using an autosomal dominant mode of inheritance with age-dependent penetrance for AD. The age curve employed in the analysis was calculated from the overall pedigree data (Haynes et al. 1986); however, the results did not change significantly when family-specific age curves were used for several of the families. In order to simulate the previous study, initially a gene frequency of 0.0001 was incorporated for the AD locus. D21S16 was analyzed in the individual families using the LIPED program (Ott 1984; Hodge et al. 1979) while LINKAGE was used to analyze the complex D21S1/D21S11 marker. This marker detects four polymorphisms which can be combined into a haplotype for the linkage analysis. Haplotypes can be constructed by hand in some cases, but this frequently results in loss of data, as not all individuals can be uniquely haplotyped (Pericak-Vance et al. 1986a). This is particularly true in LOAD pedigrees where, due to the late age-of-onset, many family members are missing and/or deceased. In order to circumvent this problem the MLINK subprogram of the LINKAGE package (Lathrop and Lalouel 1984; Lathrop et al. 1985) was used in the D21S1/D21S11 analysis, with the recombination fraction between the four sites fixed at 0.0 (Pericak-Vance et al. 1986a). Because the sites are in disequilibrium (St George-Hyslop et al. 1987), individual frequencies were calculated for each of the possible haplotypes.

LOD scores (logarithm_{10} of the odds of linkage) for the markers were calculated for each pedigree for each of the recombination fractions (θ males = θ females), 0.001, 0.05, 0.10, 0.20, 0.30, and 0.40. The results were tabulated and then summed over the various pedigrees. A LOD score $\geqslant +3$ is accepted as significant evidence for linkage while a LOD score $\leqslant -2$ is accepted as significant evidence for exclusion of linkage (Morton 1956). The resulting two-point LOD scores between AD and D21S1/D21S11 and D21S16 are given in Table 1. Linkage is excluded between AD and D21S1/D21S11 up to 11 centrimorgans (cM) ($\theta \leqslant 0.11$, $z < -2.0$). This exclusion region includes the amyloid gene (Tanzi et al. 1985). The highest individual LOD score ($\hat{z} = 0.90$ at $\hat{\theta} = 0.0$) is found in family 372, whose M met EOAD criteria. The results of the linkage analysis between AD and D21S16 are inconclusive. While the overall score is positive ($\theta = 0.0$, $\hat{z} = 1.32$), the majority of the positive information ($\hat{z} = 0.60$) came from family 372, the EOAD family. D21S16 is considerably less informative (PIC = 0.07) than the haplotype D21S1/D21S11 marker (Willard et al. 1985).

The analyses were repeated varying the disease gene frequency *(p)* and the including mutation (μ) in the model. Varying the gene frequency should allow for the possibility that the AD gene entered the pedigree through married-in individuals, and the use of mutation would aid in circumventing the confounding occurrence of sporadic AD. The range of the estimates used in the analyses were $p = 0.0001$ to 0.06 (Larsson et al. 1963) and $\mu = 0.0$ to 0.00013. The *LOD* scores from these various tests were consistently negative for D21S1/D21S11, confirming the previous findings.

Table 1. Two-point LOD scores are given for linkage of Alzheimer disease with the DNA markers D21S1/D21S11 and D21S16. LOD scores for D21S1/D21S11 were calculated using the program LINKAGE with an age-of-onset correction determined from the overall pedigree data (Haynes et al. 1986). Gene frequencies *(p)* of 0.0001 were assumed (St George-Hyslop et al. 1987). The limit of exclusion ($z < -2$; Hodge et al. 1979) found was 11 cM on either side of D21S1/D21S11. The highest individual score was in family 372, the early-onset AD family (M = 49). The program LIPED was used to analyze D21S16. The results for this marker, which is considerably less informative (PIC = 0.07; Lathrop and Lalouel 1984), were inconclusive. The use of family-specific age curves for AD did not significantly alter the linkage results. In addition, varying p (0.0001–0.06) and including mutation (μ = 0.0–0.00013) in the analysis produced consistently negative results for AD and D21S1/D21S11. The results for D21S16 remained inconclusive

	Recombination fraction (θ)					
Family	0.001	0.05	0.10	0.20	0.30	0.40
	Alzheimer's disease vs D21S1/D21S11					
191	−0.281	−0.227	−0.177	−0.098	−0.043	−0.011
285	−2.400	−0.775	−0.486	−0.217	−0.086	−0.020
401	−0.367	−0.277	−0.204	−0.102	−0.041	−0.009
180	−2.611	−1.230	−0.771	−0.338	−0.132	−0.031
164	−0.408	−0.297	−0.216	−0.108	−0.045	−0.011
300	−4.000	−1.395	−0.855	−0.376	−0.155	−0.040
203	−0.398	−0.314	−0.241	−0.128	−0.055	−0.013
302	−0.062	−0.052	−0.044	−0.029	−0.017	−0.017
372	+0.899	+0.811	+0.718	+0.515	+0.296	+0.093
317	0.000	0.000	0.000	0.000	0.000	0.000
420	0.000	0.000	0.000	0.000	0.000	0.000
333	+0.284	+0.246	+0.208	+0.135	+0.072	+0.024
208	−0.139	−0.113	−0.089	−0.050	−0.022	−0.005
Total	−9.484	−3.622	−2.158	−0.795	−0.227	−0.041
	Alzheimer's disease vs D21S16					
191	−0.063	−0.053	−0.043	−0.026	−0.012	−0.003
285	0.000	0.000	0.000	0.000	0.000	0.000
401	+0.251	+0.206	+0.163	+0.089	+0.037	+0.008
180	+0.357	+0.295	+0.235	+0.131	+0.055	+0.013
164	−0.184	−0.143	−0.109	−0.058	−0.025	−0.006
300	+0.318	+0.273	+0.228	+0.142	+0.068	+0.018
203	−0.246	−0.183	−0.133	−0.065	−0.025	−0.006
302	+0.102	+0.086	+0.070	+0.041	+0.019	+0.005
372	+0.601	+0.535	+0.465	+0.318	+0.170	+0.049
317	0.000	0.000	0.000	0.000	0.000	0.000
420	0.000	0.000	0.000	0.000	0.000	0.000
333	+0.203	+0.172	+0.141	+0.085	+0.040	+0.010
208	0.000	0.000	0.000	0.000	0.000	0.000
Total	+1.312	+1.166	+1.000	+0.648	+0.397	+0.090

Throughout all analyses, linkage could not be established between AD and D21S1/D21S11. The results for D21S16 remained inconclusive.

Finally, multipoint analysis using the LINKMAP subprogram of LINKAGE was employed in order to maximize the available information. The multipoint approach (interval mapping) increases the power of the analysis, and decreases the amount of data needed to find a significant linkage result. The distance relationship of the markers in the analysis was input as previously reported (St George-Hyslop et al. 1987). The multipoint results support the two-point findings, excluding up to 11 cM distal from D21S1/D21S11, as well as the area between the two markers, and from complete linkage to D21S16.

These data fail to support linkage of autosomal dominant LOAD to the D21S1/ D21S11 region of chromosome 21 as reported for the EOAD families. The finding of a positive score of $\hat{z} = 0.90$ at $\hat{\theta} = 0.0$ in our earliest onset family tends to support the EOAD linkage data. Thus, LOAD appears to represent a separate entity from EOAD.

Conclusion

The failure to detect linkage of autosomal dominant LOAD to the region of chromosome 21 where the EOAD gene was localized, together with the exclusion of linkage to a portion of that same region, strongly suggests more than one etiology for familial Alzheimer's disease. These differences between EOAD and LOAD are consistent with observations of both clinical and neurochemical differences between early- and late-onset AD (Seltzer and Sherwin 1983; Filley et al. 1986). These findings indicate the need for the screening of additional chromosomal areas for linkage to LOAD. The eventual localization of LOAD will provide the basis for additional studies aimed at determining the basic defect in this common form of familial AD.

References

Bartlett RJ, Pericak-Vance MA, Yamaoka L, Gilbert J, Herbstreith M, Hung W-Y, Lee JE, Mohandas T, Bruns G, Laberge C, Thibault M-C, Ross D, Roses AD (1987) A new probe for the diagnosis of myotonic muscular dystrophy. Science 235: 1648–1650

Breitner JCS, Folstein MJ (1984) Familial Alzheimer dementia: a prevalent disorder with specific clinical features. Psychol Med 14: 63–80

Breitner JCS, Silverman JM, Mohs RC, Davis KL (1988) Familial aggregation in Alzheimer's disease: comparison of risk among relatives of early- and late-onset cases, and among male and female relatives in successive generations. Neurology 38: 207–212

Chomczynski P, Qasba PK (1985) Alkaline transfer of DNA to gene screen plus membrane. New England Nuclear Publication

Congress US, Office of Technology Assessment (1987) Losing a million minds: confronting the tragedy of Alzheimer disease and other dementias. U.S. Government Printing Office, Washington, D.C., OTA-BA-323

Filley CM, Kelley J, Heaton RK (1986) Neuropsychologic features of early and late onset Alzheimer disease. Arch Neurol 43: 574–576

Folstein MF, Powell D (1984) Is Alzheimer's disease inherited: a methodologic review. Integr Psychiatry 2: 163–175

Haynes CS, Pericak-Vance MA, Dawson DV (1986) Analysis of Huntington disease linkage and age-of-onset distributions. Genet Epidemiol [Suppl] 1: 236–239

Heyman A, Wilkinson WE, Stafford JA, Helms MJ, Sigmon AH, Weinberg T (1984) Alzheimer's disease: a study of epidemiologic aspects. Ann Neurol 15: 335–341

Hodge SE, Morton LA, Tideman S, Kidd KK, Spence MA (1979) Age-of-onset correction available for linkage analysis (LIPED). Am J Hum Genet 31: 761–762

Lander ES, Botstein D (1986) In: Mapping complex genetic traits in humans: new methods using a complete RFLP linkage map. Cold Spring Harbor Symposia on Quantitative Biology. Cold Spring Harbor Laboratory, Cold Spring Harbor, pp 49–62

Larsson T, Sjogren T, Jacobson G (1963) Senile dementia: a clinical, sociomedical and genetic study. Acta Psychiatr Scand [Suppl 167] 39

Lathrop GM, Lalouel JM (1984) Easy calculations of lod scores and genetic risks on small computers. Am J Hum Genet 36: 460–465

Lathrop GM, Lalouel JM, Julier C, Ott J (1985) Multi locus linkage analysis in humans: detection of linkage and estimation of recombination. Am J Hum Genet 37: 482–498

Mohs RC, Breitner JCS, Silverman JM, Davis K (1987) Alzheimer's disease: morbid risk among first degree relatives approximates 50% by age 90. Arch Gen Psychiatry 44: 405–408

Morton NE (1956) Detection and estimation of linkage between genes for elliptocytosis and RH blood type. Am J Genet 7: 277

Nee LE, Polinsky RJ, Eldridge R, Weingartner H, Smallberg S, Ebert M (1983) A family with histologically confirmed Alzheimer's disease. Arch Neurol 40: 203–208

Ott J (1984) Estimation of the recombination fraction in human pedigree: efficient computation of the likelihood for human linkage studies. Am J Hum Genet 27: 588–597

Pericak-Vance MA, Meyers DA, Gusella JF, Folstein SE, Conneally PM (1986a) Genetic analysis workshop IV: Huntington disease linkage analysis, data description. Genet Epidemiol [Suppl] 1: 193–196

Pericak-Vance MA, Yamaoka LH, Assinder RIF, Hung W-Y, Bartlett RJ, Stajich JM, Gaskell PC, Ross DA, Sherman S, Fey GH, Humphries S, Williamson R, Roses AD (1986b) Tight linkage of apolipoprotein C2 to myotonic dystrophy on chromosome 19. Neurology 36: 1418–1423

Seltzer R, Sherwin I (1983) A comparison of clinical features in early and late-onset primary degenerative dementia. One entity or two? Arch Neurol 40: 143–146

St George-Hyslop PH, Tanzi RE, Polinsky RJ, Haines JL, Nee L, Watkins PC, Meyers RH, Feldman RG, Pollen D, Drachman D, Growdon J, Bruni A, Foncin J-F, Salmon G, Fromhelt P, Amaducci L, Sorgi S, Placentini S, Stewart GD, Hobbs W, Conneally PM, Gusella JF (1987) The genetic defect causing familial Alzheimer's disease maps on chromosome 21. Science 235: 885–890

Tanzi RE, Watkins PC, Gibbons K, Faryniarz A, Wallace M, Hallewell R, Conneally PM, Gusella J (1985) A genetic linkage map of human chromosome 21. Eighth International Workshop on Human Gene Mapping. Cytogenet Cell Genet 40: 760

Weitkamp LR, Nee L, Keats B, Polinsky RJ, Guttormsen S (1983) Alzheimer disease: Evidence for susceptibility loci on chromosomes 6 and 14. Am J Hum Genet 35: 443–453

Willard H, Skolnick M, Pearson P, Mandel JL (1985) Human gene mapping by recombinant DNA techniques: report on polymorphic DNA segments. Eighth International Workshop on Human Gene Mapping. Cytogenet Cell Genet 40: 360–390

Genetic Linkage Analysis in Two Large Belgian Alzheimer Families with Chromosome 21 DNA Markers

C. Van Broeckhoven, W. Van Hul, H. Backhovens, P. Raeymaekers, G. Van Camp, P. Stinissen, A. Wehnert, G. De Winter, J. Gheuens, and *A. Vandenberghe*

Summary

We previously reported two large Belgian Alzheimer families, AD/A and AD/B, with autosomal dominant transmission of the disease and early onset of the disease symptoms (< 35 years). Both pedigrees were used to examine the distance between the FAD and APP gene, using informative haplotypes of two DNA polymorphisms of the APP cDNA. Furthermore, we analysed possible linkage of both families with chromosome 21 using the markers D21S16 and D21S1/S11 and several other 21 probes. We found positive *LOD* scores with D21S13. Pulse field gel electrophoresis helped us to prove that D21S13 and D21S16 are closely related and may in fact be regarded as one locus in the linkage analysis of Alzheimer families. Linkage data indicate that the FAD gene is most likely located near D21S13/S16, closer to the centromere.

Introduction

At least 50% of all patients with senile dementia are clinically diagnosed Alzheimer cases (Terry and Katzman 1983). In as much as 40% of these cases there is strong evidence of a previous family history of the disease (Heston et al. 1981), indicating the involvement of a genetic predisposing factor in this neurodegenerative disorder. Several families are now known in which the disease segregates according to a clear autosomal dominant inheritance pattern (Cook et al. 1979; Goudsmit et al. 1981; Nee et al. 1983). Such families can be used to study the linkage relationship between the genetic defect causing Alzheimer's disease and different polymorphic DNA markers (Botstein et al. 1980).

The first linkage results came from St George-Hyslop et al. (1987) proving the existence of a familial Alzheimer gene (FAD) on chromosome 21. They found positive linkage of FAD with two anonymous DNA markers, D21S16 and D21S1/S11, located on the proximal long arm of chromosome 21 (Watkins et al. 1987). Simultaneously the gene for the amyloid precursor protein (APP), a component of senile plaques found in brain tissue from patients with Alzheimer's disease, was localised in the same region of chromosome 21 (Kang et al. 1987; Tanzi et al. 1987a). Close proximity of the FAD gene and the APP gene led to the suggestion that the amyloid protein gene was the primary site of the genetic defect in familial Alzheimer dementia. However, this hypothesis was eliminated very rapidly by illustrating the occurrence of recombination events between both genes in several families (Van Broeckhoven et al. 1987; Tanzi et al. 1987b). A *LOD* score of $z < -2$ at a recombination fraction of $\theta = 0.07$ excluded the FAD gene from the immediate vicinity of the APP gene (Van Broeckhoven et al. 1987). Combined linkage data indicated that the most likely position of the FAD gene was proximal of D21S1/S11 (St George-Hyslop et al. 1987; Tanzi et al. 1987b).

Although the amyloid precursor protein gene is not identical with the familial Alzheimer gene, the existence of an altered APP gene expression in Alzheimer brain pathology cannot yet be excluded. The possiblity of a long-range effect of the FAD gene defect on the APP gene expression remains open for discussion.

Results and Discussion

We recently reported an informative BglII polymorphism recognised by a subclone of the APP cDNA clone spanning the coding region for the A4 polypeptide (Van Broeckhoven et al. 1987; Table 1). Simultaneously Tanzi et al. (1987b) reported three different RFLPs derived from both the 5′ and 3′ end of the APP cDNA clone.

Table 1. Polymorphic DNA markers on chromosome 21. The chromosome 21 DNA markers, their allele lenghths and frequencies (Van Broeckhoven et al. 1987; Tanzi et al. 1987b; Stewart et al. 1985; Watkins et al. 1985; Davies et al. 1984)

Locus	Restriction enzyme	Alleles 1 and 2 (kb)	Allele frequencies
APP	BglII	9.6/6.9	0.36/0.64
APP	EcoRI	6.6/6.1	0.37/0.63
D21S16	XbaI	7.3/6.4	0.10/0.90
D21S1	BamHI	7.1/6.3	0.20/0.80
	MspI	7.6/5.0	0.38/0.62
D21S11	EcoRI	2.9/1.9	0.28/0.68
	TaqI	5.5/4.0	0.35/0.65
D21S13	TaqI	7.0/6.0	0.71/0.29

In an attempt to determine the genetic distance between the FAD gene and the APP gene, we first increased the information from the APP locus as a polymorphic marker by calculating haplotype frequencies between the BglII RFLP and the most informative EcoRI RFLP (Table 1) reported by Tanzi et al. (1987b). Lack of significant linkage disequilibrium between both polymorphisms allowed us to establish informative haplotypes at the APP gene.

Secondly, we examined the Alzheimer families AD/A and AD/B, with both APP RFLPs and calculated *LOD* scores for linkage to FAD using these APP haplotypes. The pedigree of the families is illustrated in Fig. 1. Very early onset of the disease symptoms (< 35 years) and availability of DNA of patients in two generations make these Alzheimer pedigrees very useful for linkage analysis studies. *LOD* scores were calculated using MLINK of the LINKAGE package (Lathrop et al. 1985) assuming a

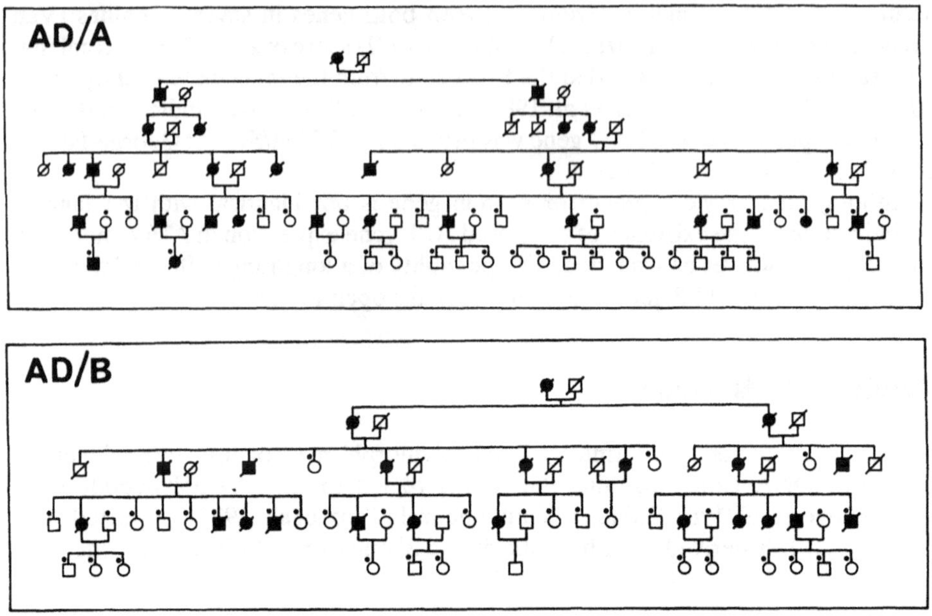

Fig. 1. Pedigrees of Alzheimer families. *Circle,* female; *square,* male; *diagonal line,* deceased; *filled symbols,* affected individual; *black dots,* cases available for genetic analysis

gene frequency of 0.0001 for the FAD gene defect (St George-Hyslop et al. 1987). Combined likage data for the two families are shown in Table 2. A *LOD* score of $-\infty$ at a recombination fraction of $\theta = 0.0$ indicates the presence of crossovers between the APP locus and the FAD defect in each family. If we take the average recombination rate for the human genome, the total *LOD* scores exclude ($z < -2$), now a segment of 1.3 10^7 bp on either side of the APP locus separating the FAD defect from the APP gene by a fairly large distance.

The existence of a FAD gene on the proximal long arm of chromosome 21 follows from the linkage results obtained by St George-Hyslop et al. (1987). They analysed four families with early onset of the disease (< 60 years) with several 21 DNA markers

Table 2. Combined *LOD* scores for linkage of the APP gene to FAD. Haplotype frequencies for the APP locus were estimated from those observed in 59 unrelated normal individuals where coupling phase of the individual RFLP alleles could be unequivocally determined. Considering alleles 1 and 2 for the RFLPs in the order EcoRI and BglII, the haplotype frequencies used were as follows: "111" 0.11, "121" 0.29, "211" 0.26, "221" 0.32, and all others 0.02

Pedigree	Recombination fraction (θ)							Exclusion limit
	0.00	0.01	0.05	0.10	0.20	0.30	0.40	($z < -2$)
AD/A	$-\infty$	−1.96	−1.04	−0.54	−0.09	+0.03	+0.03	
AD/B	$-\infty$	−6.79	−3.71	−2.11	−0.76	−0.24	−0.04	
Total	$-\infty$	−8.75	−4.75	−2.65	−0.85	−0.21	−0.02	$\theta = 0.13$

Table 3. *LOD* scores for linkage of the FAD gene to D21S16 and D21S1/S11. Allele frequencies are shown in Table 1. In the case of the locus D21S1/S11, information from only three enzymes was used since D21S11 showed complete linkage disequilibrium in both our families. Haplotype frequencies were estimated from those observed in 66 unrelated individuals and compared with the values published by St George-Hyslop et al. (1987). Since there were no significant discrepancies between both calculations, we used the frequencies observed in our population. Considering alleles 1 and 2 for the RFLPs in the order MspI, BamHI and EcoRI, the haplotype frequencies are "121" 0.23, "222" 0.41, "212" 0.20, and all others 0.16

Marker locus	Pedigree	Recombination fraction (θ)							Exclusion limit
		0.00	0.01	0.05	0.10	0.20	0.30	0.40	($z < -2$)
S16	AD/A	−5.10	−2.25	−1.15	−0.65	−0.24	−0.08	−0.02	
	AD/B	−0.91	−0.81	−0.54	−0.35	−0.15	−0.05	−0.01	
	Total	−6.01	−3.06	−1.69	−1.00	−0.39	−0.13	−0.03	θ = 0.03
S1/S11	AD/A	−∞	−0.99	−0.35	−0.09	+0.09	+0.10	+0.04	
	AD/B	−∞	−8.42	−4.26	−2.56	−1.08	−0.43	−0.12	
	Total	−∞	−9.41	−4.61	−2.65	−0.99	−0.33	−0.08	θ = 0.12

and found positive *LOD* scores with D21S16 and D21S1/S11. We examined both our families for linkage of FAD with these probes (Table 1). The *LOD* scores are summarised in Table 3. The total *LOD* scores for either of the two probes remain negative. The value $-\infty$ at recombination fraction $\theta = 0.0$ and the exclusion limit ($z < -2$) of $\theta = 0.12$ for D21S1/S11 indicate that this marker is not tightly linked to the FAD defect in the two families examined. No definite crossovers were observed between FAD and D21S16.

The absence of positive *LOD* scores may be due to the absence of a FAD gene on chromosome 21, adding support to the idea of genetic heterogeneity in Alzheimer's disease, to linkage between FAD and distant markers or to lack of *informativeness* of the markers used in the analysis. The latter possibility is supported by the following arguments. D21S16 is a weakly informative probe due to the low frequency of its minor allele. The D21S1/S11 locus is a composite of two loci, D21S1 and D21S11, detecting two polymorphisms each. Although haplotypes can be used for the four RFLPs, the informativeness of the marker is limited by the occurrence of linkage disequilibrium between the RFLPs detected (St George-Hyslop et al. 1987).

Genetic heterogeneity between Alzheimer families with early and late onset of the disease was suggested by Roses and his group at the 9th Human Gene Mapping conference (Paris, September 1987). They presented linkage data of an extensive study of essentially late-onset families (> 60 years) with both of these markers. Their results indicated that late-onset Alzheimer families are not tightly linked to the D21S1/S11 locus with exclusion limits ranging up to $\theta = 0.16$. D21S16 was not very informative in their families.

Both pedigrees AD/A and AD/B were further analysed with several other 21 DNA markers. We found a suggestive *LOD* score in family AD/A with the probe D21S13 (Davies et al. 1984). LOD scores for linkage for FAD with D21S13 are shown in Table 4. A maximal LOD score of +1.43 at $\theta = 0.05$ was obtained with no crossovers in either family.

Table 4. *LOD* scores for linkage of FAD with D21S13. The polymorphism used for D21S13 and its allele frequencies are shown in Table 1. Recombination fraction at which the peak *LOD* score occurred was calculated using the program ILINK of the LINKAGE package (Davies et al. 1987)

Pedigree	Recombination fraction (θ)							Peak *LOD* score ($\hat{z}$)
	0.00	0.01	0.05	0.10	0.20	0.30	0.40	
AD/A	+1.45	+1.59	+1.71	+1.60	+1.15	+0.63	+0.18	
AD/B	−0.35	−0.33	−0.28	−0.22	−0.12	−0.06	−0.06	
Total	+1.10	+1.26	+1.43	+1.38	+1.03	+0.57	+0.16	+1.43 ($\hat{\theta} = 0.05$)

D21S13 is located in the 21q11.1–21q21.2 region (Neve et al. 1986), closer to the centromere than D21S1/S11 (Van Keuren et al. 1986). Therefore, we examined the linkage relation of D21S13 to D21S16 and D21S1/S11, the first two linked markers. D21S13 is tightly linked to D21S16 ($\hat{z} = 6.33$ at $\theta = 0.0$) with no crossovers observed in over 100 meioses tested (Backhovens et al. in preparation). Subsequently close proximity of both markers was proven by pulse field gel electrophoresis (Van Hul et al., in preparation). A preliminary pulse field map around D21S13/S16 is illustrated in Fig. 2. These results indicate that D21S16 and D21S13 map at the same position on chromosome 21 and may in fact be regarded as one locus in the linkage analysis program. As opposed to D21S16, D21S13 is a very polymorphic probe which will be more useful in the linkage analysis of Alzheimer families.

The positive *LOD* scores obtained with D21S13, although not conclusive, indicate that at least in family AD/A the genetic defect is located on chromosome 21. The results obtained with D21S13 also support the hypothesis that the absence of positive linkage with D21S16 and D21S1/S11 reflects merely absence of information, with D21S16 being a close but uninformative marker and D21S1/S11 a more informative but distant marker.

On the chromosome 21q map D21S13 is located proximal of D21S1/S11 at a recombination fraction of $\theta = 0.12°$, APP is distal of D21S1/S11 at $\theta = 0.04$ (Backhovens et al., in preparation). Taking into account these map positions and the exclusion limits calculated for FAD around all loci tested, a more proximal position of the FAD gene closer to D21S13/S16 comes forward. Linkage analysis of several more Alzheimer families with both D21S13 and D21S16 is needed to prove this preliminary localisation of the familial Alzheimer gene.

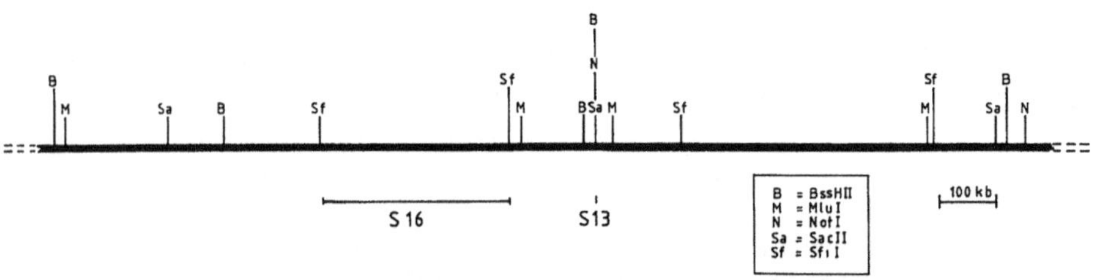

Fig. 2. Pulse field map of the D21S13/S16 locus. Positions of D21S13 and D21S16 indicated by *arrows* below the map were deduced from restriction fragments recognised by both probes on the same pulse field blots generated with five different rare cutter enzymes. Fragment sizes were estimated with respect to yeast markers

References

Botstein D, White RL, Skolnick M, Davis RW (1980) Construction of a genetic linkage map in man using restriction fragment length polymorphisms. Am J Hum Genet 32: 314–331

Cook RH, Ward BE, Austin JH (1979) Studies in aging of the brain: IV. Familial Alzheimer disease: Relation to transmissible dementia. aneuploidy, and microtubular defects. Neurology 29: 1402–1412

Davies KE, Harper K, Bonthron D, Krumlauf R, Polkey A, Pembrey ME, Williamson R (1984) Use of a chromosome 21 cloned DNA probe for the analysis of non-disjunction in Down syndrome. Hum Genet 66: 54–56

Goudsmit J, White BJ, Weitkamp LR, Keats BJB, Morrow CH, Gajdusek DC (1981) Familial Alzheimer's disease in two kindreds of the same geographic and ethnic origin. J Neurol Sci 49: 79–89

Heston LL, Mastri AR, Anderson VE, White J (1981) Dementia of the Alzheimer type. Arch Gen Psychiatry 38: 1085–1090

Kang J, Lemaire H-G, Unterbeck A, Salbaum JM, Masters CL, Grzeschik K-H, Multhaup G, Beyreuther K, Müller-Hill B (1987) The precursor of Alzheimer's disease amyloid A4 protein resembles a cell-surface receptor. Nature 325: 733–736

Lathrop GM, Lalouel JM, Julier C, Ott J (1985) Multilocus linkage analysis in humans: detection of linkage and estimation of recombination. Am J Hum Genet 37: 482–498

Nee LE, Polinsky RJ, Eldridge R, Weingartner H, Smallberg S, Ebert M (1983) A family with histologically confirmed Alzheimer's disease. Arch Neurol 40: 203–208

Neve RL, Stewart GD, Newcomb P, Van Keuren ML, Patterson D, Drabkin HA, Kurnit DM (1986) Human chromosome 21-encoded cDNA clones. Gene 49: 361–369

Stewart GD, Harris P, Galt J, Ferguson-Smith MA (1985) Cloned DNA probes regionally mapped to human chromosome 21 and their use in determining the origin of nondisjunction. Nucl Acids Res 13: 4125–4132

St George-Hyslop PH, Tanzi RE, Polinsky RJ, Haines JL, Nee L, Watkins PC, Myers RH, Feldman RG, Pollen D, Drachman D, Growdon J, Bruni A, Foncin J-F, Salmon D, Frommelt P, Amaducci L, Sorbi S, Piacentini S, Stewart GD, Hobbs WJ, Conneally PM, Gusella JF (1987) The genetic defect causing familial Alzheimer's disease maps on chromosome 21. Science 235: 885–890

Tanzi RE, Gusella JF, Watkins PC, Bruns GAP, St George-Hyslop P, Van Keuren ML, Patterson D, Pagan S, Kurnit DM, Neve RL (1987) Amyloid β-protein gene: cDNA, mRNA distribution, and genetic linkage near the Alzheimer locus. Science 235: 880–884

Tanzi RE, St George-Hyslop PH, Haines JL, Polinsky RJ, Nee L, Foncin J-F, Neve RL, McClatchey AI, Conneally PM, Gusella JF (1987) The genetic defect in familial Alzheimer's disease is not tightly linked to the amyloid β-protein gene. Nature 329: 156–157

Terry RD, Katzman R (1983) Senile dementia of the Alzheimer type. Ann Neurol 14: 497–506

Van Broeckhoven C, Genthe AM, Vandenberghe A, Horsthemke B, Backhovens H, Raeymaekers P, Van Hul W, Wehnert A, Gheuens J, Cras P, Bruyland M, Martin JJ, Salbaum M, Multhaup G, Masters CL, Beyreuther K, Gurling HMD, Mullan MJ, Holland A, Barton A, Irving N, Williamson R, Richards SJ, Hardy JA (1987) Failure of familial Alzheimer's disease to segregate with the A4-amyloid gene in several European families. Nature 329: 153–155

Van Keuren ML, Watkins PC, Drabkin HA, Jabs EW, Gusella JF, Patterson D (1986) Regional localization of DNA sequences on chromosome 21 using somatic cell hybrids. Am J Hum Genet 38: 793–804

Watkins PC, Tanzi RE, Cheng SV, Gusella JF (1987) Molcular genetics of human chromosome 21. J Med Genet 24: 257–270

Watkins PC, Tanzi RE, Gibbons KT, Tricoli JV, Landes G, Eddy R, Shows TB, Gusella JF (1985) Isolation of polymorphic DNA segments from human chromosome 21. Nucl Acids Res 13: 6075–6088

Alternative cDNA Clones of Amyloid β Protein Precursor Gene Encode Proteinase Inhibitor

D. Goldgaber, J. W. Teener, and *D. C. Gajdusek*

Summary

The amyloid beta protein precursor (APP) gene encodes several different mRNAs that share identical sequences, including the 43 amino acid long amyloid beta protein region. The region that is distinct is encoded by two exons 168 bp and 57 bp long. These two exons are both spliced out in one form of APP mRNA, the 168 bp long exon is utilized in a second form, and both exons are utilized in a third form. In addition, alternative polyadenylation sites are used in generation of the third form of APP mRNA. The deduced amino acid sequence of the 168 bp long exon has approximately 50% homology with Kunitz type protease inhibitors, with all six cysteine residues conserved. Both exons are highly conserved in evolution and are found in the genomes of monkey, dog, rat and mouse. The overexpression of the APP gene encoding the protease inhibitor domain may lead to interference with the normal processing of the amyloid protein precursor and result in the formation of the amyloid beta protein.

Introduction

The isolation and characterization of cDNA clones encoding amyloid β protein as part of a larger precursor protein strongly suggested an abnormality in the processing of this precursor in patients with Alzheimer's disease (Goldgaber et al. 1987). The processing of proteins is a multistep cascade event involving proteolysis at one or more stages. A proper control of proteolysis is crucial in the processing of proteins.

The overexpression of the amyloid β protein precursor (APP) gene, proposed earlier as a prerequisite for the amyloid β protein formation (Goldgaber et al. 1987), has now been documented in both Down's syndrome (Tanzi et al. 1987) and in Alzheimer's disease (Cohen et al. 1988; Higgins et al. 1988; Schmechel et al. 1988).

Amyloid β precurser and proteinase inhibitor

In order to understand the structure and expression of the APP gene we have isolated and sequenced APP cDNA clones from a normal human fibroblast cDNA library and from a normal human brain stem cDNA library. These clones could be divided into two groups according to their open reading frames (ORF; Fig. 1). One group consists

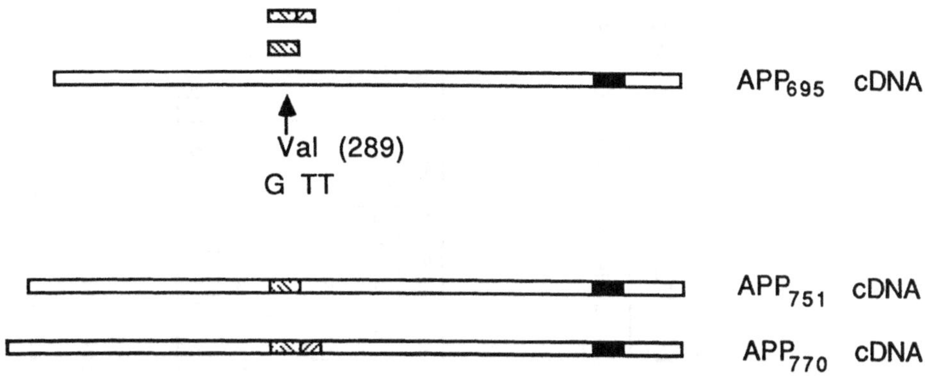

Fig. 1. A schematic representation of APP open reading frames (ORF). Clones with ORF APP_{751} and APP_{770} were isolated from the normal human fibroblast and normal human brain stem cDNA libraries; clones with ORF APP_{695} were isolated from the brain cDNA libraries. *Open box,* open reading frame; *black box,* amyloid beta protein region; *hatched boxes,* 168 bp and 225 bp inserts; *arrow pointing up* indicates GTT codon for valine at position 289

of clones with ORF of 695 amino acids described by Kang and colleagues (Kang et al. 1987) and the second with larger alternative ORFs, APP_{751} and APP_{770}, identified recently in clones isolated from transformed cell cDNA libraries (Ponte et al. 1988; Tanzi et al. 1988; Kitaguchi et al. 1988). The nucleotide sequences of the new ORFs are identical to that of APP_{695}, except for a 168 bp or 225 bp insert between G and TT of the GTT codon for valine at position 289. The 225 bp insert contained the entire 168 bp insert followed by 57 additional base pairs (Fig. 2). The inserts did not interrupt the ORF and new polypeptides of 751 and 770 amino acids could be deduced from these clones.

Computer analysis of the deduced polypeptides revealed about 50% identity between the amino acid sequence encoded by the inserts and the Kunitz family of small serine proteinase inhibitors (Laskowski and Kato 1980). Six cysteine residues were found in conserved positions. The reactive site was gly-pro-cys-arg-ala, with arginine in the P_1 position (Fig. 3). These results were in agreement with earlier reports on APP cDNA clones isolated from transformed cell cDNA libraries (Ponte et al. 1988; Tanzi et al. 1988; Kitaguchi et al. 1988). The reactive site residue P_1, generally corresponds to the specificity of the cognate enzyme. Inhibitors with P_1 arginine tend to inhibit trypsin-like enzymes.

This Kunitz-type proteinase inhibitor is the second serine proteinase inhibitor found to be associated with the amyloid β protein. The first one, α_1-antichymotrypsin, was found in extracellular deposits of amyloid in brains of patients with Alzheimer's disease (Abraham et al. 1988). It was also found that α_1-antichymotrypsin was overexpressed in brains of patients with Alzheimer's disease.

The finding of alternative APP cDNA clones encoding both the amyloid β protein and a proteinase inhibitor in normal human cDNA libraries raises a number of questions about the relationship, if any, between the inhibitor and the processing of the precursor of amyloid β protein. The physiological function of proteinase inhibitors

```
      *
GPCRA                    168 bp
EVCSEQAETGPCRAMISRWYFDVTEGKCAPFFYGGCGGNRNNFDTEEYCMAVCGSAI                         57 a.a.

                         225 bp
EVCSEQAETGPCRAMISRWYFDVTEGKCAPFFYGGCGGNRNNFDTEEYCMAVCGSAMSQSLLKTTQEPLARDPVKL      76 a.a.
```

Fig. 2. 57 amino acid sequence deduced from the 168 bp insert and 76 amino acid sequence deduced from the 225 bp insert in a one-letter code. Letters GPCRA above amino acid sequence show reactive site of the inhibitor with arginine marked by *asterisk* at the P_1 position

```
                                    P1
57 a.a. insert   E V C S E Q A E T G P C R A M I S R W Y F D V T E G K C A P F F Y G G C G G N R N N F D T E E Y C M A V C G S A I
ITI    Horse     A A C N L P I V Q G P C R A F I R L W A F D A A Q G K C V L F T Y G G C R G N G N K F Y S Q K E C K E Y C G I P G
ITI    Pig       S A C S L P I V Q G P C R A F I R L W A F D A A Q G K C V L F N Y G G C Q G N G N K F Y S Q K E C K E Y C G V P G
BPIP   Bovine    D F C L E P I Y T G P C K A R I I R Y F Y N A K A G L C Q T F V Y G G C R A K R N N F K S A E D C M R T C G G A I
SBPI   Bovine    D F C L E P P Y T G P C K A A M I R Y F Y N A K A G F C E T F V Y G G C R A K S N N F K S A E D C M R T C G G A
ITI    Human     D S C Q L G Y S A G P C M G M T S R Y F Y N G T S M A C E T F Q Y G G C M G N G N N F V T E K E C L Q T C R T V A

                     C         C                   C           C                 C   C
```

Fig. 3. Comparison of the 57 amino acid insert from APP cDNA clones with the sequences of Kunitz family of small serine protease inhibitors from Protein Sequence Database: National Research Foundation, Washington, D.C. ITI, inter-α-tripsin inhibitor; BPIP, basic protease inhibitor precursor; SBPI, serum basic protease inhibitor; P_1 indicates basic amino acid residue arginine in the active site. *Underlined letters* below compared sequences indicate highly conserved cysteine residues

in general is elimination, or control, of proteolysis (Laskowski and Kato 1980). The overexpression of both α_1-antichymotrypsin and APP in brains of patients with Alzheimer's disease is, so far, the only abnormality associated clearly with amyloid formation. The nature of this association is not yet known.

References

Abraham CR, Selkoe DJ, Potter H (1988) Immunochemical identification of the serine protease inhibitor α_1-antichymotrypsin in the brain amyloid deposits of Alzheimer's disease. Cell 52: 487–501

Cohen ML, Golde TE, Usiak MF, Younkin LH, Younkin SG (1988) In situ hybridization of nucleus basalis neurons shows increased β-amyloid mRNA in Alzheimer's disease. Proc Natl Acad Sci USA 85: 1227–1231

Goldgaber D, Lerman MI, McBride OW, Saffiotti U, Gajdusek DC (1987) Characterization and chromosomal localization of a cDNA encoding brain amyloid of Alzheimer's disease. Science 235: 877–880

Higgins GA, Lewis DA, Bahmanyar S, Goldgaber D, Gajdusek DC, Young WG, Morrison JH, Wilson MC (1988) Differential regulation of amyloid-β-protein mRNA expression within hippocampal neuronal subpopulations in Alzheimer's disease. Proc Natl Acad Sci USA 85: 1297–1301

Kang J, Lemaire HG, Unterbeck A, Salbaum JM, Masters CL, Grzeschik K-H, Multhaup G, Beyreuther K, Muller-Hill B (1987) The precursor of Alzheimer's disease amyloid A4 protein resembles a cell-surface receptor. Nature 325: 733–736

Kitaguchi N, Takahashi Y, Tokushima Y, Shiojiri S, Ito H (1988) Novel precursor of Alzheimer's disease amyloid protein shows protease inhibitory activity. Nature 331: 530–532

Laskowski M, Kato I (1980) Protein inhibitors of proteinases. Rev Biochem 49: 593–626

Ponte P, Gonzales-DeWhitt P, Schilling J, Miller J, Hsu D, Greenberg B, Davis K, Wallace W, Lieberburg I, Fuller F, Cordell B (1988) A new A4 amyloid mRNA contains a domain homologous to serine proteinase inhibitors. Nature 331: 525–527

Schmechel DE, Goldgaber D, Burkhart DS, Gilbert JR, Gajdusek DC, Roses AD (1988) Cellular localization of messager RNA encoding amyloid-beta-protein in normal tissue and in Alzheimer's disease. Alzheimer Dis Assoc Dis J 2: 96–111

Tanzi RE, Gusella JF, Watkins PC, Bruns GA, St George-Hyslop P, Van Keuren ML, Patterson D, Pagan S, Kurnit DM, Neve RL (1987) Amyloid beta protein gene: cDNA, mRNA distribution, and genetic linkage near the Alzheimer's locus. Science 235: 880–884

Tanzi RE, McClatchey AI, Lamperti ED, Villa-Komaroff L, Gusella JF, Neve RL (1988) Protease inhibitor domain encoded by an amyloid precursor mRNA associated with Alzheimer's disease. Nature 331: 528–530

Precursor of Alzheimer's Disease (PAD) A4 Amyloid Protein

C. L. Masters, G. Multhaup, J. M. Salbaum, A. Weidemann, T. Dyrks, C. Hilbich, P. Fischer, G. König, J. Beer, D. Bunke, U. Mönning, S. Fuller, R. Martins, G. Simms, B. Rumble, and *K. Beyreuther*

Summary

Alzheimer's disease affects 1% of the population of the Western world and 100% of aged individuals with Down's syndrome. It is characterized by neuronal dysfunction and depositions of amyloid A4 protein (β-protein) in the form of intracellular neurofibrillary tangles, extracellular plaques and cerebrovascular amyloid. Amyloid A4 is a self-aggregating protein that consists of 42–43 residues. "Reverse genetics" based on the sequence of amyloid A4 protein has indicated that the amyloid protein is encoded as part of a larger protein by a gene on chromosome 21. Recent cloning studies have indicated that the amyloid precursor gene encodes at least three alternatively spliced products.

We suggest that amyloid formation may arise as a consequence of membrane damage. Accordingly, amyloid formation would be a secondary event, yet could cause selective neuronal dysfunction in Alzheimer's disease. We also suggest that if amyloid deposition occurs at clinical target sites, such as in neurons or between synapses, amyloid formation could be a crucial event for the clinical expression of dementia.

The localization of the amyloid precursor in rat brain at or near the surface of neurons is in agreement with such a concept and leads to the proposal of a function of the precursor A4 protein in cell-cell interactions.

Introduction

Alzheimer's disease (AD) is the commonest cerebral degenerative disorder causing amyloid deposits in the brain and dementia. The disease is age-related in a most unusual fashion: in Down's syndrome (DS) amyloidogenesis occurs between the ages of 10–30; in familial AD (FAD) onset tends to occur between 30–60, whereas in sporadic AD onset is later, in the 60–80 age group. The development of the clinical features of AD is linked to the amount of deposition of amyloid in the limbic areas and cerebral cortex. The amyloid is found in three locations: intracellular deposits in neurons in the form of neurofibrillary tangles (NFT) and extracellular deposits in the neuropil as amyloid plaque cores (APC) and congophillic angiopathy (ACA). The major protein component isolated from NFT, APC and ACA is a self-aggregating small polypeptide of 4–4.5 kd, the A4 protein (Masters et al. 1985 a, b; Beyreuther et al. 1986; Glenner and Wong 1984 a, b). The same A4 subunit is found in the NFT isolated from neurons in the Guam Parkinsonism-dementia complex (Guiroy et al. 1987).

Precursor of the A4 Molecule (PreA4)

Since the A4 molecule is small and unlikely to be a primary translational product, we predicted (Masters et al. 1985 a) that it would be derived from a larger precursor. This precursor (PreA4) has now been characterized with respect to both nucleotide sequence and deduced amino acid sequence from the analysis of a full-length cDNA encoding a primary translational product of 695 residues (Kang et al. 1987). RNA blot hybridization reveals two transcripts of 3.4 and 3.2 kb in fetal cortex (Kang et al. 1987), indicating that more than one translation product is encoded by the PAD gene (precursor of Alzheimer's disease amyloid A4 protein). The PAD gene is located on chromosome 21 (Kang et al. 1987; Goldgaber et al. 1987; Tanzi et al. 1987 a; Robakis et al. 1987), within the band 21q21 (Blanquet et al. 1987; Robakis et al. 1987; Van Broeckhoven et al. 1987; Zabel et al. 1988) in or near the 21q21–21q22.1 boundary segment, the triplication of which may be sufficient for the phenotypic expression of DS.

The genetic locus which controls expression of FAD has also been mapped to chromosome 21 (St George-Hyslop 1987 a) but is separable from the coding region of the PAD gene (Van Broeckhoven et al. 1987; Tanzi et al. 1987 b). The postulated duplication of the PAD gene in AD, analogous to that seen in Down's syndrome (DS), has not yet been demonstrated (Delabar et al. 1987, St George-Hyslop et al. 1987 b; Podlisny et al. 1987; Tanzi et al. 1987 c; Van Broeckhoven et al. 1987). There are at least three alternatively spliced products of the PAD gene: the originally described protein with 695 residues ($PreA4_{695}$), and two other larger proteins of 751 residues ($PreA4_{751}$) and 770 residues ($Pre\ A4_{770}$; Kang et al. 1987; Ponte et al. 1988; Tanzi et al. 1988; Kitaguchi et al. 1988). The two longer forms carry an additional domain with protease inhibitor function. The 695-residue amyloid A4 precursor is an integral, glycosylated membrane protein of 92 kD which spans the bilayer once (Dyrks et al. 1988). It consists of three extracellular domains that follow a transient signal sequence of 17 residues, a transmembrane domain and a 47-residue cytoplasmic domain. It has the typical structural features of a cell-surface receptor.

The PAD Promoter

We have cloned and characterized the promoter of the amyloid A4 protein precursor gene, which we hereafter refer to as PAD (precursor of Alzheimer's disease A4 amyloid protein gene) to address questions on the transcriptional control of the amyloid A4 precursor gene (Salbaum et al., submitted for publication). The PAD promoter strongly resembles the promoters of "housekeeping" genes. It lacks a typical TATA box and shows a high GC content of 72% in a DNA region that confers promoter activity to a reporter gene in an in vivo assay. Transcription initiates at multiple sites. Sequences homologous to the consensus binding sites of transcription factor AP-1/Fos and the heat-shock control element binding protein were found upstream of the RNA start sites. Six copies of a nine base pair-long, GC-rich element are located between position −200 and −100. A protein-DNA interaction could be mapped to this element. The 3.8 kb of the 5 region of the PAD gene includes two Alu-type repetitive sequences. These findings suggest that four mechanisms may participate in the transcription regulation of the PAD gene. These are the stress-related heat-shock element; the oncogene related AP-1/Fos binding site; the potential protein binding at the GC-rich element; and the possible methylation of the CpG region. A disturbance in the regulation of PAD gene products over a longer period of time could well contribute to the rate of amyloid formation. Control of PAD gene expression in the clinical conditions of Down's syndrome and familial and sporadic AD might have therapeutic potential.

Elevated levels of PreA4, presumably the result of overexpression, are found in DS but not in AD (Rumble et al., manuscript in preparation). Selective overexpression of PreA4 mRNA in certain neuronal populations is suggested by some in situ hybridization studies (Cohen et al. 1988; Higgins et al. 1988) but not others (Lewis et al. 1988). Northern blots of cortical mRNA also fail to demonstrate a gene-dosage effect in AD (Godert, 1987).

The amyloid A4 sequence corresponds to residues 597–638/639 of $PreA4_{695}$ (Kang et al. 1987). If the amyloid is a proteolytic breakdown product of the precursor, cleavage has to occur in the 3rd extracellular domain that spans residues 290–624 of $PreA4_{695}$ and within the transmembrane domain (residues 625–648). Amyloid formation may arise as a consequence of membrane damage. Accordingly, amyloid formation would be a secondary event but yet could still cause selective neuronal dysfunction in AD. We suggest that if amyloid deposition occurs at clinical target sites, such as in neurons or between synapses, amyloid formation could be a crucial event for the clinical expression of dementia (Dyrks et al. 1988)

PreA4 and Amyloid A4 Precursor-Product Relationship

Since the precursor-product relationship for PreA4 and amyloid A4, and the specific biochemical events leading to the release of the amyloidogenic peptide are not established, we have studied the in vitro expression of the full-length cDNA copy of the 695-residue PreA4 (Dyrks et al. 1988) and of the 770-residue PreA4 (unpublished). We have also analysed the transmembrane orientation and biogenesis of the in vitro translation product. We constructed, cloned and expressed DNA fragments that encode the putative signal peptide and two of the three putative extracellular domains of the PreA4 proteins, as well as DNA fragments that encode the part of the precursor corresponding to the amyloidogenic fragment together with the putative transmembrane and cytoplasmic domains. Thus, we were able to identify and determine the size of the putative signal peptide and the aggregational properties of the part of the molecule that includes the amyloid sequence.

We have been able to demonstrate that the precursor of the AD-specific amyloid A4 protein is an integral, glycosylated membrane protein which spans the bilayer once (Dyrks et al. 1988). The carboxy-terminal domain of 47 residues was located at the cytoplasmic side of the membrane. The three domains following the transient signal sequence of 17 residues face the opposite side of the membrane. The C-terminal 100 residues of the precursor comprising the amyloid A4 part and the cytoplasmic domain have a high tendency to aggregate, and proteinase K treatment results in peptides of the size of amyloid A4. This finding supports the concept that there is a precursor-product relationship between precursor and amyloid A4.

The experimentally determined relative molecular mass of 91500 for $PreA4_{695}$ and 103000 for $PreA4_{770}$ determined for the in vitro synthesized proteins in the presence and absence of membranes is substantially higher than the theoretical value calculated from the cDNA-derived protein sequence for the PreA4s of 78.6 kd and 88.6 kd, respectively (Dyrks et al. 1988; Kang et al. 1987; Kitaguchi et al. 1988). An explanation for this unexpected electrophoretic mobility on SDS gels would be reduced SDS binding of the very acidic second extracellular domain that includes 45 negatively charged Asp and Glu residues in the PreA4 sequence 188–290. In vitro synthesis of the 303 N-terminal residues of PreA4 which contain this negatively charged domain resulted in a protein of relative molecular mass of 39000 instead of the calculated 33700. Since the same mass difference of 15% between calculated and experimentally determined molecular mass was found for the two entire precursors, the postulated reduction in SDS binding may be responsible for this abnormal migration in the gel.

The $PreA4_{695}$ sequence includes two N-glycosylation sites in the third domain at positions 467–469 and 496–498 and a N-glycosylation negative Asn-Pro-Thr sequence located in the cytoplasmic domain. Translation of the entire precursor in the presence of membranes leads to the removal of the 17-residue-long signal sequence and the addition of two carbohydrate chains due to N-glycosylation. Competitive inhibition of carbohydrate transfer with N-glycosylation-acceptor-tripeptides showed a 2-kd mass change, a value compatible with two carbohydrate moieties being added.

From our in vitro translation studies, we conclude that there is not a simple PreA4-amyloid relationship. Protease treatment of the full-length in vitro translation products does not result in amyloid A4 formation. In view of our finding that the precursor fragment beginning with the amyloid A4 sequence does aggregate, we conclude that besides proteolytic cleavage, other events, such as post-translational modification, are important.

A4 Protein Deposition

The diagnosis of AD is difficult in the absence of a specific marker for disease. Immunocytochemical techniques are more sensitive and are quite specific for the demonstration of A4 protein deposition (Davies et al. 1988). Immunocytochemistry is proving of great value in distinguishing the A4 amyloid of AD from the PrP amyloid of Creutzfeld-Jakob disease (CJD), kuru and the Gerstmann-Sträussler syndrome (GSS). We have also used immunocytochemistry on population-based surveys of amyloid A4 protein deposition to estimate the time it takes to develop these lesions (Rumble et al., in preparation; Davies et al. 1988). Our estimate of 30 years is in agreement with the age of the amyloid judged by the rate of racemization (Shapira et al. 1988).

The PAD gene is expressed in brain and in peripheral tissues such as muscle and epithelial cells (Tanzi et al. 1987 a; Goedert 1987; Shivers et al. 1988; Bahmanyar et al. 1987; Zimmermann et al. 1988). In contrast, the pathological hallmarks of AD,

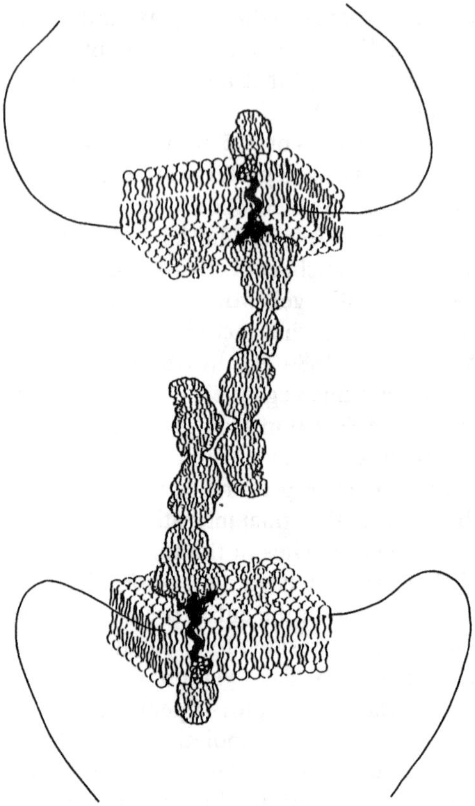

Fig. 1. Hypothetical models for the homotypic interaction of $PreA4_{695}$ and $PreA4_{751/770}$ on apposing neural cell processes (presynaptic and postsynaptic). *Darkened amyloidogenic region* (A4 sequence) corresponds to the stem-like structure that anchors the molecules in the lipid membrane

amyloid depositions in the form of NFT, APC and ACA, are strictly confined to the brain. Using immunocytochemistry PreA4 is detected in brain sections as patches on or near the plasma membrane of neuronal cell bodies and their proximal dendrites (Shivers et al. 1988). These data suggest a role for the precursor in cell contact (Fig. 1). Further support for such a concept comes from the variable presence of the additional domain in the sequence of the alternatively spliced forms of the amyloid A4 precursor that functions as a serine protease inhibitor (Kitaguchi et al. 1988). This domain is inserted between the 2nd and 3rd extracellular domains of $PreA4_{695}$, either in the form of 56 residues (Ponte et al. 1988; Tanzi et al. 1988) or of 75 residues (Kitaguchi et al. 1988). A clue to the function of the inhibitor domain of $PreA4_{751}$ and $PreA4_{770}$ may be that the glia-derived neurite-promoting factor also includes a protease inhibitor domain which is thought to control protease-dependent neurite extension (Gloor et al. 1986). By analogy, $PreA4_{751}$ and $PreA4_{770}$ could control protease- dependent processes required for both brain plasticity and tissue regeneration, since the corresponding mRNAs are found in brain and in peripheral organs (Tanzi et al. 1988; Kitaguchi et al. 1988). However, the existence of $PreA4_{695}$ that lacks the protease inhibitor domain, as well as the multidomain structure of the whole PreA4, suggests that more than protease inhibitor function is specified by the members of this protein family.

Conclusion

In both the unconventional virus diseases (scrapie, CJD, kuru and GSS) and the AD-related conditions (DS, FAD, sporadic AD, Guam Parkinsonism-dementia complex, and normal aging) there is now ample evidence for neuronal membrane glycoproteins which, in some manner, are converted into an amyloidogenic species. The amyloid which is deposited in these infectious diseases (Masters et al. 1981) is now known to be composed of the PrP protein (Bolton et al. 1982; Prusiner et al. 1983; Bendheim et al. 1984; Hope et al. 1988), a host-encoded protein (Oesch et al. 1985) which copurifies with infectivity. The scrapie-associated fibril (SAF; Merz et al. 1981) is also amyloid in nature but distinguishable structurally from the fibrils which constitute the extracellular plaques and vascular deposits. The neuronal origin of PrP (Kretzschmar et al. 1986) suggests that a similar process underlies amyloidogenesis in both AD and these infectious diseases. Since the PrP gene (Prn-p) is probably the same as the Sinc (scrapie incubation period) gene (Carlson et al. 1986; Westaway et al. 1987), a fundamental role of PrP might lie in the replicative cycle of the infectious agent. The conversion of a protease-sensitive neuronal membrane glycoprotein into a protease-resistant subunit which aggregates into amyloid fibrils is a key step in the pathogenesis of these diseases. The genetic elements controlling this event may prove to be of fundamental importance in unravelling the nature not only of the infectious agent but also the diseases which appear as premature forms of aging.

Acknowledgements. Financial support from the Deutsche Forschungsgemeinschaft, the BMFT of the F. R. G., the Thyssen Foundation, the Boehringer Ingelheim Fonds, the Fonds der chemischen Industrie of the F. R. G., the Humboldt Foundation, the Alzheimer's Disease and Related Disorders Association and the NH and MRC of Australia is gratefully acknowledged.

References

Bahmanyar S, Higgins GA, Goldgaber D, Lewis DA, Morrison JH, Wilson MC, Shankar SK, Gajdusek DC (1987) Localization of amyloid β protein messenger RNA in brains from Alzheimer's disease patients. Science 237: 77–80

Bendheim PE, Barry RA, DeArmond SJ, Stites DP, Prusiner SB (1984) Antibodies to a scrapie prion protein. Nature 310: 418–421

Beyreuther K, Multhaup G, Simms G, Pottgiesser J, Schroeder W, Martins RN, Masters CL (1986) Neurofibrillary tangles of Alzheimer's disease and "aged" Down's syndrome contain the same protein as the amyloid of plaque cores and blood vessels. Discussions in Neurosci 3: 68–79, 143–157

Blanquet V, Goldgaber D, Turleau C, Créau-Goldberg N, Delabar J, Sinet PM, Roudier M, de Grouchy J (1987) The β amyloid protein (AD-AP) cDNA hybridizes in normal and Alzheimer individuals near the interface of 21q21 and q22.1. Ann Génét 30: 68–69

Bolton DC, McKinley MP, Prusiner SB (1982) Identification of a protein that purifies with the scrapie prion. Science 218: 1309–1311

Carlson GA, Kingsbury DT, Goodman PA, Coleman S, Marshall ST, DeArmond S, Westaway D, Prusiner SB (1986) Linkage of prion protein and scrapie incubation time genes. Cell 46: 503–511

Cohen ML, Golde TE, Usiak MF, Younkin, LH, Younkin SG (1988) In situ hybridization of nucleus basalis neurons shows increased β-amyloid mRNA in Alzheimer disease. Proc Natl Acad Sci USA 85: 1227–1231

Davies L, Wolska B, Hilbich C, Multhaup G, Martins R, Simms G, Beyreuther K, Masters CL (1988) A4 amyloid protein deposition and the diagnosis of Alzheimer's disease: prevalence in aged brains determined by immunocytochemistry compared with conventional neuropathologic techniques. Neurology (in press)

Delabar J-M, Goldgaber D, Lamour Y, Nicole A, Huret J-L, de Grouchy J, Brown P, Gajdusek DC, Sinet P-M (1987) β amyloid gene duplication in Alzheimer's disease and karyotypically normal Down syndrome. Science 235: 1390–1392

Dyrks T, Weidemann A, Multhaup G, Salbaum JM, Lemaire H-G, Kang J, Müller-Hill B, Masters CL, Beyreuther K (1988) Identification transmembrane orientation and biogenesis of the amyloid A4 precursor of Alzheimer's disease. EMBO J 7: 949–957

Glenner GG, Wong CW (1984a) Alzheimer's disease: initial report of the purification and characterization of a novel cerebrovascular amyloid protein. Biochem Biophys Res Comm 120: 885–890

Glenner GG, Wong CW (1984b) Alzheimer's disease and Down's syndrome: sharing of a unique cerebrovascular amyloid fibril protein. Biochem Biophys Res Comm 122: 1131–1135

Gloor S, Odink K, Guenther J, Nick H, Monard D (1986) A glia-derived neurite promoting factor with protease inhibitory activity belongs to the protease nexins. Cell 47: 687–693

Goedert M (1987) Neuronal localization of amyloid beta protein precursor mRNA in normal human brain and in Alzheimer's disease. EMBO J 6: 3627–3632

Goldgaber D, Lerman MI, McBride OW, Saffiotti U, Gajdusek DC (1987) Characterization and chromosomal localization of a cDNA encoding brain amyloid of Alzheimer's disease. Science 235: 877–880

Guiroy DC, Miyazaki M, Multhaup G, Fischer P, Garruto RM, Beyreuther K, Masters CL, Simms G, Gibbs CJ Jr, Gajdusek DC (1987) Amyloid of neurofibrillary tangles of Guamanian parkinsonism-dementia and Alzheimer disease share identical amino acid sequence. Proc Natl Acad Sci USA 84: 2073–2077

Higgins GA, Lewis DA, Bahmanyar S, Goldgaber D, Gajdusek DC, Young WG, Morrison JH, Wilson MC (1988) Differential regulation of amyloid-β-protein mRNA expression within hippocampal neuronal subpopulations in Alzheimer disease. Proc Natl Acad Sci USA 85: 1297–1301

Hope J, Multhaup G, Reekie LJD, Kimberlin RH, Beyreuther K (1988) Molecular pathology of scrapie-associated fibril protein (PrP) in mouse brain affected by the ME7 strain of scrapie. Eur J Biochem 172: 271–277

Kang J, Lemaire H-G, Unterbeck A, Salbaum JM, Masters CL, Grzeschik K-H, Multhaup G, Beyreuther K, Müller-Hill B (1987) The precursor of Alzheimer's disease amyloid A4 protein resembles a cell-surface receptor. Nature 325: 733–736

Kitaguchi N, Takahashi Y, Tokushima Y, Shiojiri S, Ito H (1988) Novel precursor of Alzheimer's disease amyloid protein shows protease inhibitory activity. Nature 311: 530–532

Kretzschmar HA, Prusiner SB, Stowring LE, DeArmond SJ (1986) Scrapie prion proteins are synthesized in neurons. Am J Pathol 122: 1–5

Lewis DA, Higgins GA, Young WG, Goldgaber D, Gajdusek DC, Wilson MC, Morrison JH (1988) Distribution of precursor amyloid-β-protein messenger RNA in human cerebral cortex: relationship to neurofibrillary tangles and neuritic plaques. Proc Natl Acad Sci USA 85: 1691–1695

Masters CL, Gajdusek DC, Gibbs CJ Jr (1981) Creutzfeldt-Jakob disease virus isolation from the Gerstmann-Sträussler syndrome. With an analysis of the various forms of amyloid plaque deposition in the virus-induced spongiform encephalopathies. Brain 104: 559–587

Masters CL, Simms G, Weinman NA, Multhaup G, McDonald BL, Beyreuther K (1985a) Amyloid plaque core protein in Alzheimer disease and Down syndrome. Proc Natl Acad Sci USA 82: 4245–4249

Masters CL, Multhaup G, Simms G, Pottgiesser J, Martins RN, Beyreuther K (1985b) Neuronal origin of a cerebral amyloid: neurofibrillary tangles of Alzheimer's disease contain the same protein as the amyloid of plaque cores and blood vessels. EMBO J 4: 2757–2763

Merz PA, Somerville RA, Wisniewski HM, Iqbal K (1981) Abnormal fibrils from scrapie-infected brain. Acta Neuropathol 54: 63–74

Oesch B, Westaway D, Wälchli M, McKinley MP, Kent SBH, Aebersold R, Barry RA, Tempst P, Teplow DB, Hood LE, Prusiner SB, Weissmann C (1985) A cellular gene encodes scrapie PrP 27–30 protein. Cell 40: 735–746

Podlisny MB, Lee G, Selkoe DJ (1987) Gene dosage of the amyloid β precursor protein in Alzheimer's disease. Science 238: 669–671

Ponte P, Gonzalez-DeWhitt P, Schilling J, Miller J, Hsu D, Greenberg B, Davis K, Wallace W, Lieberburg I, Fuller F, Cordell B (1988) A new A4 amyloid mRNA contains a domain homologous to serine proteinase inhibitors. Nature 331: 525–527

Prusiner SB, McKinley MP, Bowman KA, Bolton DC, Bendheim PE, Groth DF, Glenner GG (1983) Scrapie prions aggregate to form amyloid-like birefringent rods. Cell 35: 349–358

Robakis NK, Ramakrishna N, Wolfe G, Wisniewski HM (1987) Molecular cloning and characterization of a cDNA encoding the cerebrovascular and neuritic plaque amyloid peptides. Proc Natl Acad Sci USA 84: 4190–4194

Shapira R, Austin GE, Mirra SS (1988) Neuritic plaque amyloid in Alzheimer's disease is highly racemized. J Neurochem 50: 69–74

Shivers BD, Hilbich C, Multhaup G, Salbaum M, Beyreuther K, Seeburg PH (1988) Alzheimer's disease amyloidogenic glycoprotein: expression pattern in rat brain suggests role in cell contact. EMBO J 7: 1365–1370

St George-Hyslop PH, Tanzi RE, Polinsky RJ, Haines JL, Nee L, Watkins PC, Myers RH, Feldman RG, Pollen D, Drachman D, Growdon J, Bruni A, Foncin J-F, Salmon D, Frommelt P, Amaducci L, Sorbi S, Piacentini S, Stewart GD, Hobbs WJ, Conneally PM, Gusella JF (1987a) The genetic defect causing familial Alzheimer's disease maps on chromosome 21. Science 235: 885–890

St George-Hyslop PH, Tanzi RE, Polinsky RJ, Neve RL, Pollen D, Drachman D, Growdon J, Cupples LA, Née L, Myers RH, O'Sullivan D, Watkins PC, Amos JA, Deutsch CK, Bodfish JW, Kinsbourne M, Feldman RG, Bruni A, Amaducci L, Foncin J-F, Gusella JF (1987b) Absence of duplication of chromosome 21 genes in familial and sporadic Alzheimer's disease. Science 238: 664–666

Tanzi RE, Gusella JF, Watkins PC, Bruns GAP, St George-Hyslop P, van Keuren ML, Patterson D, Pagan S, Kurnit DM, Neve RL (1987a) Amyloid β protein gene: cDNA, mRNA distribution, and genetic linkage near the Alzheimer locus. Science 235: 880–884

Tanzi RE, St George-Hyslop PH, Haines JL, Polinsky RJ, Nee L, Foncin J-F, Neve RL, McClatchey AI, Conneally PM, Gusella JF (1987b) The genetic defect in familial Alzheimer's disease is not tightly linked to the amyloid β-protein gene. Nature 329: 156–157

Tanzi RE, Bird ED, Latt SA, Neve RL (1987c) The amyloid β protein gene is not duplicated in brains from patients with Alzheimer's disease. Science 238: 666–669

Tanzi RE, McClatchey AI, Lamperti ED, Villa-Komaroff L, Gusella JF, Neve RL (1988) Protease inhibitor domain encoded by an amyloid protein precursor mRNA associated with Alzheimer's disease. Nature 311: 528–530

Van Broeckhoven C, Genthe AM, Vandenberghe A, Horsthemke B, Backhovens H, Raeymaekers P, Van Hul W, Wehnert A, Gheuens J, Cras P, Bruyland M, Martin JJ, Salbaum M, Multhaup G, Masters CL, Beyreuther K, Gurling HMD, Mullan MJ, Holland A, Barton A, Irving N, Williamson R, Richards SJ, Hardy JA (1987) Failure of familial Alzheimer's disease to segregate with the A4-amyloid gene in several European families. Nature 329: 153–155

Westaway D, Goodman PA, Mirenda CA, McKinley MP, Carlson GA, Prusiner SB (1987) Distinct prion proteins in short and long scrapie incubation period mice. Cell 51: 651–662

Zabel BU, Salbaum JM, Multhaup G, Masters CL, Bohl J, Beyreuther K (1988) Sublocalization of the gene for the precursor of Alzheimer's disease amyloid A4 protein on chromosome 21. Human Gene Mapping (in press)

Zimmermann K, Herget T, Salbaum JM, Schubert W, Hilbich C, Cramer M, Masters CL, Multhaup G, Kang J, Lemaire H-G, Beyreuther K, Starzinski-Powitz A (1988) Localization of the putative precursor of Alzheimer's disease-specific amyloid at nuclear envelopes of adult human muscle. EMBO J 7: 367–372

Cloning of the Beta Amyloid Peptide Gene in Alzheimer's Disease

J. N. Octave, F. de Sauvage, A. F. Macq, J. M. Maloteaux, C. G. Rasool, M. P. Vitek, A. J. Blume, J. M. Brucher, T. de Barsy, A. Trouet, and *E. C. Laterre*

Summary

We have isolated and sequenced clones from the brain cDNA libraries derived from three patients with sporadic Alzheimer's disease (AD). Our results indicate that AD β-amyloid peptide (AD-BAPP) clones have sequences which do not differ from those found in BAPP cDNAs isolated from a normal fetus and a normal adult brain. We have noted that the sequence of the non-AD partial BAPP cDNA isolated by Goldgaber et al. differs from the sequences of our AD-BAPP cDNAs. The inverted dinucleotide would translate into serine instead of tyrosine at position 687 in BAPP and thereby create a putative glycosylation site at the C-terminus of the postulated BAPP. Such a difference might affect the processing of BAPP. However, as only one sequence from non-AD brains differs among the five human BAPP cDNAs now reported, the significance of such heterogeneity is unclear.

Among several AD-BAPP clones isolated in cDNA libraries constructed from three patients with AD, we never observed the insertion of 168 bp between position 865 and 866 which has been recently reported in cultured cells. This suggests that even if different populations of BAPP mRNA are present in normal and AD brain, as a result of an alternative splicing of a single transcriptional unit, the BAPP which contains a serine protease inhibitor activity is not widely expressed in AD.

Our results suggest that there are no mutations in or about the 42 amino acid sequence of the BAPP, and that the accumulation of amyloid consistently found in AD may results from altered translation of the mRNA or from altered post-translational processing of BAPP.

Introduction

In 1907, Alois Alzheimer reported the case of a 51-year-old woman who showed rapidly increasing memory and orientation impairment. After 4.5 years of illness, the patient died and the anatomophathological examination of her brain showed very characteristic changes in neurofibrils and the deposition of a peculiar substance in the cerebral cortex (Alzheimer 1907).

Since that time, the origin of the altered substances found in the centre of the so-called senile plaques has been debated. Congo red stains the central core and a typical birefringence characterizes the amyloid substance on polarization microscopy. The amyloid core of the senile plaques is surrounded by degenerating cellular material, increased numbers of microglial cells containing fibrils and lipofuscin aggregates.

In 1985, Masters et al. reported isolating a peptide from senile plaques containing amyloid deposits. This peptide contained about 40 amino acids (aa) and was named the A4 peptide (A for amyloid and 4 because the peptide has a molecular weight of 4 kD). The aa sequence of the NH_2-terminus reveals that this peptide is identical to the beta amyloid peptide (BAP) found a few years earlier by Glenner and Wong (1984), who were interested in vascular amyloid deposition.

In 1987, Kang and collaborators synthesized an oligonucleotide corresponding to the aa 10 to 16 of the BAP and screened a cDNA library obtained from a fetal human brain. The cloning of the BAP revealed some important information. First, the BAP is expressed in a brain which does not show any lesion of AD. Second, BAP seems to be the result of the proteolysis of a larger protein containing 695 aa. This beta amyloid peptide precursor (BAPP) resembles a glycosylated cell-surface receptor whose role is still unknown. Third, the BAPP gene is on chromosome 21.

In about 10% of cases Alzheimer's disease is inherited as an autosomal dominant trait. The chromosomal localization of the defective gene in familial Alzheimer's disease (FAD) has been discovered by using genetic linkage to DNA markers on chromosome 21 (St George-Hyslop et al. 1987a). Furthermore, the gene coding for the BAPP gene has been mapped to the same approximate region of chromosome 21 as that coding for the genetic defect in FAD (Tanzi et al. 1987a), raising the possibility that the BAPP gene product, which could be important in the pathogenesis of AD, is also the site of the inherited defect in FAD. However, restriction fragment length polymorphisms (RFLPs) of the BAP gene have been identified, and the pattern of segregation of the BAP gene in several FAD pedigrees has been determined (Tanzi et al. 1987b; Van Broeckhoven et al. 1987). The detection of several recombination events with FAD suggests that the BAP gene is not the site of the inherited defect underlying this disorder.

In Down's syndrome (DS), amyloid-containing plaques are found in adult brains and the trisomic chromosome 21 is responsible for the overexpression of the BAP gene (Delabar et al. 1987). A third copy of the BAP gene was reported to be in the DNA of some patients with AD (Delabar et al. 1987). However, subsequent studies have found the number of BAP genes to be the same in normal subjects and patients with AD (Furuya et al. 1988; Murdoch et al. 1988; Podlisny et al. 1987; St George-Hyslop et al. 1987b). Additionally, similar levels of BAP mRNA are found on Northern blots of normal and AD brain RNAs (Tanzi et al. 1987a). Thus, quantitative increases in amyloid gene numbers and mRNA levels have become less likely explanations for the increased amyloid deposition in AD.

Recently, a second BAPP mRNA that encodes an additional internal domain with a sequence characteristic of a Kunitz-type serine protease inhibitor has been reported in cultured cells (Ponte et al. 1988; Tanzi et al. 1988; Kitaguchi et al. 1988). This new BAPP mRNA could arise by alternative splicing of a single transcriptional unit.

Increased amyloid deposition in AD might result from differently processing BAPP whose aa sequences vary, as a consequence of an alternative splicing. In order to gain further insight into this possibility, we cloned and characterized BAP cDNAs from three brain libraries of sporadic AD patients. Cloning and characterizing such cDNAs is important since BAP has been isolated and sequenced only from deposits within

AD brains, whereas the three BAPP cDNA clones reported to date have been isolated from libraries constructed from non-diseased brain mRNA.

Data on the Subjects

One of the three clones reported here was from a cDNA library provided by Clontech. This library was derived from the hippocampus of a 67-year-old male patient with sporadic AD. According to the vendor, the diagnosis was achieved through an evaluation of the clinical profile prior to death and the observation of senile plaques in the brain upon post-mortem autopsy.

The second clone was derived from a man (B.P.) who was 64 years old when he died. Alzheimer's disease was diagnosed three years before his death. There were no other known cases of dementia in his family. Memory loss was marked and there was a progressive intellectual deterioration. The patient was diabetic and also presented Parkinson-like hypokinesia of gait. The evolution of the disease was followed by clinical as well as psychological tests. The post-mortem anatomopathological examination confirmed AD by the presence of a large number of senile plaques, neurofibrillary tangles and granulovacuolar alterations in the cerebral cortex (Fig. 1).

The third clone was derived from a man (G.J.) who was 54 years old when he died. The patient was a right-handed technician. The first symptoms were a progressive loss of memory and a disorientation in time. He was examined for the first time at the age of 52: severe ideomotor, ideational, dressing and constructional apraxias were noted with anosognosia. There was agraphia and a failure to understand speech. Memory

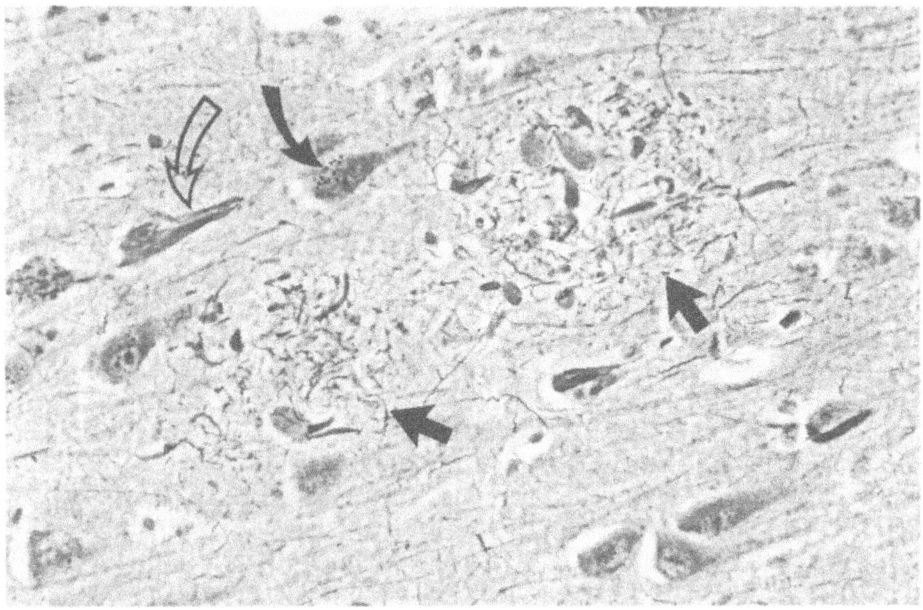

Fig. 1. Anatomopathological examination of the right Ammon's horn from the brain of a patient with AD (B.P., 64 years old). *Arrows* indicate neurofibrillary tangles (⇦), granulovacuolar alterations (➘), and senile plaques (➡)

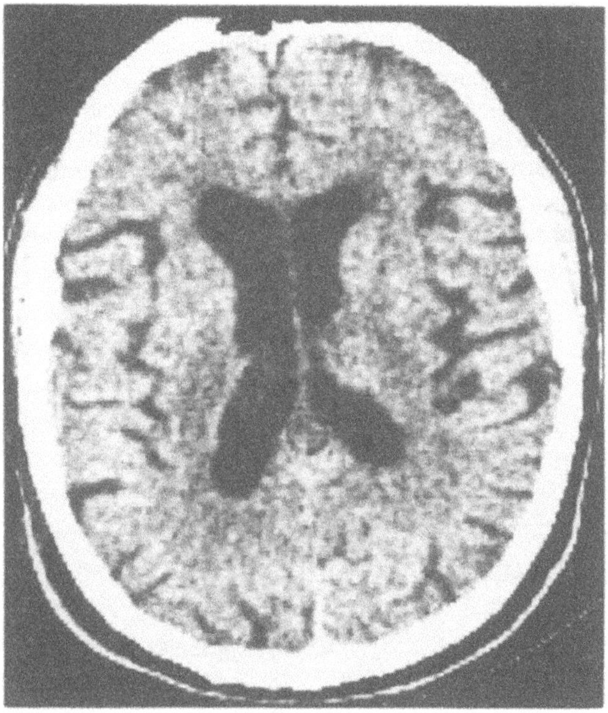

Fig. 2. C.T. scan of the brain of an AD patient (G.J. 52 years old) showing diffuse atrophy of the cerebral cortex and slight enlargement of the lateral ventricles

was severely impaired. The patient rapidly developed a typical presenile AD with aphasia, acalculia and alexia. A CT scan showed cortical atrophy with slight enlargement of the cerebral ventricles (Fig. 2). The diagnosis was confirmed by anatomopathological examination which revealed the presence of senile plaques with amyloid core.

Construction and Screening of cDNA Libraries

The brains of the first (B.P.) and the second patient (G.J.) were recovered 12 and 3 h after death, respectively. One hemisphere of the cerebral cortex was fixed for anatomopathological examination. The remaining brain tissue was dissected on ice, and tissue samples from different areas were immediately frozen in liquid nitrogen and stored at −80 °C until the preparation of RNA.

RNA from frontal cerebral cortex was prepared by homogenization of the tissue in 9 volumes of 5 *M* guanidinium thiocyanate and centrifugation for 24 h at 150000 *g* on a 5.7 *M* cesium chloride cushion, as described by Chirgwin et al. (1979). The quality of RNA prepared from post-mortem human brain was controlled by in vitro translation. Total RNA (10 μg) derived from the cerebral cortex of our first patient (B.P.) was incubated for 90 min at 26° C with a rabbit reticulocyte lysate in a total volume of 25 μl containing 5 μCi [^{35}S]methionine. At the end of the incubation, 2 μl was recovered in order to count the total radioactivity and 2 μl was precipitated with 10% TCA. In the absence or the presence of cerebral cortex RNA, 0,6% and 12% of the radioactivity was precipitated by TCA. The radiolabeled proteins were analysed by polyacrylamide gel electrophoresis in the presence of SDS. The results presented in Fig. 3a indicate that no proteins were synthesized in the absence of RNA but that the RNA isolated from the brain of B.P. was able to produce high molecular weight proteins.

mRNA was isolated by oligo-dT cellulose chromatography, with a recovery of 10 to 20 μg of poly-A+/mg of total RNA. cDNA was synthesized in the presence of reverse transcriptase, RNAse H and DNA polymerase, using Amersham enzymes and protocols. After methylation of the cDNA with *Eco*RI methylase, addition of *Eco*RI

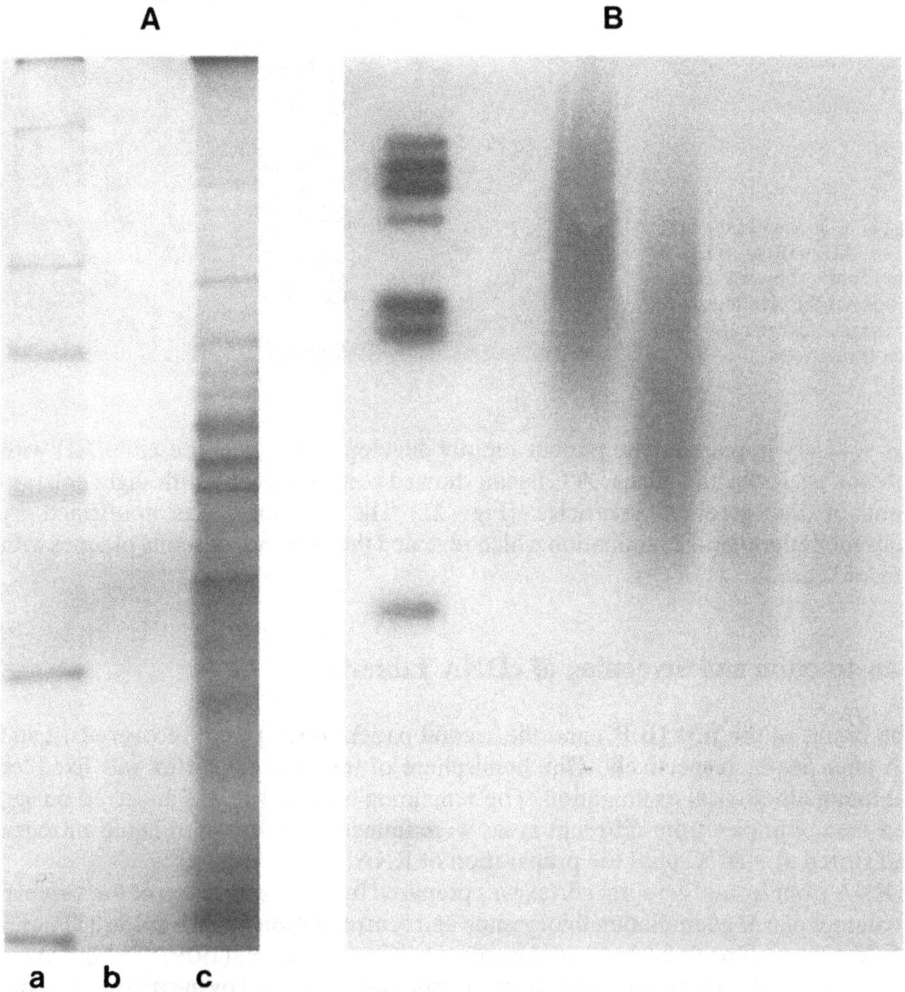

Fig. 3A, B. RNA isolation and cDNA synthesis. **A** In vitro translation of the cerebral cortex RNA isolated from the patient B.P. *a* Molecular weight markers: 220, 92.5, 69, 46, 30, and 14.3 kd. *b* Translation without RNA. *c* Translation of 10 μg cerebral cortex RNA. **B** Size fractionation of labeled cDNA on a Biogel A 50 m column. DNA size markers: 23130, 9416, 6557, 4361, 2322, 2027, 564, and 125 bp

Table 1. cDNA libraries constructed from Alzheimer's disease (AD) brains

Patient	ng cDNA	Plaque formation units	Recombinants %
B.P.	100	990000	96
G.J.	150	4150000	91
Clontech		810000	87

linkers, digestion with *Eco*RI, and size fractionation on agarose A 50 m column, the cDNA fragments were inserted in the *Eco*RI site of the lambda gt 11 vector. After in vitro packaging, the percentage of recombinants was determined by plating the phages on Y 1088 *E. coli* cells in the presence of 1 m*M* X gal. and 5 m*M* IPTG as previously described (Octave et al. 1987). The size fractionation presented in Fig. 3b indicates that long cDNA fragments were synthesized. The characteristics of the two cDNA libraries we have constructed and those of the Clontech library are given in Table 1.

For the screening of the cDNA libraries, we synthesized an oligonucleotide probe (AMYCON) which corresponds to amino acids 9–25 of BAP.

cDNA inserts from recombinant lambda clones were subcloned in the EcoRI site of pUC 19. Sanger-type DNA sequencing of subclones using oligonucleotides which correspond to different portions of the cDNA was as described by Davis et al. (1986).

Isolation and Characterization of cDNA Clones

Six million clones of the cDNA library provided by Clontech were screened with the AMYCON probe. Of the putative positives, LED-701 had the larger insert (approximately 1.6 kb), containing an internal EcoRI site. Following EcoRI digestion, Southern blot analyses showed that ^{32}P-end labeled AMYCON hybridized to a 0.6 kb fragment of LED-701. The two fragments were subcloned into pUC19 and sequenced according to the method of Sanger (Sanger et al. 1977). Comparison of this sequence to that from fetal brain BAPP-cDNA showed that they were identical (Fig. 4 a, b).

The shorter fragment of LED-701 was used for the screening of 500000 clones of our cDNA library constructed from the patient B.P. Of the six positives, B-13A1 had the largest insert, approximately 2.5 kb, containing an internal EcoRI site. The EcoRI fragments were subcloned in pUC19 and sequenced. The results presented in Fig. 4 a, c indicate that, from the position 363 to the position 2633, the sequence is identical to the fetal BAPP-cDNA, containing the BAP coding sequence, the BAPP termination codon and part of the 3′ non-coding sequence of the mRNA.

The shorter fragment of B-13A1 was used for the screening of 200000 clones of our second cDNA library constructed from patient G.J. One clone (G-25A1) containing the BAP coding sequence, the BAPP termination codon and the 3′ non-coding sequence was isolated. The sequence from position 660 to position 2941 was identical to the fetal BAPP-cDNA (Fig. 4 a, d).

It is important to note that all the clones isolated from the AD libraries have sequences which do not differ from those found in BAPP cDNAs isolated from a normal fetus and a normal adult brain.

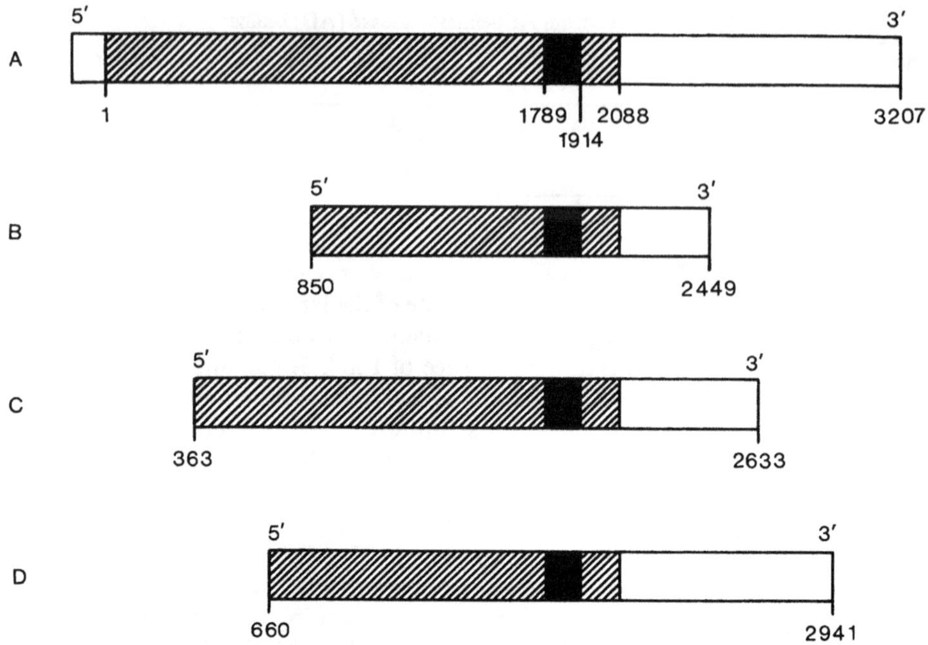

Fig. 4A–D. Schematic representation of various BAPP cDNAs. **A** Human fetal brain cDNA isolated by Kang et al. **B** Human AD brain cDNA isolated from the commercial library. **C** Human AD brain cDNA isolated from patient B.P. **D** Human AD brain cDNA isolated from patient G.J. Nucleotide sequence numbers are given below the boxes representing the non-coding sequences (□), the BAPP (▨), and the BAP (■)

Discussion

RFPs identified on the BAPP gene have been reported not to be genetic markers of FAD in several American and European families (Van Broeckhoven et al. 1987; Tanzi et al. 1987b), indicating that in FAD, the genetic defect is not localized on the BAPP gene. It remains clear, however, that one of the principal histological characteristics of Alzheimer's disease is the presence of amyloid-containing plaques in the cerebral cortex of affected patients. The increased amyloid deposition containing the BAP, in both familial and sporadic cases, could result from an abnormal processing of a BAPP precursor obtained by alternative splicing of a single transcriptional unit. Examples of brain-specific alternative RNA splicing have previously been reported (Nawa et al. 1984; Amara et al. 1982; Martinez et al. 1987), and an alternative splicing of the BAPP transcriptional unit has been recently proposed (Ponte et al. 1988, Tanzi et al. 1988; Kitaguchi et al. 1988).

Dementia refers to deterioration of mental functions and can be due to different organic diseases. Among the degenerative forms of dementia, AD is characterized by different ages of onset and a variety of clinical features, which could correspond to different subtypes, although the lines of clinical distinction remain rarely sharply drawn. There are no biological or ante-mortem markers allowing clear-cut distinctions between clinical subtypes, and AD is currently a diagnosis of exclusion which has to be confirmed by anatomopathological examination.

Therefore, it is very important to know the clinical history of the patients as well as the post-mortem diagnosis in order to make further comparisons of the results obtained at the molecular level.

In this paper, we report on two patients with known clinical histories and confirmed diagnoses of AD. We have isolated and sequenced clones from the brain cDNA libraries derived from these two patients as well as from a third patient, all with sporadic AD. Our results indicate that AD-BAPP clones have sequences which do not differ from those found in BAPP-cDNAs isolated from a normal fetus and a normal adult brain (Kang et al. 1987; Goldgaber et al. 1987; Robakis et al. 1987). We have noted that the sequence of the non-AD partial BAPP-cDNA isolated by Goldgaber et al. differs from the sequences of our AD-BAPP-cDNAs. The inverted dinucleotide would translate into serine instead of tyrosine at aa position 687 in BAPP, and thereby create a putative glycosylation site at the C-terminus of the postulated BAPP. Such a difference might affect processing of BAPP. However, as only one sequence from non-AD brains differs among the five human BAPP-cDNAs now reported, the significance of such heterogeneity is unclear.

Among several AD-BAPP clones isolated in cDNA libraries constructed from three patients with AD, we never observed the insertion of 168 bp between position 865 and 866 which has been recently reported in cultured cells (Ponte et al. 1988; Tanzi et al. 1988; Kitaguchi et al. 1988). This suggests that even if different populations of BAPP-mRNA are present in normal and AD brain, as a result of an alternative splicing of a single transcriptional unit, the BAPP which contains a serine protease inhibitor activity is not widely expressed in AD.

Our results suggest that there are no mutations in or about the 42 aa sequence of the BAP, and that the accumulation of amyloid consistently found in AD may result from altered translation of the mRNA or from altered post-translational processing of BAPP.

Acknowledgments. The excellent technical assistance of A. Cuignet and B. Tasiaux-Doumont is acknowledged. This work was supported by the Belgian Fonds de la Recherche Scientifique Médicale grants no. 3.4560.88 and 3.4553.87 and the Fondation Médicale Reine Elisabeth and a research grant from the Loterie Nationale, Belgium

References

Alzheimer A (1907) Über eine eigenartige Erkrankung der Hirnrinde. Allg Z Psychiatr 64: 146–148

Amara SG, Jonas V, Rosenfeld MG, Ong ES, Evans RM (1982) Alternative RNA processing in calcitonin gene expression generates mRNAs encoding different polypeptide products. Nature 298: 240–244

Chirgwin JM, Przybyla AE, MacDonald RJ, Rutter WJ (1979) Isolation of biological active ribonucleic acid from sources enriched in ribonuclease. Biochemistry 48: 5294–5299

Davis LG, Dibner M, Battey J (1986) Basic methods in molecular biology. Elsevier, New York

Delabar J-M, Goldgaber D, Lamour Y, Nicole A, Huret J-L, de Grouchy J, Brown P, Gajdusek DC, Sinet P-M (1987) Beta-amyloid gene duplication in Alzheimer's disease and karyoty pically normal Down syndrome. Science, 235: 1390–1392

Furuya H, Sasaki H, Goto I, Wong C, Glenner G, Sakaki Y (1988) Amyloid beta-protein duplication is not common in Alzheimer's disease: analysis by polymorphic restriction fragments, Biochem Biophys Res Comm, 150: 75–81

Glenner GG, Wong CW (1984) Alzheimer's disease: initial report of the purification and characterization of a novel cerebrovascular amyloid protein. Biochem Biophys Res Comm 120: 885–890

Goldgaber D, Lerman MI, Bride WO, Saffiotti U, Gajdusek DC (1987) Characterization and chromosomomal localization of a cDNA encoding brain amyloid of Alzheimer's disase. Science 235: 877–880

Kang J, Lemaire HG, Unterbeck A, Salbaum JM, Masters CL, Grzeschik KH, Multhaup G, Beyreuter K, Muller-Hill B (1987) The precursor of Alzheimer's disease amyloid A4 protein resembles a cell-surface receptor. Nature 325: 733–736

Kitaguchi N, Takahashi Y, Tokushima Y, Shiojiri S, Ito H (1988) Novel precursor of Alzheimer's disease amyloid protein shows protease activity, Nature, 331: 530–532

Martinez R, Mathey-Prevot B, Bernards A, Baltimore D (1987) Neuronal $pp60^{c\text{-}src}$ contains a six amino acid insertion relative to its non-neuronal counterpart. Science, 237: 411–416

Masters CL, Simms G, Weiman MA, Multhaup G, McDonald, BL, Beyreuther K (1985) Amyloid plaque core protein in Alzheimer disease and Down's syndrome. Proc Natl Acad Sci USA 82: 4245–4249

Murdoch G, Manuelidis L, Kim J, Manuelidis E (1988) Beta-amyloid dosage in Alzheimer's disease. Nucleic Acids Res 16: 357

Nawa H, Kotani H, Nakanishi S (1984) Tissue-specific generation of two preprotachykinin mRNAs from one gene by alternative RNA splicing. Nature 312: 729–734

Octave JN, de Sauvage F, Maloteaux JM, Laterre EC, Trouet A (1987) Construction of lambda GT 11 cDNA libraries from post-mortem human brains. In: Peeters H (ed) Protides of biological fluids, Vol 35. Pergamon Press, Oxford, pp 67–70

Podlisny MB, Lee G, Selkoe D (1987) Gene dosage of the amyloid beta precursor protein in Alzheimer's disease. Science 238: 669–671

Ponte P, Gonzalez-De Whitt P, Schilling J, Miller J, Hsu D, Greenberg B, Davis K, Wallace W, Lieberburg I, Fuller F, Cordell B (1988) A new A4 amyloid mRNA contains a domain homologous to serine proteinase inhibitors. Nature 331: 525–527

Robakis NK, Ramakrishna N, Wolfe G, Wisniewski HM (1987) Molecular cloning and characterization of a cDNA encoding the cerebrovascular and the neuritic plaque amyloid peptides. Proc Nat Acad Sci USA 84: 4190–4194

Sanger F, Nicklen S, Coulson AR (1977) DNA sequencing with chain-terminating inhibitors, Proc Natl Acad Sci USA 74: 5463–5467

St George-Hyslop PH, Tanzi RE, Polinski RJ, Haines JL, Nee L, Watkins PC, Myers RH, Feldman RG, Pollen D, Drachman D, Growdon J, Bruni A, Foncin J-F, Salmon D, Frommelt P, Amaducci L, Sorbi S, Piacentini S. Gusella JF (1987a) The genetic defect causing Alzheimer's disease maps on chromosome 21. Science 235: 885–889

St George-Hyslop P, Tanzi RE, Polinsky R, Neve R, Pollen D, Drachman D, Growdon J, Cupples L, Nee L, Meyers R, O'Sullivan D, Watkins P, Amos J, Deutsch C, Bodfish J, Kinsbourne M, Feldman R, Bruni A, Amaducci L, Foncin J-F, Gusella JF (1987b) Absence of duplication of chromosome 21 genes in famil̇ial and sporadic Alzheimer's disease, Science 238: 664–666

Tanzi RE, Gusella JF, Watkins PC, Bruns GAP, St George-Hyslop B, Van Keuren ML, Patterson D, Pagan S, Kurnit DM, Neve RL (1987a) Amyloid beta protein gene: cDNA mRNA distribution and genetic linkage near the Alzheimer locus. Science 235: 880–884

Tanzi RE, St George-Hyslop PH, Haines JL, Polinsky RJ, Nee L, Foncin J-F, Neve RL, McClatchey AI, Conneally PM, Gusella JF (1987b) The genetic defect in familial Alzheimer's disease is not tightly linked to the amyloid beta protein gene; Nature 329: 156–157

Tanzi RE, McClatchey AI, Lamperti ED, Villa-Komaroff L, Gusella JF, Neve RL (1988) Protease inhibitor domain encoded by an amyloid protein precursor mRNA associated with Alzheimer's disease. Nature 331: 528–530

Van Broeckhoven C, Genthe AM, Vandenberghe A, Horsthemke B, Backhovens H, Raeymaekers P, Van Hul W, Wehnert A, Gheuens J, Cras P, Bruyland M, Martin JJ, Salbaum M, Multhaup G, Masters CL, Beyreuther K, Gurlind HMD, Mullan MJ, Holland A, Barton A, Irving N, Williamson R, Richards SJ, Hardy JA (1987) Failure of Alzheimer's disease to segregate with the A4 amyloid gene in several European families. Nature 329: 153–155

Molecular Analysis of Patients with Alzheimer's Disease

J.-M. Delabar, Z. Rahmani, J.-L. Blouin, A. Nicole, N. Creau-Goldberg, I. Ceballos, Y. Lamour, M. Roudier, P. Davous, and *P.-M. Sinet*

Summary

The possibility of a genetic link between Alzheimer's disease (AD) and Down's syndrome (DS) is supported by the similarity of the neuropathological and neurochemical changes found in the brain of AD patients and middle-aged DS patients. To test this hypothesis we performed gene dosage experiments with DNA sequences that we found duplicated in DS patients with partial trisomy. Various parameters which could modify the results of gene dosage have been tested. Among these parameters, RNase treatment was shown to introduce significant variations: in fibroblasts from one AD patient that we have studied extensively, dosage of the β-amyloid gene and the protooncogene ETS2 gave the same values for RNase-untreated DNA and increased copy number for RNase-treated DNA from fibroblasts. DS models for AD suggest that overexpression of one or a few chromosome 21 genes leads to AD pathology. Thus it is potentially interesting to study chromosome 21 gene expression in AD. RNA quantification experiments were run on fibroblast cultures from five AD patients, three age-matched controls and two DS patients: mRNA for CuZn superoxide dismutase was significantly increased in four AD patients and two DS patients as compared to actin RNA. A *t*-test common to the five blots showed a significant increase ($p < 0.001$). For ETS2 sequences qualitative results were obtained: the level of ETS2 RNA was higher in AD patients and DS patients than in controls. For AD patients these results could be explained by variations of the regulation of gene expression, either at the transcriptional level or through the control of the stability of RNA. However, the observed increase is similar in DS and AD patients. Furthermore, in one AD patient gene dosage and RNA level quantification were performed on the same fibroblasts; increased values were found for both ETS2 DNA sequences and ETS2 RNA sequences. Therefore these results are also compatible with duplication of some chromosome 21 sequences in some AD patients.

Possible Genetic Links Between Down's Syndrome and Alzheimer's Disease

Onset of the clinical signs of dementia in aged Down's syndrome (DS) patients is a matter of controversy; these signs seem to occur in around 50% of the patients. But all the brains from trisomy 21 patients over 30 years of age which have been examined share many, if not all, histopathological features found in the brains of patients with

Alzheimer's disease (AD): neuritic plaques and neurofibrillary tangles are observed in both conditions. Antibodies against paired helical filaments (PHFs) from AD patients are also specific for PHFs found in DS patients (Mattiace et al. 1987). Moreover the cerebral amyloid proteins from DS patients and AD patients show the same amino acid composition (Glenner and Wong 1984). The regions of the brain which are involved in AD are specific and they are also modified in DS patients: for example, degeneration of the locus coeruleus appears highly selective in AD and in DS with no fewer neurons in the adjacent regions (Ingram et al. 1987). Yates et al. (1981) reported a reduction of the enzymes choline-acetyltransferase and acetylcholinesterase in the affected brains of DS patients; this decrease is a characteristic of AD. The neuropathological and neurochemical changes in aged DS patients are, therefore, similar to those found in AD patients. The possibility of a genetic link between these two diseases is also supported by dermatoglyphic studies. In a study of 50 patients with presumed senile dementia of the AD type, Weinreb (1985) reported an increased frequency of ulnar loops, a pattern commonly found in DS patients. Furthermore, a high frequency of palmar Sydney line and a transversality index equal or superior to 31 have been found in AD patients (N. Okra-Podrabinek et al. 1988).

Gene dosage experiment

Such links between DS and AD might be explained by the presence of duplicated sequences on chromosome 21 in AD. To test this hypothesis we performed gene-dosage experiments with DNA sequences that we have found duplicated in DS patients with partial trisomy. In the first set of experiments we studied the leukocyte DNA of six patients with sporadic AD (Delabar et al. 1986, 1987). Gene dosage was performed with normal controls, DS patients and AD patients. Results indicated an increased copy number for APP sequences in two patients (with the probe COL5A2 as reference) and an increased copy number for ETS2 sequences in six patients (with the probe COL1A2 as reference). Recently four articles (St George-Hyslop et al. 1987; Tanzi et al. 1987; Podlisny et al. 1987; Furuya et al. 1988) have appeared which show no duplication of the amyloid gene (APP) in the DNA of AD patients as compared with normal controls. To elucidate this contradiction we have studied various parameters which could modify the results of gene dosage. The most striking variations were obtained by comparing fibroblast DNA from a normal control, one AD patient and one DS patient. Gene dosage was first performed on fibroblast DNA which was not treated by RNase: there was no significant difference between normal and AD patient DNA for the content of APP or ETS2 sequences. The same DNAs were treated with RNase before a second deproteinisation step and subjected again to gene-dosage analysis. Two different DNA preparations with the same protocol were used for the control and the patients. They showed an increased gene copy number ($P < 0.001$) for both APP and ETS2 sequences (Table 1), in agreement with the first study performed on leukocyte DNA from the same patient. These results show the sensitivity of the gene-dosage method to various factors; they are compatible with a duplication of the APP and ETS2 sequences in the DNA of this patient. These data are preliminary; this protocol must be applied to the study of fibroblast and blood DNA from other AD patients.

Table 1. Gene dosage for a patient with Alzheimer's disease (AD2) as compared with an age-matched control (C7) and a patient with Down's syndrome (DS). DNA was extracted from fibroblasts with or without treatment by RNase. Results are expressed as m ± S. D. for *(n)* measurements

Probe/ref. probe no. RNase	APP/COL5A2 $\bar{x}$ SD *n*	ETS2/COL1A2
C7 (control)	2 ± 0.47 (15)	2 ± 0.25 (10)
AD2 (Alzheimer's)	1.57 ± 0.27 (10)	1.84 ± 0.2 (5)
DS (Down's)	2.51 ± 0.7 (5)	2.03 ± 0.16 (5)
RNase treatment		
C7	2 ± 0.38 (11)	2 ± 0.39 (11)
AD2	3.05 ± 0.84 (13)[a]	3.12 ± 0.66 (12)[a]
DS	2.86 ± 0.32 (6)[a]	3.74 ± 1.17 (6)[a]

[a] Means or the values for AD of DS patients are significantly different from the control with $P < 0.001$

mRNA quantification

The existence of a genetic link between DS and AD could also imply that some genes carried by chromosome 21 are overexpressed in cells from AD patients. A modification in the genome of these patients might also imply that changes in expression could be observed in different tissues and not only in the brain. To investigate this hypothesis we are performing quantification experiments of the amounts of mRNA coded by various chromosome 21 genes. For this study primary fibroblast cultures were established from five AD patients and three age-matched controls; fibroblasts from two DS patients were also included in the investigation. We present here preliminary results on the quantification of the message coding for CuZn SOD using as a reference probe a cDNA coding for actin (Lieman-Hurwitz et al. 1982). Five different Northern blots were run with varying amounts of RNA: on each, gel samples from one control, one AD patient and one DS patient were deposited (Fig. 1). After successive hybridization with CuZn SOD cDNA and actin cDNA the autoradiographs were analysed by densitometry (exposure time was chosen to obtain peak values inside a predetermined linear range). Four of the five AD patients were found to present a significantly increased amount of CuZn SOD mRNA, compared with controls, although less pronounced than in DS patients (Table 2). Increased CuZn SOD mRNA levels in trisomic 21 fibroblasts are secondary to a gene-dosage effect. The ratio between trisomy 21 and control values is in most cases larger than the theoretical value of 1.5. Such a deviation from the theoretical value has been observed by others at the mRNA level (Sherman 1983) as well as at the protein level (Villano et al. 1981). Our results on CuZn SOD mRNA quantification in fibroblasts from AD patients suggest that an increase in CuZn SOD enzymatic activity might be observed in the same fibroblasts. Such an increase has been previously reported for the comparison between one AD patient and one normal control and one DS patient (Thienhaus 1986). Further studies are required to determine whether the observed changes are secondary to a gene-dosage effect or, more likely, to a pathological change in the regulation of mRNA synthesis or stability, which might reflect a specific genetic defect in these patients.

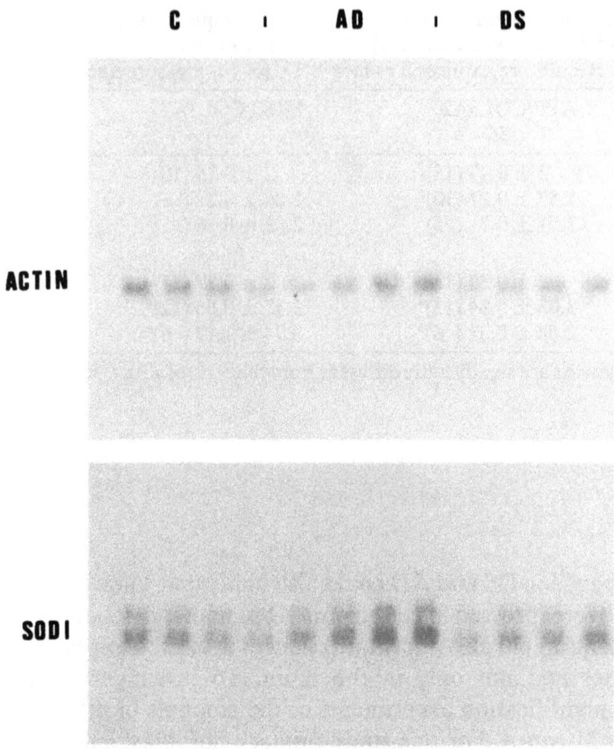

Fig. 1. Northern blot analysis of the amount of mRNA coding for CuZn superoxide dismutase in fibroblast cell cultures from the forearm skin of: aged control (C), sporadic AD patient (AD), and Down's syndrome patient (DS). Total RNA was loaded in four different amounts on an 8% agarose, 2.2 *M* formaldehyde gel and blotted on a Zetabind nylon membrane. Hybridization conditions were as described previously (Delabar et al. 1986). The reference probe was an actin cDNA (gift from J. L. Mandel)

Table 2. Cu-Zn SOD mRNA quantification

	C[a]	AD/C	AD	AD/DS	DS	DS/C
C_1, AD_1, DS_1	1 ± 0.41 (4)	$P < 0.05$	2.07 ± 0.74 (4)	$P < 0.001$	4.32 ± 0.72 (4)	$P < 0.001$
C_1, AD_2, DS_2	1 ± 0.42 (4)	NS	1.2 ± 0.7 (4)	NS	3.4 ± 1.23 (3)	$P < 0.02$
C_2, AD_3, DS_2	1 ± 0.22 (4)	$P < 0.05$	3.43 ± 1.75 (4)		11.59 ± 3.26 (3)	
C_3, AD_4, DS_1	1 ± 0.16 (4)	$P < 0.05$	2.46 ± 1.01 (3)	NS	3.47 ± 0.93 (3)	$P < 0.01$
C_1, AD_5, DS_1	1 ± 0.12 (4)	$P < 0.02$	2.04 ± 0.55 (4)	NS	2.14 ± 0.16 (4)	$P < 0.01$

[a] C, control; AD, Alzheimer's disease patient; DS, Down syndrome patient. For each patient *(n)* slots have been analysed. Results are given as mean value ± SD. Values were compared using the *t*-test. NS, not significant

Conclusion

It has been proposed that duplication of some chromosome 21 gene sequences could be the cause of the AD-type lesions seen in the brain of DS patients (Delabar 1986; Schweber 1985). To explain the lesions in AD a mutation carried by chromosome 21 was involved to account for the genetic linkage of FAD with this chromosome (St George-Hyslop et al. 1987). We can also infer from our results and from the correlation between trisomy 21 and AD-type lesions that duplication of chromosome 21 sequences is a characteristic common to DS and some AD patients. These duplications are visible only in specifically prepared specimens of DNA. We suggest, therefore, that the DNA of AD patients might contain different kinds of duplications which differ among patients: a duplication in early FAD near the FAD locus and duplications of other chromosome 21 sequences in some other AD cases.

Duplications of regulatory genes could also induce an overexpression of some genes carried by chromosome 21.

References

Delabar J-M, Lamour Y, Gegonne A, Davous P, Roudier M, Nicole A, Ceballos I, Amouyel P, Stehelin D, Sinet P-M (1986) Rearrangement of chromosome 21 in Alzheimer's disease. Ann Genet 29: 226–228

Delabar J-M, Sinet P-M, Chadefaux B, Nicole A, Gegonne A, Stehelin D, Creau-Goldberg N, Turleau C, de Grouchy J (1987) Submicroscopic duplication of chromosome 21 and trisomy 21 phenotype (Down's syndrome). Hum Genet 76: 225–229

Delabar J-M, Goldgaber D, Lamour Y, Nicole A, Huret J-L, de Grouchy J, Brown P, Gajdusek DC, Sinet P-M (1987) Amyloid gene duplication in Alzheimer's disease and karyotypically normal Down's syndrome. Science 235: 1390–1392

Furuya H, Sasaki H, Goto I, Wong CW, Glenner GG, Sakaki Y (1988) Amyloid β-protein gene duplication is not common in Alzheimer's disease: analysis by polymorphic restriction fragments. Biochem Biophys Res Commun 150: 75–81

Glenner GG, Wong WC (1984) Alzheimer's disease and Down's syndrome: sharing of a unique cerebrovascular amyloid fibril protein. Biochem Biophys Res Commun 122: 1131–1135

Ingram VM, Aslamy Z, Jhavery S, Miller CH, Moore HM, Blanchard BJ, Parry DE (1987) Neuropathology in Alzheimer's and Down's diseases: the locus coeruleus. 17th Meeting of the Society of Neurosciences, New Orleans, Abstract 7–12

Lieman-Hurwitz J, Dafni N, Lavie V, Groner Y (1982) Human cytoplasmic superoxide dismutase cDNA clone: a probe for studying the molecular biology of Down syndrome. Proc Natl Acad Sci USA 79: 2808–2811

Mattiace LA, Sparkman DR, White CL (1987) Alzheimer paired helical filament immunoreactivity in Down Syndrome brain. 17th Meeting of the Society of Neurosciences, New Orleans, Abstract 316, 4

Niebuhr E (1974) Down's syndrome. The possibility of a pathogenic segment on chromosome no. 21. Humangenetik 21: 99–101

Okra-Podrabinek N, Roudier M, Lamour Y, de Grouchy J (1988) Dermatoglyphic patterns in senile dementia of Alzheimer's type. Ann Genet 31: 91–96

Podlisny MB, Lee G, Selkoe DJ (1987) Gene dosage of the β-amyloid precursor protein in Alzheimer's disease. Science 238: 669–671

Sherman L, Dafni N, Lieman-Hurwitz J, Groner Y (1983) Nucleotide sequence and expression of human chromosome 21-encoded superoxide dismutase mRNA. Proc Natl Acad Sci USA 80: 5465–5469

Schweber M (1985) A possible unitary genetic hypothesis for Alzheimer's disease and Down's syndrome. Molecular structure of the number 21 chromosome and Down's syndrome. Ann NY Acad Sci 450: 223–238

St George-Hyslop PH, Tanzi RE, Polinsky RJ, Haines JL, Nee L, Watkins PC, Myers RH, Feldman RG, Pollen D, Drachman D, Growdon J, Bruni A, Foncin J-F, Salmon D, Frommelt P, Amaducci L, Sorbi S, Piacentini S, Stewart GD, Hobbs WJ, Conneally PM, Gusella JF (1987) The genetic defect causing familial Alzheimer's disease maps on chromosome 21. Science 235: 885–890

St George-Hyslop PH, Tanzi RE, Polinsky RJ, Neve RL, Pollen D, Drachman D, Growdon J, Cupples LA, Nee L, Myers RH, O'Sullivan D, Watkins PC, Amos JA, Deutsch CK, Bodfish JW, Kinsbourne M, Feldman RG, Bruni A, Amaducci L, Foncin J-F, Gusella JF (1987) Absence of duplication of chromosome 21 genes in familial and sporadic Alzheimer's disease. Science 238: 664–666

Tanzi RE, Bird ED, Latt SA, Neve RL (1987) The amyloid β-protein gene is not duplicated in brains from patients with Alzheimer's disease. Science 238: 666–669

Thienhaus OJ, Cliffe C, Zemlan FO, Bosmann HB (1986) Superoxide dismutase, chromosome 21, and Alzheimer's disease. Biol Psychiatry 21: 1101–1109

Villano BC del, Tischfield JA (1981) Quantitation of human cuprozinc superoxide dismutase (SOD-1) by radioimmunoassay and its possible significance in disease. Methods Enzymol 74: 359–370

Weinreb HJ (1985) Fingerprint patterns in Alzheimer's disease. Arch Neurol 42: 50–54

Yates CM, Ritchie IM, Simpson J, Maloney AFJ, Gordon A (1981) Noradrenaline in Alzheimer type dementia and Down syndrome. Lancet II: 39–40

Paired Helical Filaments (PHF): Update 1988

H.M. Wisniewski, and *K. Iqbal*

Summary

We have developed a laboratory test which quantitates the immunoreactivity towards the Alzheimer paired helical filament (PHF) protein and PHF cross-reactive proteins in cerebrospinal fluid (CSF) from patients with Alzheimer's disease (AD). This PHF reactivity is present in higher concentration in CSF from AD than from non-AD controls. The method employed for detection of this reactivity is enzyme-linked immunosorbent assay. By analyzing a greater number of CSF samples from patients with AD and non-AD controls, the sensitivity and specificity of this test can be evaluated to determine its clinical usefulness as a laboratory diagnostic test for AD. The clinical trials on this diagnostic test have now been started. However, it can already be predicted that there will be both some false positives and some false negatives. Data from a large group of cases are therefore necessary to define the specificity of the diagnostic test, which hopefully will be available in the near future.

Neurofibrillary changes occur in many pathological conditions

Neurons with neurofibrillary changes are found, in varying numbers, in many and unrelated human diseases (Wisniewski et al. 1979). Recently, we found (Wisniewski et al. 1987 a) that in hydrocephalic brains, neurons with neurofibrillary changes made of paired helical filaments (PHF) tangles are commonly found. The topographic distribution of the tangles bearing neurons was similar to that seen in Alzheimer's disease (AD), indicating topographic (irrespective of etiology) susceptibility to PHF formation. It was also noticed that, as in Alzheimer's disease, there were neurons next to each other in the same area, one affected by neurofibrillary changes and the other looking normal. However, it appears that there are factors other than hydrocephalus which contribute to the PHF formation, because 41% (24 of 59 studied) of the cases which were comparable in all important characteristics (i. e., same degree of hydrocephalus, etiology, age, duration) develop Alzheimer neurofibrillary tangles (ANT).

Recently we looked for Alzheimer neuropathology in mentally retarded people age 23 and up. In this group we found a high proportion of people who had neurofibrillary changes without the presence of neuritic (senile) plaques (Barcikowska et al. 1988: Popovitch et al. 1988). A history of epilepsy or central nervous system (CNS) trauma appears to increase the chance of developing PHF.

As indicated above, neurofibrillary changes occur in many and unrelated pathological conditions. In some of the diseases few neurons with tangles are found while in others, such as postencephalitic Parkinsonism, dementia pugilistica and Guam-Parkinson dementia syndrome, there are many neurons with neurofibrillary changes. In postencephalitic Parkinsonism, in areas affected by neurofibrillary changes virus was present. In Guam-Parkinson dementia syndrome, environmental neurotoxins (aluminum, cycad intoxication) were implicated as a cause of the disease (Spencer et al. 1987). Since the report by Goodman (1953) it has been known that there is no constant proportionate relationship between the number of plaques and the number of neurons with neurofibrillary changes. To emphasize this point he described a 48-year-old man who, within 8 months, developed dementia and died. Neuropathological examination revealed, in the absence of argentophilic plaques, enormous numbers of nerve cells with neurofibrillary degeneration in various parts of the brain. Of interest is the fact that Prussian blue preparations revealed heavy precipitation of an iron substance within the cytoplasm of the nerve cells, oligodendroglia, and in the walls of the capillaries and arterioles. The other case was a 61-year-old woman who died 1 year after the onset of mental symptoms. According to Goodman, "the microscopic picture afforded a striking contrast to the previous case. There were myriads of plaques thorughout the cortex but only one cell showing Alzheimer neurofibrillary degeneration was seen." Recently. Terry et al. (1987) reported that, in a large series of patients (60) over age 74, a significant minority (30%) lacked neocortical tangles. According to Terry et al. (1987) "SDAT with neocortical ANT is the same disease as SDAT without them, although the presence of such tangles is associated with a tendency towards greater severity." In other words cases where, by and large, only plaques are present are diagnosed as AD/SDAT. What about cases with neurofibrillary changes only? Goodman included such cases in the group of AD. We (Popovitch et al. 1987) described a 28-year-old male with pyramidal and extrapyramidal signs and severe dementia with widespread and extensive neurofibrillary changes and Lewy bodies. This case was classified as a young adult form of dementia with neurofibrillary changes and Lewy bodies.

In our (HMW) opinion cases with PHF containing neurons only should not be diagnosed as AD/SDAT. However, cases with dementia and very many plaques and few, if any, neurons with neurofibrillary tangles should be classified as AD/SDAT. It should be noted, however, that cases with very many neurons with neurofibrillary tangles are less common and occur in younger people. As was stressed by Terry et al. (1987), cases without neocortical ANT and many plaques are not uncommon and occur in older individuals. According to Matsuyama and Nakamura (1978), in routine autopsy material of people with no indication of mental illness, neurofibrillary changes in parahippocampal gyrus, hippocampal formation, and median occipital temporal gyrus and plaques in occipito temporal gyrus and parahippocampal gyrus start to appear approximately at the same time (30–39 years of age). However, the incidence of neuritic (senile) plaques was much lower than that of neurofibrillary changes. Using immunocytochemical techniques with antibodies against A4 amyloid protein, Davies et al. (1988) studied 120 brains for the presence of plaques. In their material, up to the fifth decade no patients were positive. In the sixth decade 20% were positive. This percentage rose to 28% in the seventh, 43% in the eighth, and 81% in the ninth decade.

In studying Down's syndrome brains we also found that plaques and tangles start to appear approximately at the same age (15–20 years). However, the incidence of neuritic plaques was much higher than neurons with tangles, suggesting a gene-dose effect on formation of plaques (Wisniewski et al. 1987b). PHF with the twist about 80 nm were found only in the human central nervous system. Kawasaki et al. (1987), however, reported PHF in upper cervical ganglia in a 76-year-old non-demented man.

Polypeptide Compositional Analysis of PHF

Biochemical studies on (PHF) have been slowed by the difficulty of obtaining sufficient quantities of isolated PHF from autopsied AD/SDAT brains, the heterogeneity of PHF, and the sparing solubility of the tangles. The polypeptide composition of isolated PHF is heterogeneous – 2–3 major bands in 45 kD-62 kD region, a ladder of minor bands especially in this region and in the high molecular weight area, and even protein which is excluded from the SDS-polyacrylamide gel are seen (Grundke-Iqbal et al. 1981, 1984, 1985; Iqbal et al. 1984). The 45 kD-62 kD PHF polypeptides have been identified as microtubule-associated polypeptides tau by their co-electrophoresis on SDS polyacrylamide gels and by their immunoreactivity with tau (Grundke-Iqbal et al. 1986a, 1986b). Furthermore, both monoclonal and affinity purified polyclonal antibodies to tau have been shown to immunocytochemically label PHF (Brion et al. 1985; Delacourte and Defossez 1986; Grundke-Iqbal et al. 1986a, 1986b; Kosik et al. 1986; Wood et al. 1986). More recently cross-reactivity between PHF and ubiquitin, an 8.2 kD protein ubiquitous to all tissues, and some ubiquitin in isolated PHF hase been found (Mori et al. 1987; Perry et al. 1987a, 1987b). However, the exact amount of ubiquitin and, for that matter, also of tau in PHF remain to be determined. Recently PHFS isolated with and without pronase were compared by scanning transmission electron microscopy (STEM) to determine their mass per unit length (Goedert et al. 1988; Wishik et al. 1988a, 1988b). These studies suggest that the subunit molecular mass of PHF is 120 kD before pronase and 100 kD after pronase treatment. The material removed by pronase was identified as protein tau. Further studies of the 100 kD protein identified peptide fragments of 9.5 and 12 kD which turned out to also be fragments of tau, which is tightly bound within the pronase-resistant core of the PHF. According to these authors the tightly bound stub of tau accounts for some 10% of the pronase-resistant core of the PHF. However, the identity of the remaining 90% of the PHF core is unknown, but there is no evidence to suggest that it is tau or A4 protein.

Tau in PHF is altered (Grundke-Iqbal et al. 1988b). One of these alterations of the tau in PHF is phosphorylation which is different from that seen in normal human brains (Grundke-Iqbal et al. 1986b). Other alterations of tau, including its possible ubiquitination, are yet to be established.

The group of Masters and Beyreuther (1985) have claimed that PHF are made from the amyloid beta-peptide (A4 protein). However, neither our laboratory nor any other laboratory has been able to reproduce these findings. To the contrary, employing monoclonal antibodies to the beta-peptide and immunocytochemical labelling, we have observed that the beta-peptide is present in neuronal cytoplasm but is not associated with the neurofibrillary tangles (Grundke-Iqbal et al. 1988a).

Antibodies to several other polypeptides, including the neurofilament heavy subunit (Gambetti et al. 1980; Gambetti et al. 1983; Anderton et al. 1982; Sternberger et al. 1985) and the microtubule associated protein MAP_2 (Kosik et al. 1984), have been shown to immunolabel tangles in tissue sections. However, no biochemical evidence for the presence of these polypeptides or their fragments in PHF has been reported to date.

As indicated above, to date the amino acid sequence of PHF core polypeptides has not been determined. This is probably because of the heterogeneous polypeptide composition and posttranslational modifications of the polypeptides making the PHF. Isolation of individual polypeptides or peptides from purified PHF required for obtaining information on amino acid sequencing is a difficult task, but one which must be undertaken to understand the biochemistry of this lesion.

Immunochemical Studies of PHF

While polypeptide compositional analysis has been moving slowly, more satisfying progress has been made in the immunochemical studies of PHFs. Both polyclonal and monoclonal antibodies to PHF have been obtained (Grundke-Iqbal et al. 1981, 1984, 1988a; Wang et al. 1984). Based on these studies we have developed a laboratory test which quantitates the immunoreactivity towards the Alzheimer PHF protein and PHF cross-reactive proteins in cerebrospinal fluid (CSF) from patients with AD (Mehta et al. 1985; Iqbal et al. 1988). This PHF reactivity is present in higher concentration in CSF from AD than from non-AD controls. The method employed for detection of this reactivity is enzyme linked immunosorbent assay (ELISA). Briefly, microtiter plates containing plastic wells are first coated with PHF proteins. A mixture of CSF and mouse monoclonal antibodies to PHF is incubated in the wells and then washed off. Next, the wells are exposed to a goat anti-mouse antibody to which the enzyme alkaline phosphatase has been coupled. The enzyme labelled antibody reacts with mouse monoclonal antibody to PHF. Lastly, they are filled with a colorless solution of paranitrophenyl phosphate that changes to yellow in the presence of alkaline phosphatase activity. The absorbance of the contents of each well is read in a spectrophotometer-microtiter plate reader. This is a competitive assay; high PHF immunoreactivity results in less color at the end of the test. Thus, CSF from AD shows less color compared with that from non-AD controls. The amount of PHF immunoreactivity in unknown CSF is determined from the standard curve made using serial dilutions of known concentrations of PHF proteins. It is also usual to include a reference-positive sample on each plate. The latter compensates for slight day-to-day variations in test conditions. Hence, CSF from AD contains increased amounts of PHF and or PHF-cross-reactive proteins which inhibit the reaction between PHF and its corresponding antibody. Our preliminary studies revealed that CSF from 27 of 29 AD patients had 20%–50% inhibition whereas 25 of 27 non-AD controls had inhibition between 0%–20%. By evaluating a greater number of CSF samples from patients with AD and non-AD controls, the sensitivity and specificity of this test can be evaluated to determine its clinical usefulness as a laboratory diagnostic test for AD.

The clinical trials on this diagnostic test have now been started. However, it can already be predicted that there will be both some false-positive and some false-negative cases. As indicated above, the test is based on PHF immunoreactivity and it is known that a small number of nondemented aged individuals show the same degree of Alzheimer neuropathology as the AD-SDAT cases (Tomlinson 1986). These neuropathologically but not clinically expressed AD-SDAT cases are at high risk for developing dementia and are likely to show positive on the test. On the other hand, AD-SDAT cases which are known to have mostly plaques and minimal tangles (Terry et al. 1987) might show negative on the test. Data from a large group of cases are therefore necessary to define the specificity of the diagnostic test which hopefully will be available in the near future.

References

Anderton BH, Breinburg D, Downes MJ, Green PJ, Tomlinson BE, Ulrich J, Wood JN (1982) Monoclonal antibodies show that neurofibrillary tangles and neurofilaments share antigenic determinants. Nature 298: 84–86

Barcikowska M, Kozlowski PB, Kujawa M, Rudelli R, Silverman W, Zigman W, Wisniewski HM (1988) Neuritic plaques, neurofibrillary tangles and congophilic angiopathy in the elderly mentally retarded population. Morphometric and clinicopathological study. J Neuropathol Exp Neurol 47: 339

Brion JP, Passareiro H, Nunez J, Flament-Durand J (1985) Mise en evidence immunologique de la proteine tau au niseau des lesions degenerescence neurofibrillaires de la maladie d'Alzheimer. Arch Biol (Brux) 95: 220–235

Davies L, Wolska B, Simms G, Kakulas BA, Masters CL (1988) Prevalence of the A4 amyloid protein of Alzheimer's disease in aged brains. Neurology [Suppl 1] 38: 265

Delacourte A, Defossez A (1986) Alzheimer's disease: tau proteins, the promoting factors of microtubule assembly are major components of paired helical filaments. J Neurol Sci 76: 173–186

Gambetti P, Shecket G, Ghetti B, Hirano A, Dahl D (1983) Neurofibrillary changes in human brain. An immunocytochemical study with a neurofilament antiserum. J Neuropathol Exp Neurol 42: 69–79

Gambetti P, Velasco ME, Dahl D, Bignami A, Roesmann U, Sindely SD (1980) Neurofibrillary tangles in Alzheimer disease: an immunohistochemical study. In: Amaducci L, Davison AN, Antuono P (eds) Aging of the brain and dementia. Aging, vol 13. Raven Press, New York, pp 55–63

Goedert M, Wischik CM, Crowther RA, Walker JE, Klug A (1988) Cloning and sequencing of the cDNA encoding a core protein of the paired helical filament of Alzheimer disease: identification as the microtubule-associated protein tau. Proc Nat Acad Sci USA 85: 4051–4055

Goodman L (1953) Alzheimer disease. A clinico-pathologic analysis of twenty-three cases with a theory on pathogenesis. J Nerv Ment Dis 117: 97–130

Grundke-Iqbal I, Iqbal K, Merz P, Wisniewski HM (1981) Isolation and properties of Alzheimer neurofibrillary tangles. J Neuropathol Exp Neurol 40: 312

Grundke-Iqbal I, Iqbal K, Quinlan M, Tung YC, Zaidi MS, Wisniewski HM (1986a) Microtubule-associated protein tau: a component of Alzheimer paired helical filaments. J Biol Chem 261: 6084–6089

Grundke-Iqbal I, Iqbal K, Tung YC, Quinlan M, Wisniewski HM, Binder LI (1986b) Abnormal phosphorylation of the microtubule associated protein tau in Alzheimer cytoskeletal pathology. Proc Nat Acad Sci 83: 4913–4917

Grundke-Iqbal I, Iqbal K, Tung YC, Wang GP, Wisniewski HM (1984) Alzheimer paired helical filaments: immunochemical identification of polypeptides. Acta Neuropathol (Berl) 62: 259–267

Grundke Iqbal I, Wang GP, Iqbal K, Tung KC, Wisniewski HM (1985) Alzheimer paired helical filaments: identification of polypeptides with monoclonal antibodies. Acta Neuropathol (Berl) 68: 279–283

Grundke-Iqbal I, Kim KS, Iqbal K, Wisniewski HM (1988a) Amyloid immunoreactivity and neurofibrillary tangles co-exist in the same neuron in Alzheimer disease (AD-SDAT). J Neuropathol Exp Neurol 47: 355

Grundke-Iqbal I, Vorbrodt AW, Iqbal K, Tung YC, Wang GP, Wisniewski HM (1988b) Microtubule associated polypeptides tau are altered in Alzheimer paired helical filaments. Mol Brain Res 4: 43–52

Iqbal K, Wang GP, Wisniewski HM, Grundke-Iqbal I (1988) Paired helical filament immunoreactivity in CSF. Alzheimer Dis Assoc Dis J (in press)

Iqbal K, Zaidi T, Thompson CH, Merz PA, Wisniewski HM (1984) Alzheimer paired helical filaments: bulk isolation, solubility and protein composition. Acta Neuropathol (Berl) 62: 167–177

Kosik KS, Duffy LK, Dowling MM, Abraham C, McCluskey A, Selkoe DJ (1984) Microtubule-associated protein 2: Monoclonal antibodies demonstrate the selective importance of certain epitopes into Alzheimer neurofibrillary tangles. Proc Nat Acad Sci USA 81: 7941–7945

Kosik KS, Joachim CL, Selkoe DJ (1986) The microtubule associated protein, tau, is a major antigenic component of paired helical filaments in Alzheimer's disease. Proc Nat Acad Sci USA 83: 4044–4048

Kawasaki H, Murayama S, Tomonaga M, Izumiyama, Shimada H (1987) Neurofibrillary tangles in human upper cervical ganglia. Morphological study with immunohistochemistry and electron microscopy. Acta Neuropathol (Berl) 75: 156–169

Masters CL, Multhaup G, Sims C, Poltigiesser K (1985) Neuronal origin of a cerebral amyloid: neurofibrillary tangles in Alzheimer's disease contain the same protein as the amyloid of plaques and cores and blood vessels. EMBO J 4: 2757–2763

Matsuyama H, Nakamura S (1978) Senile changes in the brain in the Japanese: incidence of Alzheimer's neurofibrillary change and senile plaques. In Katzman R, Terry RD, Bick KL (eds) Alzheimer's disease: senile dementia and related disorders. Aging, vol 7. Raven, New York, pp 287–313

Mehta PD, Thal L, Wisniewski HM, Grundke-Iqbal I, Iqbal K (1985) Paired helical filament antigen in CSF. Lancet I: 35

Mori H, Kondo J, Ihara Y (1987) Ubiquitin is a component of paired helical filaments in Alzheimer's disease. Science 235: 1641–1644

Perry G, Friedman R, Shaw G, Chau V (1987a) Ubiquitin is detected in neurofibrillary tangles and senile plaque neurites of Alzheimer disease brains. Proc Nat Acad Sci USA 84: 3033–3036

Perry G, Mulvihill P, Manetto V, Fried V, Smith H, Grundke-Iqbal I, Iqbal K, Autilio-Gambetti L, Gambetti P (1987b) Ubiquitin epitopes in Alzheimer paired helical filaments: a study with monoclonal antibodies to ubiquitin and paired helical filaments. J Cell Biol 105: 203a

Popovitch ER, Wisniewski HM, Kaufman MA, Grundke-Iqbal I, Wen GY (1987) Young-adult form of dementia with neurofibrillary changes and Lewy bodies. Acta Neuropathol (Berl) 74: 97–104

Popovitch ER, Wisniewski HM, Wen GY (1988) Alzheimer's neuropathology in mentally retarded people aged 45–64. J Neuropathol Exp Neurol 47: 339

Spencer PS, Hugon J, Ludolph A, Nunn PB, Ross SM, Roy DN, Schaumberg HH (1987) Discovery and partial characterization of primate motor-system toxins. In: Selective neuronal death. Ciba Foundation Symposium 126. Wiley, Chichester, pp 221–238

Sternberger NH, Sternberger LA, Ulrich J (1985) Aberrant neurofilament phosphorylation in Alzheimer disease. Proc Nat Acad Sci USA 82: 4274–4276

Terry RD, Hansen LA, DeTeresa R, Davies P, Tobias H, Katzman R (1987) Senile dementia of the Alzheimer type without neocortical neurofibrillary tangles. J Neuropathol Exp Neurol 46: 262–268

Tomlinson BE (1986) Dementia and the deposition of amyloid in the brain. In: Neuropathology [Suppl] 3: 1–12

Wang GP, Grundke-Iqbal I, Kascsak RJ, Iqbal K, Wisniewski HM (1984) Alzheimer neurofibrillary tangles: monoclonal antibodies to inherent antigen/s. Acta Neuropathol (Berl) 62: 268–275

Wischik CM, Novak M, Edwards PC, Klug A, Trchelaar W, Crowther RA (1988a) Structural characterization of the core of the paired helical filament of Alzheimer disease. Proc Nat Acad Sci USA 85: (in press)

Wischik CM, Novak M, Thgersen HC, Edwards PC, Runswick MJ, Jaker R, Walker JE, Milstein C, Roth M, Klug A (1988b) Isolation of a fragment of tau derived from the core of the paired helical filament of Alzheimer disease. Proc Natl Acad Sci USA 85: 4506–4510

Wisniewski HM, Popovitch ER, Kaufman MA, Wisniewski KE (1987a) Neurofibrillary changes in advanced hydrocephalus. A clinicopathological study. J Neuropathol Exp Neurol 46: 340

Wisniewski HM, Rabe A, Wen GY, Wisniewski KE (1978b) Gene dose effect on early formation of neuritic plaques in Down syndrome (DS). J Neuropathol Exp Neurol 46: 334
Wisniewski K, Jervis GA, Moretz RC, Wisniewski HM (1979) Alzheimer neurofibrillary tangles in diseases other than senile and presenile dementia. Ann Neurol 5: 288–294
Wood JG, Mirra SS, Pollock NJ, Binder LI (1986) Neurofibrillary tangles of Alzheimer's disease share antigenic determinants with the axonal microtubule-associated protein tau. Proc Natl Acad Sci USA 83: 4040–4043

Studies of the Beta-Amyloid Precursor Protein in Brain and the Pathological Transformation of Tau into the Neurofibrillary Tangle

K. S. Kosik, and *D. J. Selkoe*

Summary

We report our ongoing work to characterize the molecular nature of neurofibrillary tangles and senile plaques. The work on the senile plaque focuses on identifying at the protein level the beta-amyloid precursor protein using antibodies to various synthetic peptides predicted from the cDNA sequence. Two independently raised antibodies to the carboxy terminal domain of the precursor protein both recognize an approximately 120 kD protein on immunoblots present in a membrane fraction from multiple tissues. The antibodies also stain some granular material in the senile plaques that is distinct from the amyloid core fibrils and the dystrophic neurites. Work on elucidating the neuritic pathology of Alzheimer's disease has focused on the tau protein which, by immunocytochemistry, can be visualized in regions of neuropil that extend well beyond the classical distributions of the senile plaques and neurofibrillary tangles. The sequence of several tau monoclonal antibody recognition sites has been identified and demonstrates that large portions of the tau molecule are included in the neurofibrillary tangle.

Introduction

The neuronal attrition of Alzheimer's disease is associated with prominent structural changes evident by light microscopy of appropriately stained tissue sections. Neurofibrillary tangles and senile plaques represent the principal alterations, although granulovacuolar degeneration, Hirano bodies, and vascular amyloid are also frequently seen in the disease. Senile plaques contain a central amyloid core, which consists principally of the beta-amyloid protein also referred to as A4. A major advance in Alzheimer's research was the cloning and sequencing of the entire beta-amyloid precursor protein (Goldgaber et al. 1987; Kang et al. 1987; Robakis et al. 1987; Tanzi et al. 1987). The constituents of the neurofibrillary tangle have remained more problematic due to the difficulty in directly analyzing these structures. Paired helical filament (PHF) fractions prepared by any of several different isolation procedures have impurities and are not convincingly solubilized in toto. The two leading protein candidates as integral components of the PHF are tau (Brion et al. 1985a, b; Grundke-Igbal et al. 1986a; Kosik et al. 1986; Nukina and Ihara 1986; Wood et al. 1986; Yamamoto et al. 1983) and ubiquitin (Mori et al. 1987; Perry et al. 1987). What the ubiquitin is conjugated to in the PHF remains an open question. Data on the compositions of Hirano bodies and granulovacuolar degeneration rest only on immunohistochemical stains with defined antibodies. These data suggest that these structures also consist of cytoskeletal elements. Granulovacuolar degeneration is immunochemically related to tubulin (Price et al. 1985), and Hirano bodies are immunochemically related to actin, actin-associated proteins (Galloway et al. 1987a; Goldman 1983) and tau (Galloway et al. 1987b). More recently a widespread dystrophy within the neuropil has been observed (Kowall and Kosik 1987) by tau immunohistochemistry that is more extensive than either the senile plaques or the neurofibrillary tangles. Prominent, abnormal tau-immunoreactive neuropil fibers are densely present even in cortical regions without classical neurofibrillary tangle and senile plaque formation.

Neurofibrillary Tangles and Senile Plaques in Dementia

The relative importance of plaques and tangles to the clinical problem of dementia and the relationship of these structures to each other have been matters of controversy that remain unsettled. The neurofibrillary tangles are thought to be less specific because they are seen in a number of apparently unrelated diseases including: Guam Parkinson-dementia complex, postencephalitic Parkinson's disease, dementia pugilistica, long-surviving cases of subacute sclerosing panencephalitis, and certain variants of Hallervorden-Spatz disease (Eidelberg et al. 1987). The specificity with which either senile plaques or neurofibrillary tangles are associated with dementia has been raised since older individuals may meet the neuropathological criteria (Khachaturian et al. 1985) for Alzheimer's disease with few if any neurofibrillary tangles (Terry et al. 1987), and relatively younger individuals can develop Alzheimer's disease with abundant neurofibrillary tangles and few senile plaques. Most recently several cognitively intact elderly cases have been reported with senile plaques numerous enough to meet the criteria for Alzheimer's disease (Katzman et al. 1988). Similarly, it has been known for some time that while Down's syndrome individuals inevitably develop senile plaques and neurofibrillary tangles beyond the age of approximately 35, they do not inevitably develop the clinical features of Alzheimer's disease. It will be of interest to determine whether the numerous dystrophic neurites in the neuropil have a better correlation with the dementia than either senile plaques or neurofibrillary tangles.

The formation of highly stable intra- and extraneuronal protein filaments accompanies progressive neuronal degeneration in Alzheimer's disease and, to a lesser extent, in brain aging. Several lines of evidence suggest that the approximately 20 nm PHF inside neurons are distinct at the protein level from the approximately 8 nm amyloid filaments that accumulate extracellularly in plaque cores and blood vessels. PHF are immunochemically distinguished from amyloid in senile plaque cores and along vessels. Antibodies to tau stain the PHF, but not the amyloid. In the region of the senile plaque, one observes tau reaction product in the neuritic region of the plaque while the amyloid core remains unstained. Antibodies to various β-amyloid synthetic peptides and to alpha-1-antichymotrypsin (to be discussed below) stain amyloid and not PHF. The beta-amyloid sequence, found in both vascular amyloid (Glenner and Wong 1984) and senile plaque cores (Masters et al. 1985), cannot reliably be obtained from PHF, whereas the ubiquitin sequence can. The report of the beta-amyloid sequence from a PHF fraction in Guamanian Parkinson-dementia (Guiroy et al. 1987), a disease without senile plaques, is flawed by the possible contamination of vascular amyloid fibrils in the preparation. This common contaminant is suggested by the lack of correlation between the amino acid composition and the sequence obtained by Guiroy et al. (1987). The amino acid compositions of the amyloid cores and the PHF fractions differ markedly. Proline is present in PHF fractions, consistent with its relative abundance in tau, and is absent in highly purified senile plaque cores, consistent with its absence in the beta-amyloid protein. The amyloid cores, prepared by automated fluorescent sorting (Selkoe et al. 1986), are known to be highly pure because their amino acid compositions closely approximate the predicted composition based upon the known sequence of the amyloid fibrils. Two additional tentative conclusions also derive from these compositions: (a) the beta-amyloid is the most abundant component of the amyloid cores and (b) the compositions are most consistent with most of the beta-amyloid peptides in the core ending at residue 39 or 40 within the published sequence. Both of these points have important implications and will be discussed more fully below.

Senile Plaque as an Immunogen

Since the cloning of cDNAs for the beta-amyloid precursor, attempts to identify the precursor protein in brain have been made largely with antibodies raised against synthetic peptides based upon the predicted sequence, and against isolated senile plaque cores. Senile plaque cores as an immunogen have generally resulted in antisera that recognize both the plaque cores and vascular amyloid. An antiserum against the Alzheimer amyloid was used to screen a liver cDNA expression library from which three clones, all coding for alpha-1-antichymotrypsin, were detected (Abraham et al. 1988). The amyloid antiserum recognizes at least two distinct epitopes in alpha-1-antichymotrypsin. Antisera against purified alpha-1-antichymotrypsin stained Alzheimer amyloid deposits, both in situ and after detergent extraction from brain. Alpha-1-antichymotrypsin is expressed in Alzheimer brain, particularly in those areas prone to develop amyloid lesions. This serine protease inhibitor is also produced in the liver and released into the serum. The suggestion that a protease inhibitor is present within the senile plaque has gained additional importance because at least one alternative transcript of the beta-amyloid precursor protein contains a domain that shares a very high homology with the Kunitz family of protease inhibitors, which include the human plasma protein, inter-alpha-trypsin inhibitor (Kitaguchi et al. 1988; Ponte et al. 1988; Tanzi et al. 1988). It has been speculated that the inhibitor domain may serve as a promotor of neurite growth, a phenomenon which has been observed in the region around senile plaques.

Synthetic Peptides

Additional information has been derived from antibodies raised against synthetic peptides. The first of these synthetic peptides were P28 and P11. The P28 has a sequence identical to the first 28 residues of the beta-protein sequence reported by Masters et al. (1985) with a cysteine added to the carboxy terminus. P11 consists of residues 18 to 28 as reported by Wong et al. (1985). The sequence of both peptides was confirmed with an Applied Biosystems Model 470 sequenator using its standard program. Synthetic peptides have also been prepared from a threonine-rich region spanning residues 258–278 and from the carboxy terminus spanning residues 576–695. According to the membrane model of the beta-amyloid precursor protein proposed by Kang et al. (1987), the carboxy terminus is believed to be located intracellularly. On Western blots, unfractionated homogenates of cortex and other brain regions consistently show an immunoreactive approximately 120 kDa protein complex, using antibodies to the 20-residue C-terminus of the precursor. Two different anti-C terminal sera recognize these bands; absorption with the C-terminal peptide abolishes the staining of the bands. The preimmune sera also do not stain these proteins (Selkoe et al. 1988). The approximately 120 dKa protein is insoluble in physiologic buffers and is found in the Triton-soluble, membrane-enriched fraction of brain. A band of similar molecular weight is identified by anti-C in adrenal and, to a somewhat lesser extent, in several other nonneural organs that contain beta-amyloid mRNA. Fetal human brain also contains readily detectable approximately 120 kDa Triton-soluble protein. We have recently found that both of our C-terminal antisera selectively label granular, apparently extracellular material in the centers of some senile plaques; this staining is abolished by peptide absorption (Selkoe et al. 1988). One anti-C and certain other beta-amyloid antisera also identify an approximately 80 kDa protein(s) that is considered cytosolic because it is soluble in aqueous buffers. This immunoreactive protein is detected in amyloid-prone (cortex, hippocampus, striatum) but not amyloid-poor (cerebellum, pons, white matter) brain regions. Based on these early observations, we hypothesize that the approximately 120 dKa proteins, which appear on gradiant gels to be a complex of four to five closely spaced bands, represent the native β-amyloid precursor protein in human brain and other organs. The relationship of the variably detectable approximately 80 kDa proteins to the β-precursor is unclear, but we speculate that they may represent soluble fragments of the precursor that occur in higher amounts in those brain regions susceptible to amyloidosis in AD and normal aged brain. We are now attempting to purify and obtain sequence data from the approximately 120 kDa proteins and further characterize potential smaller fragments. The goal of this work is to elucidate the progressive, regionally selective processing of the β-precursor into amyloid filaments during brain aging and in AD.

Tau Protein and Neurofibrillary Tangles

Recent advances in our laboratory have provided some indirect insights into the pathogenesis of neurofibrillary tangles. These insights stem from the original observation made by ourselves and others that tau protein is a major antigenic component of the PHF (Brion et al. 1985 a, b; Grundke-Igbal et al. 1986 a; Kosik et al. 1986; Nukina and Ihara 1986; Wood et al. 1986; Yamamoto et al. 1983). Tau is a microtubule-associated protein in that it copurifies with tubulin through repeated cycles of temperature-dependent assembly/disassembly and immunocytochemically colocalizes with microtubules. It is thought to stabilize tubulin as a polymerized microtubule (Drubin and Kirschner 1986). The only other component of these structures that has been convincingly demonstrated is ubiquitin (Mori et al. 1987; Perry et al. 1987). One cytoskeletal protein that was also considered part of the PHF was the neurofilament protein (Anderton et al. 1986). A subset of monoclonal antibodies against the neurofilament protein reacted with neurofibrillary tangles and was also thought to recognize a phosphorylation site. It is exactly this subset of neurofilament antibodies that cross reacts with tau protein (Kziezak-Reding et al. 1987; Nukina et al. 1987; Yen et al. 1987). Since most other neurofilament antibodies do not stain neurofibrillary tangles, it is unlikely that the neurofilament is incorporated substantially into the PHF and the observed immunoreactivity is due to a cross-reaction with tau.

We are aware of only one neurofilament antibody that stains neurofibrillary tangles, but appears not to cross-react with tau (Gambetti et al. 1986). There is currently no good explanation for how this finding relates to the overall composition of PHF. The basis for this cross-reaction is thought to be a conserved phosphorylation site that may be present not only in tau and neurofilament, but also in a histone protein and rhodopsin, two other phosphoproteins which are known to cross-react with at least one of the antibodies (RT97) in this category. The mid-sized neurofilament (NF-M) contains the frequently repeated sequence, Lys-Ser-Pro-Val (Myers et al. 1987). A partial cDNA of the rat large neurofilament (NF-H) contains at least four or five copies of a repeating Lys-Ser-Pro-Ala-Glu in a phosphate-rich region of the protein (Robinson et al. 1986). This repeated amino acid sequence may represent a kinase recognition site. A homologous repeat occurs twice in the mouse tau sequence (Lee et al. 1988) and may be the basis for the cross-reactivity.

We have isolated cDNA clones for human tau from a human fetal brain expression library (Neve et al. 1986). The RNA species recognized by the tau clones is a 6 kilobase message that is expressed in the human brain but not in other human tissues. During development it undergoes an approximately one-half kilobase shift in size that may be related to the molecular weight shift in the protein that has been observed to occur during development. The tau gene was localized to a site on chromosome 17q21 by both "spot-blot" mapping and in situ hybridization to chromosomes (Neve et al. 1986). Recently the sequence of mouse tau has been reported and shown to contain at least one splice junction (Lee et al. 1988). We have sequenced a number of tryptic fragments from bovine tau on an Applied Biosystems gas phase sequenator and have shown the remarkable conservation of this protein.

Studies with Monoclonal Antibodies 5E2 and Tau1

Because there are several monoclonal antibodies that have been shown to react with neurofibrillary tangles, we sought to determine whether they all recognize the same site or whether their epitopes lie within spatially distinct regions of the molecule. Two monoclonal antibodies were used for this study: 5E2 and tau 1 (Kosik et al. 1987b). 5E2 was raised in our laboratory against human fetal tau and has been shown to react monospecifically with all of the heterogeneous tau isoforms in fetal and adult brain (including the 110 kDa tau band) from many mammalian species. Tau 1 was raised by Dr. Lester Binder (Binder et al. 1985) and is also monospecific for the tau isoforms.

To identify the epitopes for these antibodies we utilized the technique of Mehra et al. (1986) to create sublibraries in lambda gt11 from our tau cDNA. We were able to determine the region of these two epitopes by sequencing immunoreactive clones from the sublibrary and identifying a region of minimum overlap which contained the epitope. Both of these monoclonal antibodies recognize neurofibrillary tangles and are directed against spatially distinct regions of the tau protein. It is therefore unlikely that the reaction of tau antibodies with neurofibrillary tangles is a cross-reaction since distinct epitopes from tau are present in the tangle. The tau 1 epitope may have additional interest because of its phosphatase sensitivity (Grundke-Igbal et al. 1986b; Wood et al. 1986). Unlike other tau antibodies tau 1 appears to recognize neurofibrillary tangles only after treatment with alkaline phosphatase. It is therefore possible that an abnormal phosphorylation event occurs at the tau 1 site, which may have a role in the pathogenesis of the neurofibrillary tangle. Other independent evidence has also raised the possibility of abnormal phosphorylation in the PHF (Ihara et al. 1986). Recently we sought to measure the amount of inorganic phosphate in PHF fractions directly using the method of Stull and Buss (1977). This approach is highly problematic for the following reasons: (a) much of the PHF fraction remains insoluble under the assay conditions, (b) no PHF fraction prepared by currently available techniques is absolutely pure, and (c) the molecular weight of the PHF subunit is unknown so that the stoichiometry cannot be calculated. In attempting the determination we found that only about 3% of the SDS-insoluble PHF fraction solubilized in the 1.2 N HCl. However, this small amount of protein did have readily detectable amounts of inorganic phosphate.

Tau as Substrate for Protein Kinase C

Tau is known to be a phosphoprotein and is considered a substrate for the calcium/calmodulin-dependent protein kinase (CaM kinase) (Baudier and Cole 1987; Schulman 1987; Wood et al. 1986). Recently the possibility has been raised that tau may also serve as a substrate for protein kinase C (Baudier et al. 1987). We have identified several sites in tau that are phosphorylated by CaM kinase (Kosik et al. 1987a) and one of these sites occurs within a carboxy terminal repeated sequence. In mouse the repeat occurs three with approximately 50% homology (Lee et al. 1988). It has been postulated that the tau repeat may represent the microtubule-binding domain. Our preliminary data suggest that none of the in vitro CaM kinase sites are equivalent to the tau 1 site or to the conserved putative phosphorylation site present in NF-H, NF-M, and tau.

Antibody Alz 50

Another recently discovered aspect of the relationship between neurofibrillary tangles and tau is the tau-immunoreactivity present in the antibody Alz 50 originally described by Wolozin and Davies (1987) (Hyman et al. 1987). The immunoreactivity of Alz 50 was compared with that of the two tau monoclonal antibodies, tau 1 and 5E2, mentioned above (Nukina et al. 1988). All three antibodies react with all of the heterogeneous isoforms of tau observed in rat, bovine, and human brain. All of the antibodies react with both the fetal and the mature forms of tau. All of the antibodies continue to react with all of the tau bands after treatment with alkaline phosphatase sufficient to shift the mobility of the tau isoforms downward.

Alz 50 precipitated proteins from Alzheimer brain tissue at the molecular weight of 50–70 kDa; these precipitated proteins were reactive with the tau antibodies (Nukina et al. 1988). Alz 50 also precipitated proteins of 160–180 kDa from Alzheimer brain. It was difficult to assess the reactivity of these higher molecular weight proteins with tau since this material typically resulted in a smear over a wide molecular weight range when blotted with tau antibodies. It was clear that these higher molecular weight Alz 50 immunoprecipitated proteins were not reactive with a ubiquitin antibody that has been demonstrated to react with the conjugated form of ubiquitin (Mori et al. 1987).

While biochemically the data suggest some sequence homology between the Alz 50 antigen (designated A68) and tau, the immunocytochemical data are more perplexing. Alz 50 recognizes both neurons that do and do not contain neurofibrillary tangles (Kowall and Kosik 1987). Alz 50 immunoreactive neurons without tangles are present in neuronal populations at risk for the development of neurofibrillary tangles. The distribution of the immunoreactivity in these cells extends well into the cell body, the apical dendrite of pyramidal cells, and may even be present in dendritic spines. In contradistinction, tau-immunocytochemistry with the monoclonal antibody 5E2 does not label the apical dendrite of non-tangle-bearing neurons in Alzheimer's disease (Kowall and Kosik 1987). The Alz 50 antigen is also more resistant to fixation than any of several epitopes recognized by antibodies raised directly against tau.

Immunocytochemistry of Tau in the Neuropil

With optimal fixation tau-immunocytochemistry does reveal striking alterations that affect the neuropil in the Alzheimer disease brain (Kowall and Kosik 1987). In control brain tau-immunoreactive fiber bundles form a pattern resembling that seen with myelin stains due to its predisposition for the axon. No staining of neuronal cell bodies, glial cells, or oligodendrocytes was observed. The prominence of white matter staining suggests that tau may be especially enriched in projection systems. In Alzheimer's disease there is a pervasive disruption of the cortical axons to the extent that the normal radially deployed bundles are no longer discernible. Instead tau-immunoreactivity is displaced into the neuronal cell bodies, dendrites, and presynaptic regions. Most apparent is the tangle-associated tau-immunoreactivity which extends into the proximal portion of the apical dendrite. Most remarkable are the tau-reactive dystrophic neurites or "curly fibers" that are widely present in the neuropil and more abundant than either the senile plaques or the neurofibrillary tangles. These curly fibers are densely present even in layer I of the cortex where there are very few senile plaques and rare, if any, neurofibrillary tangles. Our preliminary data suggest that a significant number of the curly fibers may be dystrophic dendrites, which would imply a highly displaced location for the tau reaction product. Because electron micrographs of Alzheimer cortex have not revealed large numbers of PHF in regions beyond the neurofibrillary tangles and plaque neurites, it is likely that some proportion of these curly fibers may contain the straight filaments described by Perry et al. (1988).

References

Abraham CR, Selkoe DJ, Potter H (1988) Immunochemical identification of the serine protease inhibitor alpha-1-antichymotrypsin in the brain amyloid deposits of Alzheimer's disease. Cell 52: 487–501

Anderton BH, Breinburg D, Downes MJ, Green PJ, Tomlinson BE, Ulrich J, Wood JN, Kahn J (1986) Monoclonal antibodies show that neurofibrillary tangles and neurofilaments share antigenic determinants. Nature 298: 84–86

Baudier J, Cole RD (1987) Phosphorylation of tau proteins to a state like that in Alzheimer's brain is catalyzed by a calcium/calmodulin-dependent kinase and modulated by phospholipids. J Biol Chem 262: 17577–17583

Baudier J, Lee S-H, Cole RD (1987) Separation of the different microtubule-associated tau protein species from bovine brain and their mode II phosphorylation by Ca^{2+}/phospholipid-dependent protein kinase C. J Biol Chem 262: 17584–17590

Binder LI, Frankfurter A, Rebhun LI (1985) The distribution of tau in the mammalian central nervous system. J Cell Biol 101: 1371–1378

Brion JP, Couck AM,, Passareiro E, Flament-Durand J (1985a) In Traper J and Gispen WH (eds), Advances in applied neurological science: senile dementia of the Alzheimer type. Springer, Berlin, pp 164–174

Brion JP, Passariero H, Nunez J, Flament-Durant J (1985b) Immunologic determinants of tau protein are present in neurofibrillary tangles of Alzheimer's disease. Arch Biol 95: 229–235

Drubin DG, Kirschner MW (1986) Tau protein function in living cells. J Cell Biol 103: 2739–2746

Eidelberg D, Sotrel A, Joachim C, Selkoe D, Forman A, Pendlebury WW, Perl DP (1987) Adult onset Hallervorden-Spatz disease with neurofibrillary pathology. Brain 110: 993–1013

Galloway PG, Perry G, Gambetti P (1987a) Hirano body filaments contain actin and actin-associated proteins. J Neuropathol Exp Neurol 46: 262–268

Galloway PG, Perry G, Kosik KS, Gambetti P (1987b) Hirano bodies contain tau protein. Brain Res 403: 337–340

Gambetti P, Perry G, Autilio-Gambetti L (1986) Paired helical filaments: Do they contain neurofilament epitopes? Neurobiol Aging 7: 451–452

Glenner GG, Wong CG (1984) Initial report of the purification and characterization of a novel cerebrovascular amyloid protein. Biochem Biophys Res Commun 120: 885–890

Goldgaber D, Lerman MI, McBride OW, Saffiotti V, Gajdusek DC (1987) Characterization and chromosomal localization of a cDNA encoding brain amyloid of Alzheimer's disease. Science 235: 877–880

Goldman JE (1983) The association of actin with Hirano bodies. J Neuropathol Exp Neurol 42: 146–152

Grundke-Iqbal I, Iqbal K, Quinlan M, Tung Y-C, Zaidi MS, Wisniewski HM (1986a) Microtubule-associated protein tau: a component of Alzheimer paired helical filaments. J Biol Chem 261: 6084–6089

Grundke-Iqbal I, Iqbal K, Tung Y-C, Quinlan M, Wisniewski H, Binder LI (1986b) Abnormal phosphorylation of the microtubule-associated protein tau in Alzheimer cytoskeletal pathology. Proc Natl Acad Sci USA 83 4913–4917

Guiroy DC, Miyazaki M, Multhaup G, Fischer P, Garruto RM, Beyreuther K, Masters CL, Simms G, Gibbs CJ Jr, Gajdusek DC (1987) Amyloid of neurofibrillary tangles of Guamanian parkinsonism-dementia and Alzheimer disease share identical amino acid sequence. Proc Natl Acad Sci USA 84: 2073–2077

Hyman BT, Van Hoesen GW, Wolozin B, Davies P, Damasio AR (1987) Alz 50: recognition of Alzheimer-related neuronal changes before neurofibrillary tangle formation. Neurology (Abstract) [Suppl 1] 37: 225

Ihara Y, Nukina N, Miura R, Ogawara M (1986) Phosphorylated tau protein is integrated into paired helical filaments in Alzheimer's disease. J Biochem 99: 1807–1810

Kang J, Lemaire H-G, Unterbeck A, Salbaum JM, Masters CL, Grzeschik K-H, Multhaup G, Beyreuther K, Muller-Hill B (1987) The precursor of Alzheimer's disease amyloid A4 protein resembles a cell-surface receptor. Nature 325: 733–736

Katzman R, Terry R, DeTeresa R, Brown T, Davies P, Fuld P, Renbing X, Peck A (1988) Clinical, pathological, and neurochemical changes in dementia: a subgroup with preserved mental status and numerous neocortical plaques. Ann Neurol 23: 138–144

Khachaturian ZS (1985) Diagnosis of Alzheimer's disease. Arch Neurol 42: 1097–1105

Kitaguchi N, Takahashi Y, Tokushima Y, Shiojiri S, Ito H (1988) Novel precursor of Alzheimer's disease amyloid protein shows protease inhibitory activity. Nature 331: 530–532

Kosik KS, Joachim CL, Selkoe DJ (1986) Microtubule-associated protein tau (τ) is a major antigenic component of paired helical filaments in Alzheimer's disease. Proc Natl Acad Sci USA 83: 4044–4048

Kosik KS, Lee G, Kennedy MB (1987a) Type II Ca^{2+}/calmodulin-dependent kinase phosphorylates tau protein in the region of the mouse repeat. Am Soc Biol Chem (Abstract) Philadelphia

Kosik KS, Neve R, Lee G, Binder LI (1987b) The tau 1 epitope is not in the carboxy terminus of a tau cDNA fusion protein. Soc Neurosci Abstr 230, 10

Kowall NW, Kosik KS (1987) Axonal disruption and aberrant localization of tau protein characterize the neuropil pathology of Alzheimer's disease. Ann Neurol 22: 639–643

Ksiezak-Reding H, Dickson DW, Davies P, Yen S-H (1987) Recognition of tau epitopes by anti-neurofilament antibodies that bind to Alzheimer neurofibrillary tangles. Proc Natl Acad Sci USA 84: 3410–3414

Lee G, Cowan N, Kirschner M (1988) The primary structure and heterogeneity of tau protein from mouse brain. Science 239: 285–288

Masters CL, Simms G, Weinman NA, Multhaup G, McDonald BL, Beyreuther K (1985) Amyloid plaque core protein in Alzheimer disease and Down syndrome. Proc Natl Acad Sci USA 82: 4245–4249

Mehra V, Sweetser D, Young RA (1986) Efficient mapping of protein antigenic determinants. Proc Natl Acad Sci USA 83: 7013–7017

Mori H, Kondo J, Ihara Y (1987) Ubiquitin is a component of paired helical filaments in Alzheimer's disease. Science 235: 1641–1644

Myers MW, Lazzarini RA, Lee VM-Y, Schlaepfer WW, Nelson DL (1987) The human mid-size neurofilament subunit: a repeated protein sequence and the relationship of its gene to the intermediate filament gene family. EMBO J 6: 1617–1626

Neve RL, Harris P, Kosik KS, Kurnit DM, Donlon TA (1986) Identification of cDNA clones for the human microtubule-associated protein tau and chromosomal localization of the genes for tau and microtubule-associated protein 2. Molecul Brain Res 271–280

Nukina N, Ihara Y (1986) One of the antigenic determinants of paired helical filaments is related to tau protein. J Biochem B99: 1541–1544

Nukina N, Kosik KS, Selkoe DJ (1987) Recognition of Alzheimer paired helical filaments by monoclonal neurofilament antibodies is due to crossreaction with tau protein. Proc Natl Acad Sci USA 84: 3415–3419

Nukina N, Kosik KS, Selkoe DJ (1988) The monoclonal antibody, Alz 50, recognizes tau proteins in Alzheimer's disease brain. Neurosci Lett 87: 240–246

Perry G, Friedman R, Shaw G, Chau V (1987) Ubiquitin is detected in neurofibrillary tangles and senile plaque neurites of Alzheimer disease brains. Proc Natl Acad Sci USA 184: 3033–3036

Perry G, Mulvihill P, Manetto V, Autilio-Gambetti L, Gambetti P (1988) Immunocytochemical properties of Alzheimer straight filaments. J Neurosci 7: 3736–3738

Ponte P, Gonzalez-DeWhitt P, Sabilling J, Miller J, Hsu D, Greenberg B, Davis K, Wallace W, Lieberburg I, Fuller F, Cordell B (1988) A new A4 amyloid mRNA contains a domain homologous to serine proteinase inhibitors. Nature 331: 525–527

Price DL, Struble RG, Altschuler RJ, Casanova MF, Cork LC, Murphy DB (1985) Aggregation of tubulin in neurons in Alzheimer's disease. J Neuropathol Exp Neurol 44: 366

Robakis ND, Wisniewski HM, Jenkins EC, Devine-Gage EA, Houck GE, Yao X-L, Ramakrishna N, Wolfe G, Silverman WP, Brown WT (1987) Chromosome 21q21 sublocalisation of gene encoding β-amyloid peptide in cerebral vessels and neuritic (senile) plaques of people with Alzheimer disease and Down syndrome. Lancet I: 384–385

Robinson PA, Wion D, Anderton BH (1986) Isolation of a cDNA for the rat heavy neurofilament polypeptide (NF-H). FEBS Lett 209: 203–205

Schulman H (1987) Phosphorylation of microtubule-associated proteins by a Ca^{2+}/calmodulin-dependent protein kinase. J Cell Biol 99: 11–19

Selkoe DJ, Abraham CR, Podlisny M, Duffy LK (1986) Isolation of low molecular weight proteins from amyloid plaque fibers in Alzheimer's disease. J Neurochem 46: 1820–1834

Selkoe DJ, Podlisny MB, Vickers E (1988) Processing of the β-amyloid precursor protein in human brain: search for regional differences. (Abstract, Amer Assoc Neuropathol, June 1988). J Neuropathol Exp Neurol (in press)

Stull JT, Buss JE (1977) Phosphorylation of cardiac troponin by cyclic adenosine 3′:5′-monophosphate-dependent protein kinase. J Biol Chem 252: 851–857

Tanzi RE, Gusella JF, Watkins PC, Bruns GAP, St George-Hyslop PH, Van Keuren ML, Patterson D, Pagan S, Kurnit DM, Neve RL (1987) Amyloid β protein gene: c-DNA, mRNA distribution, and genetic linkage near the Alzheimer locus. Science 235: 880–884

Tanzi RE, McClatchey AI, Lamperti ED, Villa-Komaroff L, Gusella JF, Neve RL (1988) Protease inhibitor domain encoded by an amyloid protein precursor mRNA associated with Alzheimer's disease. Nature 331: 528–530

Terry RD, Hansen LA, Deteresa R, Davies P, Tobias H, Katzman R (1987) Senile dementia of the Alzheimer type without neocortical neurofibrillary tangles. J Neuropathol Exp Neurol 46: 262–268

Wolozin B, Davies P (1987) Alzheimer-related neuronal protein A68: specificity and distribution. Ann Neurol 22: 521–526

Wong CW, Quaranta V, Glenner GG (1985) Neuritic plaques and cerebrovascular amyloid in Alzheimer disease are antigenically related. Proc Natl Acad Sci USA 82: 8729–8732

Wood JG, Mirra SS, Pollock NJ, Binder LI (1986) Neurofibrillary tangles of Alzheimer's disease share antigenic determinants with the axonal microtubule-associated protein tau. Proc Natl Acad Sci USA 83: 4040–4043

Yamamoto H, Fukunaga K, Tanaka E, Miyamoto E (1983) Ca^{2+}- and calmodulin-dependent phosphorylation of microtubule-associated protein 2 and tau factor, and inhibition of microtubule assembly. J Neurochem 41: 1119–1125

Yen S-H, Dickson DW, Crowe A, Butler M, Shelanski ML (1987) Alzheimer's neurofibrillary tangles contain unique epitopes and epitopes in common with the heat-stable microtubule associated proteins, tau and MAP2. Am J Pathol 126(1): 81–91

Etiology Versus Pathogenesis: The Causes of Post-Translational Modifications of Host-Specified Brain Proteins to Amyloid Configuration

D. C. Gajdusek

Since amyloid is deposited as neurofibrillary tangles, plaques, and vascular amyloid in brains of all the very aged (> 90 years), and this amyloid is biochemically the same as that in Alzheimer's disease, Down's syndrome, and Guamanian amyotrophic lateral sclerosis/Parkinsonism-dementia (ALS/PD), we know that no abnormal hereditable gene is necessary for such deposition. By isolating the gene for the precursor to this amyloid we are surely tracking pathogenesis of normal aging. Alzheimer's disease, Down's syndrome, and Guamanian ALS/PD. The same applies to isolating the gene for the normal host precursor protein for the much different amyloid of the scrapie-associated fibrils of unconventional viruses (scrapie-kuru-Creutzfeldt-Jakob disease) and the amyloid plaques of these diseases.

This is elucidating not the cause, but the pathogenesis, in the hope that it will reflect back toward the causes. In the case of Alzheimer's disease this is usually environmental, but occasionally a hereditable, autosomal dominant gene, as in familial Alzheimer's disease. It is a prezygotic chromosomal duplication in Down's syndrome or an environmental deficiency-toxin in Guamanian ALS/PD. For the transmissible virus dementias the process is infectious, in which the "virus" appears to be an autocatalytic nucleation and crystallization agent for acceleration and augmentation of the amyloid configurational change of the host precursor protein and its polymerization and precipitation as amyloid insoluble fibrils. This may require proteolytic degradation of the precursor to get underway.

To become an autocatalytic nucleating agent accelerating the crystallization and precipitation requires a conformational change of the amyloid subunit polypeptide from that which it presents within the precursor protein. This degradation of the precursor and oligomeric assembly of the structurally altered polypeptide produces a *fibril amyloid enhancing factor,* which we call a "virus."

Amyloid enhancing factor is a low molecular weight glycoprotein found in systemic amino acid (AA) amyloid tissues and in amyloid fibrils. Amyloidosis may be induced in mice and hamsters by nonspecific activation of inflammatory response and production of amyloid AA precursor protein with injections of casein, silver nitrate, or lipopolysaccharide. The administration of amyloid enhancing factor shortens the lag time for such experimentally induced amyloidosis in mice and hamsters from 2 weeks to 4 days. It accelerates, therefore, the predeposition phase of amyloid production. With its tendency to complex with itself or other molecules, the amyloid enhancing factor could serve as a nucleus for fibrillar growth and deposition, thereby accelerating its own production and the amyloid formation. Fibril amyloid enhancing factor is a microfibril of amyloid AA which acts as a nucleant for polymerization of its monomer into amyloid fibrils and for production of itself by the degradation of host precursor protein.

The same type of autocatalytic nucleation and polymerization phenomenon could occur in the transmissible and the nontransmissible amyloidosis of the brain. In the nontransmissible brain amyloidosis of Alzheimer's disease, normal aging, Down's syndrome, and Guamanian parkinsonism-dementia, the 42 amino acid subunit (A4 or amyloid beta protein) polymerized to form the amyloid of the neurofibrillary tangles, amyloid plaque core, and congophilic angiopathy could, in oligomeric form or fibril microfragments themselves, form a nucleus that enhances the further amyloid deposition. In the transmissible virus dementias of kuru, Creutzfeldt-Jakob disease, and scrapie, the pathogenetic process is an infection in which the "virus" appears to be autocatalytic nucleation, crystallization, and a configurational change of a host-specified precursor protein to amyloid. This virus nucleant further accelerates and augments the polymerization and precipitation as insoluble amyloid fibrils of the structurally altered host polypeptide. Proteolytic degradation of the precursor and change in secondary and tertiary structure of the polypeptide may be needed to initiate amyloid fibril formation.

References

Axelrad MA, Kisilevsky R (1980) Biological characterizations of amyloid enhancing factor. In: Glenner GG, Costa PP, de Freitas AF (eds) Amyloid and amyloidosis. Excerpta Medica, Amsterdam, pp 527–533

Axelrad MA, Kisilevsky R, Willmer J, Chen SJ, Skinner M (1982) Further characterization of amyloid-enhancing factor. Lab Invest 47: 139–146

Beyreuther K, Multhaup G, Simms G, Pottgiesser J, Schroeder W, Martins RN, Masters CL (1986) Neurofibrillary tangles of Alzheimer's disease and "aged" Down's syndrome contain the same protein as the amyloid of plaque cores and blood vessels. Disc Neurosci 3: 68–79

Castaño EM, Frangione B (1988) Human amyloidosis, Alzheimer disease and related disorders. Lab Invest 58: 122–132

Castaño EM, Ghiso J, Prelli F, Gorevic PD, Migheli A, Frangione B (1986) In vitro formation of amyloid fibrils from two synthetic peptides of different lengths homologous to Alzheimer's disease beta protein. Biochem Biophys Res Commun 141: 782–789

Cohen AS (1965) The constitution and genesis of amyloid. Int Rev Exp Pathol 4: 159–243

Glenner GG, Wong CW (1984a) Alzheimer's disease: initial report of the purification and characterization of a novel cerebrovascular amyloid protein. Biochem Biophys Res Comm 120: 885–890

Glenner GG, Wong CW (1984b) Alzheimer's disease and Down's syndrome: sharing of a unique cerebrovascular amyloid fibril protein. Biochem Biophys Res Commun 122: 1131–1135

Gorevic PD, Castaño EM, Sarma R, Frangione B (1987) Ten to fourteen residue peptides of Alzheimer's disease beta protein are sufficient for amyloid fibril formation and its characteristic X-ray diffraction pattern. Biochem Biophys Res Commun 147: 854–862

Guiroy DC, Miyazaki M, Multhaup G, Fischer P, Garruto RM, Beyreuther K, Masters CL, Simms G, Gibbs CJ, Jr, Gajdusek DC (1987) Amyloid of the neurofibrillary tangles of Guamanian parkinsonism-dementia and Alzheimer disease share identical amino acid sequence. Proc Natl Acad Sci USA 84: 2073–2077

Hardt F, Ranlov P (1968) Transfer amyloidosis. Acta Pathol Microbiol Scand 73: 549–558

Hol PR, van Andel ACJ, van Ederen AM, Draayer J, Gruys E (1985) Amyloid enhancing factor in hamster. Br J Exp Pathol 66: 689–697

Hol PR, Snel FWJJ, Niewold ThA, Gruys E (1986) Amyloid-enhancing factor (AEF) in the pathogenesis of AA-amyloidosis in the hamster. Virchows Arch (Cell Pathol) 52: 273–281

Janigan DT (1965) Experimental amyloidosis. Am J Pathol 47: 159–171

Janigan DT, Druet RL (1968) Experimental murine amyloidosis in X-irradiated recipients of spleen homogenates or serum from sensitized donors. Am J Pathol 52: 381–390

Janigan DT (1969) Pathogenetic mechanisms in protein-induced amyloidosis. Am J Pathol 55: 379–393

Keizman I, Rimon A, Sohar E, Gafni J (1972) Amyloid accelerating factor. Acta Pathol Microbiol Scand [Suppl 233] 80: 172–177

Kirschner DA, Inouye H, Duffy LK, Sinclair A, Lind M, Selkoe DJ (1987) Synthetic peptide homologous to beta protein from Alzheimer disease forms amyloid-like fibrils in vitro. Proc Natl Acad Sci USA 84: 6953–6957

Kisilevsky R, Boudreau L (1983a) Kinetics in amyloid deposition. I. The effects of amyloid-enhancing factor and splenectomy. Lab Invest 48: 53–59

Kisilevsky R, Boudreau L, Foster D (1983b) Kinetics of amyloid deposition. II. The effects of dimethylsulfoxide and colchicine therapy. Lab Invest 48: 60–67

Masters CL, Simms G, Weinman NA, Multhaup G, McDonald BL, Beyreuther K (1985a) Amyloid plaque core protein in Alzheimer disease and Down's syndrome. Proc Natl Acad Sci USA 82: 4245–4249

Masters CL, Multhaup G, Simms G, Pottgiesser J, Martins RN, Beyreuther K (1985b) Neuronal origin of a cerebral amyloid: neurofibrillary tangles of Alzheimer's disease contain the same protein as the amyloid of plaque cores and blood vessels. EMBO J 4: 2757–2763

Niewold ThA, Hol PR, van Andel ACJ, Lutz ETG, Gruys E (1987) Enhancement of amyloid induction by amyloid fibril fragments in hamster. Lab Invest 56: 544–549

Ranlov P (1967) The adoptive transfer of experimental mouse amyloidosis by intravenous injection of spleen cell extracts from casein-treated syngeneic donor mice. Acta Pathol Microbiol Scand 70: 321–335

Shirahama T, Lawless OJ, Cohen AS (1969) Heterologous transfer of amyloid – human to mouse. Proc Soc Exp Biol Med 130: 516–519

Snow AD, Kisilevsky R (1985) Temporal relationship between glycosaminoglycan accumulation and amyloid deposition during experimental amyloidosis. Lab Invest 53: 37–44

Teilum G (1964) Pathogenesis of amyloidosis. The two-phase cellular theory of local secretion. Acta Pathol Microbiol Scand 61: 21–45

Varga J, Flinn MSM, Shirahama T, Rodgers OG, Cohen AS (1986) The induction of accelerated murine amyloid with human splenic extract. Virchows Arch (Cell Pathol) 51: 177–185

Werderlin O, Ranlov P (1966) Amyloidosis in mice produced by transplantation of spleen cells from casein-treated mice. Arch Pathol Microbiol Scand 68: 1–18

Subject Index

www.ingramcontent.com/pod-product-compliance
Lightning Source LLC
Chambersburg PA
CBHW061211240926
51846CB00006B/1182

* 9 7 8 3 6 4 2 7 3 6 4 9 0 *